Study Guide and Workbook
to accompany

UNDERSTANDING PATHOPHYSIOLOGY

Sue E. Huether
Kathryn L. McCance

Prepared by

Clayton F. Parkinson, PhD
College of Health Sciences
Weber State University
Ogden, Utah

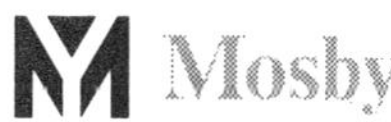

Mosby

St. Louis Baltimore Boston
Carlsbad Chicago Naples New York Philadelphia Portland
London Madrid Mexico City Singapore Sydney Tokyo Toronto Wiesbaden

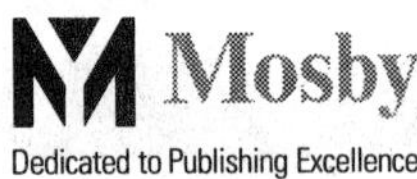

A Times Mirror
Company

Publisher: Nancy L. Coon
Senior Editor: Sally Schrefer
Developmental Editor: Gail Brower
Project Manager: Patricia Tannian
Senior Production Editor: Betty Hazelwood
Book Design Manager: Gail Morey Hudson
Manuscript Editor: Susan Warrington
Manufacturing Supervisor: Karen Lewis
Cover Art: William B. Westwood

Printed in the United States of America
Composition by Wordbench
Printing/binding by Plus Communications

Mosby–Year Book, Inc.
11830 Westline Industrial Drive
St. Louis, Missouri 63146

International Standard Book Number 0-8151-7299-0

97 98 99 / 9 8 7 6 5 4

Reviewers

SUE E. HEUTHER, RN, PhD
Associate Professor, College of Nursing
University of Utah
Salt Lake City, Utah

KATHRYN L. McCANCE, RN, PhD
Professor, College of Nursing
University of Utah
Salt Lake City, Utah

Preface

The study of pathophysiology is complex, ever expanding, and challenging. It provides correlation between normal anatomy and physiology and the processes resulting in the manifestations of disease.

This study guide is designed for students as an adjunct to *Understanding Pathophysiology* by Sue E. Huether and Kathryn L. McCance. It is intended to encourage an understanding of the consequences of pathologic processes on the structure and function of the human body.

The guide has 39 chapters, and each follows the organization of the textbook. The guide's chapters have two different formats—one for normal anatomy and physiology and another for anatomic and physiologic alterations.

For the normal anatomy and physiology chapters, it is assumed that the student possesses foundational knowledge of anatomy and physiology.

- They direct review of information, principles, and concepts that are essential for understanding the specific diseases that follow.
- Each chapter has a practice examination to give students an opportunity to assess their understanding of normality.

The chapters on alterations direct the learner's study of abnormal anatomy and physiology.

- They have foundational objectives and study objectives with both narrative and charts.
- Each chapter has a practice examination requiring factual and conceptual knowledge related to disease mechanisms.
- Each chapter has a case study linking fact and concept to reality.

The objectives for all chapters are referenced to corresponding pages in Huether and McCance's textbook. Their philosophy that students need to grasp basic laws and principles to understand how alterations occur led them to develop an understandable and conceptually integrated textbook. I am grateful to Dorian Blevins for her initial preparation of the eight chapters on alterations in children. Last, I enjoyed working with Mosby, particularly Gail Brower. All of Mosby's staff ensured that my efforts were developed into a creative, professional, and pleasing style for student learners. Without Klaus Gurgel, a sales representative for Mosby who encouraged me, the joint effort between Mosby and me would not have happened.

I wish to dedicate my efforts during the preparation of this study guide to Kimberly Jo, who makes teaching pleasurable and inspires me to search for truth and a better way to convey it to students.

Clayton F. Parkinson

Contents

PART One

BASIC CONCEPTS OF PATHOPHYSIOLOGY

CHAPTER 1

Cellular Biology

Objectives

After review of this chapter, the learner will be able to:

1. **State the functions of a typical eukaryotic cell.**
   Review page 4.

2. **Describe the function of the nucleus and identify the cytoplasmic organelles.**
   Review pages 4-5; refer to Figures 1-1 and 1-2 and Table 1-1.

3. **Describe the structure and function of the plasma membrane.**
   Review pages 5-10; refer to Figures 1-3 through 1-5 and Tables 1-2 and 1-3.

4. **Describe cellular communication.**
   Review pages 10-12; refer to Figures 1-6 and 1-7.

5. **Describe cellular catabolism and the transfer of energy to accomplish other cellular processes.**
   Refer to Figures 1-8 and 1-9.

6. **Differentiate between mediated and active transport and passive transport, between endocytosis and exocytosis, and between phagocytosis and pinocytosis.**
   Refer to Figures 1-10 through 1-16 and Table 1-4.

7. **Describe the changes in the plasma membrane that result in an action potential.**
   Review pages 20-23; refer to Figure 1-17.

8. **Identify the phases of mitosis and cytokinesis; give examples of growth factors.**
   Review pages 23-24; refer to Figure 1-18 and Table 1-5.

9. **Identify two mechanisms for tissue formation.**
   Review pages 24-27; refer to Figure 1-19.

10. **Identify the location and a major function for each type of tissue: epithelial, connective, muscle, and nervous.**
    Refer to Figures 1-21 through 1-37.

Practice Examination

1. Which are principal parts of a eukaryotic cell?

   a. fat, carbohydrate, and protein
   b. minerals and water
   c. organelles
   d. phospholipids and protein
   e. protoplasm and nucleus

2. The cell membrane is described as a fluid mosaic. Proteins have a degree of mobility within the lipid bilayer. (*More than one answer may be correct.*)

   a. The first sentence is true.
   b. The first sentence is false.
   c. The second sentence is true.
   d. The second sentence is false.
   e. The second sentence is relevant to the first.
   f. The second sentence is irrelevant to the first.

3. Which particle can penetrate cell membranes most easily?

   a. lipid-soluble, transport protein present
   b. neutral charge, water-soluble
   c. smaller, water-soluble
   d. uncharged, larger
   e. All of the above are correct.

4. In order for a cell to engage in active transport processes, it requires:

   a. mitochondria.
   b. appropriate fuel.
   c. ATP.
   d. enzymes.
   e. All of the above are correct.

5. Which is inconsistent with the others?

   a. diffusion
   b. osmosis
   c. filtration
   d. phagocytosis
   e. facilitated diffusion

6. Which can transport substances "uphill" against the concentration gradient?

   a. active transport
   b. osmosis
   c. dialysis
   d. facilitated diffusion
   e. None of the above is correct.

7. The mechanism of transport for glucose is:

   a. mediated.
   b. passive protein channel.
   c. via coupled channels.
   d. active.

8. Which statement is true for cytoplasm?

   a. It is located outside the nucleus.
   b. It provides support for organelles.
   c. It is mostly water.
   d. All of the above are true.
   e. Both a and b are true.

Match the term with its descriptor.

9. ____ anaphase
10. ____ chromatin
11. ____ metaphase
12. ____ mitochondria
13. ____ prophase
14. ____ ribosome
15. ____ telophase

a. 75-90% H_2O, lipids, and protein
b. within the nucleus, stored RNA
c. compartmentalizes cellular activity
d. single strand of DNA, nondividing cell
e. "generation plant" for ATP
f. centriole migration
g. chromatid pair alignment
h. chromatid migration
i. daughter nuclei
j. protein synthesis site

16. A major function of connective tissue is:

    a. to form glands.
    b. support and binding.
    c. covering and lining.
    d. movement.
    e. to conduct nerve impulses.

17. Which are characteristic of epithelial tissue? (*More than one answer may be correct.*)

    a. elasticity
    b. protection
    c. fills spaces between organs
    d. secretion

Match the location with the tissue type found.

18. ____ lining kidney tubules
19. ____ lining urinary bladder
20. ____ lining upper respiratory tract

a. simple squamous
b. simple cuboidal
c. simple columnar, ciliated
d. stratified squamous
e. transitional

21. Ligands that bind with membrane receptors include which of the following? (*More than one answer may be correct.*)

a. hormones
b. antigens
c. neurotransmitters
d. drugs
e. infectious agents

22. The products from the metabolism of glucose include which of the following? (*More than one answer may be correct.*)

a. kilocalories
b. CO_2
c. H_2O
d. ATP

23. Identify the correct sequence of events for initiation and conduction of a nerve impulse.

1. Sodium moves inside.
2. Potassium leaves cell.
3. Sodium permeability changes.
4. Resting potential is reestablished.
5. Potassium permeability changes.

a. 1, 3, 2, 5, 4
b. 3, 1, 5, 2, 4
c. 5, 2, 3, 1, 4
d. 4, 5, 2, 3, 1

24. Chemotaxis in tissue formation:

a. causes one cell to adhere to another.
b. involves founder cells.
c. is an attraction of migrant cells along a chemical gradient.
d. All of the above are correct.
e. None of the above is correct.

25. Cell junctions:

a. coordinate activities of cells within tissues.
b. are an impermeable part of the plasma membrane.
c. hold cells together.
d. Both a and c are correct.
e. Both b and c are correct.

CHAPTER

2

Genes and Genetic Diseases

Foundational Objectives

a. Describe the interrelationships of DNA, RNA, and proteins. Review pages 39-42; refer to Figures 2-1 through 2-5.

Memory Check!

- The gene consists of a particular sequence of nucleotides in the deoxyribonucleic acid (DNA) of the chromosome. The sequence of nucleotides in a gene determines which proteins are found in a cell, and these proteins determine both the form and function of the cell.
- Genetic information flows from DNA to RNA proteins. Three major processes are involved in the preservation and transmission of genetic information. The first is replication, or the copying of DNA to form identical daughter molecules. The second is transcription, in which the genetic message encoded within DNA is transcribed into RNA and is carried to the ribosomes, the sites of protein synthesis. The third is translation, in which the genetic message is decoded and converted into the 20-letter alphabet of protein structure. Because the sequence of nucleotides in the DNA bears a linear correspondence to the sequence of amino acids in the formed proteins, genetic information is preserved and transmitted to progeny.

b. Define general genetic terms. Review pages 42-51.

Memory Check!

Genetic Term	Definition
Progeny	Offspring
Chromosomes	Structures in the nucleus that contain DNA, which transmits genetic information; each chromosome is composed of thousands of genes arranged in linear order
Gene	DNA, the basic unit of heredity, located at a particular place on the chromosome

(Continued)

Memory Check! (cont'd)

Genetic Term	Definition
Locus	The position each gene occupies along a chromosome
Allele	One of two or more different genes that contain specific inheritable characteristics (such as eye color) and occupy corresponding positions on paired chromosomes—one gene from each parent; a different version of the same paired gene
Homozygous	A trait of an organism produced by identical or nearly identical alleles
Heterozygous	Possessing different alleles at a given chromosomal location
Karyotype	A display of human chromosomes based on their length and the location of the centromere
Genotype	The basic combination of genes of an organism
Phenotype	The expression of the gene or trait in an individual (e.g., physical appearance such as eye color)
Carrier	An individual who has a gene for disease but is phenotypically normal
Dominant traits	Traits for which one of a pair of alleles is necessary for expression (e.g., brown eyes)
Recessive traits	Traits for which two alleles of a pair are necessary for expression (e.g., blue eyes, a recessive gene on the male's X chromosome, will be expressed because the gene is not matched by a corresponding gene on the Y chromosome)
Pedigree chart	A schematic method for classifying genetic data
Expressivity	The extent of variation in phenotype for a particular genotype
Penetrance	The percentage of individuals with a specific genotype who exhibit the expected phenotype

Single-gene disorders are known to be caused by mutation in a single gene. The mutated gene may be present on one or both chromosomes of a pair.

Multifactorial disorders result when small variations in genes combine with environmental factors to produce serious defects. Multifactorial disorders tend to cluster in families.

Objectives

After review of this chapter, the learner will be able to:

1. **Characterize chromosome disorders.**
   Study pages 43-50; refer to Figures 2-10 and 2-14 through 2-16.

In **chromosome disorders**, the defect is due to an abnormality in chromosome number or structure. The structure of the genes in chromosome disorders may be normal, but the genes may be present in multiple copies or be situated on a different chromosome.

Normal somatic cells having two sets of 23 chromosomes are **diploid** (double), or 2N. Gametes with a single set of 23 chromosomes are **haploid** (single), or N. A cell with an exact multiple of the haploid number is **euploid**. Euploid numbers may be 2N, 3N (triploid), or 4N (tetraploid). Chromosome numbers that are exact multiples of N but greater than 2N are called **polyploid**. **Aneuploidy** refers to a chromosome complement that is abnormal in number but is not an exact multiple of N. An aneuploid cell may be **trisomic** (2N + 1 chromosome) or **monosomic** (2N - 1 chromosome).

Disjunction is the normal separation and migration of chromosomes during cell division. Failure of the process, or **nondisjunction**, in a meiotic division results in one daughter cell receiving both homologous chromosomes and the other receiving neither. It is the primary cause of aneuploidy. If this deviation in normal processes occurs during the first meiotic division, half of the gametes will contain 22 chromosomes and half will contain 24. If joined with a normal gamete, a gamete produced in this manner will produce either a monosomic (2N - 1) or trisomic (2N + 1) zygote.

Deviations in the normal structure of chromosomes result from the chromosome material breaking and reassembling in an abnormal arrangement. Structural abnormalities include deletion, duplication, inversion, or translocation.

In **deletion**, or loss of a portion of a chromosome, the missing segment may be a terminal portion of the chromosome resulting from a single break or an internal section resulting from two breaks. **Cri-du-chat syndrome** is such a deletion and is manifested by the "cry of the cat" in an affected child.

Duplication is the presence of a repeated gene or gene sequence. A deleted segment of one chromosome may become incorporated into its homologous chromosome.

Inversion is the reversal of gene order. The linear arrangement of genes on a chromosome is broken, and the order of a portion of the gene complement is reversed in the process of reattachment.

Translocation is the transfer of part of one chromosome to a nonhomologous chromosome. This occurs when two chromosomes break and the segments are rejoined in an abnormal arrangement.

2. **Cite examples of chromosome disorders.**
   Refer to Figures 2-11 through 2-13 and Table 2-1.

A common example of an autosomal aneuploidy disorder that results from an abnormality of chromosome number is trisomy 21, or **Down syndrome**. This disorder can result when nondisjunction of chromosome 21 occurs at meiosis, producing one gamete with an extra chromosome 21 and one gamete with no chromosome 21. Union of the extra chromosome female gamete with a normal sperm produces a 47-chromosome zygote, or trisomy 21.

The overall incidence of Down syndrome is 1 per 800 live births. The incidence increases with increasing maternal age. Clinical diagnosis of trisomy 21 is often based on facial appearance. A low nasal bridge, epicanthal folds, protruding tongue, and low-set ears are common. Mental retardation is consistent in children with Down syndrome, but its degree may vary. The average IQ is approximately 50.

Two sex chromosome aneuploidy disorders are **Turner syndrome** (female) and **Klinefelter syndrome** (male). The most common karyotype showing female phenotype is 45, X; the male karyotype is 47, XXY.

The diagnosis of Turner syndrome is suggested in the newborn by the presence of redundant neck skin and peripheral lymphedema. Later, the presence of short stature is suggestive.

Klinefelter syndrome is a common cause of infertility in men. Other manifestations include long lower extremities, sparse body hair with female distribution, and female breast development in about 50 percent of the cases. A moderate degree of mental impairment may be present.

3. Characterize single-gene disorders.
Study pages 50-58; refer to Figures 2-18, 2-23, and 2-25.

An inherited gene may be present on one or both chromosomes of a pair. The pedigree patterns of inherited traits are dependent on whether the gene is located on an autosomal chromosome, any chromosome other than a sex chromosome, or the X chromosome and whether the gene is dominant or recessive. These factors allow four basic patterns of inheritance for single-gene traits, whether normal or abnormal: autosomal dominant, autosomal recessive, X-linked dominant, and X-linked recessive.

In **autosomal dominant** inheritance of genetic defects, the abnormal allele is dominant and the normal allele is recessive. The phenotype is the same whether the allele is present in either a homozygous or heterozygous state.

Principles of autosomal dominant inheritance are (1) affected persons have an affected parent, (2) affected persons mating with normal persons have affected and unaffected offspring in equal proportion, and (3) males and females are equally affected.

In **autosomal recessive** disorders, the abnormal allele is recessive. For the trait to be expressed, a person must be homozygous for the abnormal allele. Because the dominant or normal allele masks the trait, most persons who are heterozygous for an autosomal recessive allele are phenotypically normal. When two heterozygous individuals mate and an offspring receives the recessive allele from each parent, the trait is expressed.

Characteristics of autosomal recessive inheritance are (1) the trait usually appears in siblings only, not in the parents; (2) males and females are equally likely to be affected; (3) for parents of one affected child, the recurrence risk is one in four for every subsequent birth; (4) both parents of an affected child carry the recessive allele; and (5) the parents of the affected child may be consanguineous or blood relatives.

Unlike the 44 autosomes that can be arranged in 22 homologous pairs, the two sex chromosomes in the female are XX and in the male are XY. Because the ovum must contain an X chromosome, if it is fertilized by a sperm containing an X chromosome, the progeny will be a female (XX). If the sperm contributes a Y chromosome, the progeny will be male (XY).

Traits determined by either dominant or recessive **X-linked genes** are expressed in the male. The genes on the X chromosome cannot be transmitted from father to son (fathers contribute a Y chromosome to sons) but are transmitted from father to all daughters through one X chromosome. Recessive abnormal genes on the X chromosome of a female may not be expressed because they are matched by normal genes inherited with the other X chromosome.

X-linked dominant disorders are rare. The main characteristic of this inheritance pattern is that an affected male transmits the gene to all of his daughters and to none of his sons. The affected female may transmit the gene to offspring of either sex.

In **X-linked recessive** disorders, the recessive gene located on the one X chromosome of the male is not balanced by the dominant allele on the Y chromosome and is thus expressed. Only matings between an affected male and a carrier or affected female should result in an affected female.

Males affected with an X-linked recessive disorder cannot transmit the gene to sons but transmit it to all daughters. An unaffected female who is heterozygous for the recessive gene transmits it to 50 percent of her sons and daughters.

Principles of the X-linked recessive inheritance are (1) males are predominantly affected, (2) affected males cannot transmit the gene to sons but transmit the gene to all daughters, (3) sons of female carriers have a 50 percent risk of being affected, and (4) daughters of female carriers have a 50 percent risk of being carriers.

4. Cite examples of single-gene disorders.
Study pages 51-58; refer to Figure 2-21 and Table 2-2.

One of the best-known autosomal dominant diseases is **Huntington disease**, a neurologic disorder which exhibits progressive dementia and increasingly uncontrollable movements of the limbs. A key feature of this disease is that its symptoms are not usually seen until after age 40. Thus, those who develop the disease often have had children before they are aware that they have the gene.

The severity of an autosomal dominant disease can vary greatly. An example of variable expressivity in an autosomal dominant disease is type 1 **neurofibromatosis**, or von Recklinghausen disease, which has been mapped to the long arm of chromosome 17. The expression of this gene can vary from a few harmless "cáfe au lait" spots on the skin to numerous malignant neurofibromas, scoliosis, seizures, gliomas, neuromas, hypertension, and mental retardation.

The **cystic fibrosis** gene, the cause of a lethal autosomal recessive gene, has been mapped to the long arm of chromosome 7. In this disease, defective transport of chloride ions leads to a salt imbalance that results in secretions of abnormally thick, dehydrated mucus. Some of the digestive organs, particularly the pancreas, become obstructed with mucus, resulting in malnutrition. The lung airways tend to become clogged with mucus, making them highly susceptible to bacterial infections.

The most common and severe of all X-linked recessive disorders is **Duchenne muscular dystrophy**, which affects males. This disorder is characterized by progressive muscle degeneration; individuals are usually unable to walk by age 10 or 12. The disease also affects the heart and respiratory muscles, and death due to respiratory or cardiac failure may occur before age 20. These cases are due to an absence of dystrophin, without which the muscle cell cannot survive, and muscle deterioration follows.

5. **Characterize multifactorial inheritance and cite examples.**
   Study pages 61-63; refer to Figures 2-28 and 2-29.

Not all traits are produced by single genes; some traits are the result of several genes acting together. When several genes act together, the trait is referred to as **polygenic**. When environmental factors also influence the expression of the trait, the term **multifactorial inheritance** is used. Both genes and environment contribute to variation in traits. Multifactorial disorders tend to cluster in families.

Although both height and IQ are determined by genes, they are also influenced by environment. For example, height has increased by 5 to 10 cm since the turn of the century because of improvements in nutrition and health care. Also, IQ scores can be improved by exposing children to enriched learning environments.

A number of diseases do not follow the bell-shaped distribution of polygenic and multifactorial traits. Instead, a certain threshold of liability must be crossed before the disease is expressed. A well-known example of a threshold trait is pyloric stenosis, a disorder characterized by a narrowing or obstruction of the pylorus. Chronic vomiting, constipation, weight loss, and electrolyte imbalance can result from this condition. Pyloric stenosis is much more common in males than in females. The reason for this difference is that the threshold of liability is much lower in males than in females. Thus, fewer defective alleles are required to generate the disorder in males. This also means that the offspring of affected females are more likely to have pyloric stenosis because affected females carry more disease-causing alleles than do most affected males.

Other multifactorial diseases include cleft lip and/or cleft palate, neural tube defects, clubfeet, and some forms of congenital heart disease. Hypertensive heart disease and diabetes mellitus likely can be grouped in the category of multifactorial disorders.

Practice Examination

1. Which genetic disease is caused by an abnormal karyotype?

   a. Down syndrome
   b. Huntington disease
   c. PKU
   d. neurofibromatosis
   e. cystic fibrosis

2. Which is not characteristic of Down syndrome?

   a. It is an autosomal aneuploidy.
   b. It is a genetic error of metabolism.
   c. Mental retardation is consistently expressed.
   d. Clinical diagnosis can be based on facial appearance.
   e. The karyotype is 47, XY + 21.

3. Cri-du-chat syndrome is an abnormality of chromosomal structure involving:

   a. translocation.
   b. an inversion.
   c. duplication.
   d. deletion.

4. An individual's karyotype lacks a homologous X chromosome and has only a single X chromosome present. Which statement is not true?

   a. The karyotype is 45, X.
   b. Features include ribbed neck and short stature.
   c. The karyotype is 46, XY.
   d. The disorder is a sex chromosome aneuploidy.

5. If homologous chromosomes fail to separate during meiosis, the disorder is:

   a. polyploidy.
   b. aneuploidy.
   c. disjunction.
   d. nondisjunction.
   e. translocation.

6. Cystic fibrosis has been mapped to chromosome:

   a. 17.
   b. 7.
   c. X.
   d. 16.

7. In autosomal dominant inherited disorders:

   a. affected individuals do not have an affected parent.
   b. affected persons mating with normal persons have a 50% risk of having an affected offspring.
   c. male offspring are most often affected.
   d. unaffected children born to affected parents will have affected children.

8. In X-linked recessive inherited disorders:

   a. affected males have normal sons.
   b. affected males have affected daughters.
   c. sons of female carriers have a 50% risk of being affected.
   d. the affected female may transmit the gene to both sons and daughters.

9. Which is not an autosomal dominant disease?

   a. Huntington disease
   b. neurofibromatosis
   c. Duchenne muscular dystrophy
   d. von Recklinghausen disease
   e. pyloric stenosis

10. When environmental influences cause varied phenotypic expressions of genotypes, the result is a/an:

    a. multifactorial trait.
    b. threshold liability.
    c. autosomal dominant trait.
    d. X-linked recessive trait.

11. Which likely is not a multifactorial inherited disorder?

    a. cleft palate
    b. hypertension
    c. diabetes mellitus
    d. cystic fibrosis
    e. heart disease

Match the term with the circumstance.

12. ____ recessive disorder
13. ____ multifactorial inheritance
14. ____ aneuploidy
15. ____ chromosomal aberration
16. ____ phenotype
17. ____ pedigree
18. ____ autosomal recessive inheritance

a. due to numerical or structural aberrations
b. many genes are common
c. two or more cell lines with different karyotypes
d. individual is homozygous for a gene
e. failure of homologous chromosomes to separate during meiosis or mitosis
f. outward appearance of an individual
g. a probability of .25
h. summarizes family relationships

Match the term with the circumstance.

19. ____ expressivity
20. ____ X-linked
21. ____ inversion
22. ____ dominant trait
23. ____ allele
24. ____ 47, XXY
25. ____ karyotype

a. a probability of .5
b. females are unlikely to be affected
c. species chromosomal morphology
d. expressed by one allele
e. Turner syndrome
f. different version of the same paired gene
g. Klinefelter syndrome
h. no loss or gain of genetic material, reversed order
i. extent of phenotypic variation of a particular genotype

CHAPTER

3

Altered Cellular and Tissue Biology

Foundational Objective

a. Describe processes of cellular intake and output. Review pages 14-20.

Memory Check!

- The intact, normally functioning plasma membrane is selectively or differentially permeable to substances; it allows some substances to pass while excluding others. Water and small, uncharged substances move through pores of the lipid bilayer by passive transport, which requires no expenditure of energy. This process is driven by the forces of osmosis, hydrostatic pressure, and diffusion. Larger molecules and molecular complexes are moved into the cell by active transport, which requires the expenditure of energy or ATP by the cell. In active transport, materials move from low concentrations to high concentrations. The largest molecules and fluids are ingested by endocytosis and expelled by exocytosis after cellular synthesis of smaller building blocks. When the plasma membrane is injured, it becomes permeable to virtually everything, and substances move into and out of the cells in an unrestricted manner. Notably, such substances may affect (1) the nucleus and its genetic information or (2) the cytoplasmic organelles and their varied functions. Then, there is altered cellular physiology and pathology.

Objectives

After studying this chapter, the learner will be able to:

1. **Describe the cellular adaptations occurring in atrophy, hypertrophy, hyperplasia, dysplasia, and metaplasia. Identify the condition under which each can occur.** Study pages 69-71; refer to Figures 3-1 and 3-2.

When confronted with environmental stresses that disrupt normal structure and function, the cell undergoes adaptive changes that permit survival and maintain function. An adapted cell is neither normal nor injured—it is somewhere between these two states. These changes may lead to atrophy, hypertrophy, hyperplasia, dysplasia, or metaplasia.

Cellular atrophy decreases the cell substance and results in cell shrinkage. Causes of atrophy include disuse, denervation, decreased endocrine stimulation, decreased nutrition, and ischemia. Atrophy commonly is seen in muscles that are not used or innervated.

Hypertrophy increases cell size. Hypertrophy is commonly seen in cardiac and skeletal muscle tissue. The increase in cell components is related to an increased rate of protein synthesis. Physiologic hypertrophy is observed in uterine tissue and mammary glands during pregnancy.

Hyperplasia is an increase in the number of cells of a tissue or organ. It occurs in tissues where cells are capable of mitotic division. Breast and uterine enlargement during pregnancy are examples of physiologic hyperplasia and hypertrophy that are hormonally regulated. A pathologic hyperplasia occurs when the endometrium enlarges because of excessive estrogen production. Then, abnormally thickened uterine layer may bleed excessively and frequently. Compensatory hyperplasia enables certain organs, like the liver, to regenerate after loss of substance.

Dysplasia is deranged cell growth that results in cells that vary in size, shape, and appearance of mature cells and is related to hyperplasia. Dysplasia occurs in association with chronic irritation or inflammation in the uterine cervix, oral cavity, gallbladder, and respiratory passages. Dysplasia is potentially reversible once the irritating cause has been removed. Dysplastic changes may progress to neoplastic disease.

Metaplasia is a reversible conversion from one adult cell type to another adult cell type. It allows for replacement with cells that are better able to tolerate environmental stresses. In metaplasia, one type of cell may be converted to another type of cell within its tissue class. An example of metaplasia is the substitution of stratified squamous epithelial cells for ciliated columnar epithelial cells in the airways of an individual who is a habitual cigarette smoker.

2. **Identify the mechanism of cellular injury for hypoxia, chemicals, infectious agents, immunological and inflammatory responses, genetic factors, nutritional imbalances, and physical trauma.**
   Study pages 71-77; refer to Figures 3-3 through 3-6 and Table 3-1.

Hypoxia deprives the cell of oxygen and interrupts oxidative metabolism and the generation of ATP. As oxygen tension within the cell falls, oxidative metabolism ceases and the cell reverts to anaerobic metabolism. One of the earliest effects of reduced ATP is acute cellular swelling caused by failure of the sodium-potassium membrane pump. With impaired function of this pump, intracellular potassium levels decrease and sodium and water accumulate within the cell. As fluid and ions move into the cell, there is dilatation of the endoplasmic reticulum, increased membrane permeability, and decreased mitochondrial function as extracellular calcium accumulates in the mitochondria. If the oxygen supply is not restored, there is continued loss of essential enzymes, proteins, and ribonucleic acid through the very permeable membrane of the cell. Hypoxia can result from inadequate oxygen in the air, respiratory disease, decreased blood flow due to circulatory disease, anemia, or inability of the cells to utilize oxygen. In edema, the distance for diffusion of oxygen may become too great.

Toxic chemical agents can injure the cell membrane and cell structures, block enzymatic pathways, coagulate cell proteins, and disrupt the osmotic and ionic balance of cells. Chemicals may injure cells during the process of metabolism or elimination. Carbon tetrachloride, for example, causes little damage until it is metabolized by liver enzymes to highly reactive free radicals, and then it is extremely toxic to liver cells. Carbon monoxide has a special affinity for the hemoglobin molecule and reduces hemoglobin's ability to carry oxygen.

Alcohol (ethanol) is the favorite mood-altering drug in the United States. Liver disease, nutritional disorders, and CNS impairment are serious consequences of alcohol abuse. The hepatic changes, initiated by ethanol conversion to acetaldehyde, include deposition of fat, enlargement of the liver, interruption of transport of proteins and their secretion, increase in intracellular water, depression of fatty acid oxidation, increased membrane rigidity, and acute liver cell necrosis. In the CNS, alcohol is a depressant, initially affecting subcortical structures. Consequently, motor and intellectual activity become disoriented. At high blood alcohol levels, respiratory medullary centers become depressed.

Infectious agents that survive and proliferate in the body may produce substances that injure cells and tissues. They also produce toxins and damaging hypersensitivity reactions.

Immunologic and inflammatory injury are important causes of cellular injury. Cellular membranes are injured by direct contact with cellular and chemical components of the immune and inflammatory responses. Such mediators are lymphocytes and macrophages and chemicals such as histamine, antibodies, lymphokines, complement, and proteases. Complement, a serum protein, is responsible for many of the membrane alterations that occur during immunologic injury. Membrane alterations are associated with rapid leakage of potassium out of the cell and rapid influx of water. Antibodies can interfere with membrane function by binding to and occupying receptor molecules on the plasma membrane. (Later chapters will deal with these injurious consequences as well as with hypersensitivity and autoimmune disease.)

Genetic disorders may alter the cell's nucleus and the plasma membrane's structure, shape, receptors, or transport mechanisms. (Mechanisms causing genetic abnormalities were discussed in an earlier chapter.)

Nutritional imbalances are important because cells require adequate amounts of proteins, carbohydrates, lipids, vitamins, and minerals to function normally. If inadequate or excessive amounts of nutrients are consumed and transported, pathophysiologic cellular effects can develop.

Injurious physical agents include temperature extremes, changes in atmospheric pressure, radiation, illumination, mechanical factors, noise, and prolonged vibration. Physical injury is often environmental.

The **temperature extremes** of chilling or freezing of cells cause hypothermic injury directly by creating high intracellular sodium concentrations. Vasoconstriction causes ischemic injury, infarction, and necrosis. Hyperthermic injury, excessive heat, varies depending on the nature, intensity, and duration of the heat. Burns cause extensive loss of fluids and plasma proteins.

Sudden increases or decreases in **atmospheric pressure** cause blast injury. In air blast or explosive injuries, tissue injury is due to compressive waves of air against the body. The pressure changes may collapse the thorax, rupture solid internal organs, or cause widespread hemorrhage. In immersion blast, water pressure is applied suddenly to the body, and the body is forced up out of the water. With sudden decreases in pressure, carbon dioxide and nitrogen normally dissolved in the blood leave solution and form tiny bubbles, gas emboli, which obstruct blood vessels and cause hypoxia.

Ionizing radiation is any form of radiation capable of removing orbital electrons from atoms. Ionizing radiation is emitted by x-rays, gamma rays, and alpha and beta particles. DNA is the most vulnerable target of radiation. Irradiation during mitosis produces chromosome aberrations.

The harmful effects of **illumination** in fluorescent lighting include eye strain, obscured vision, and possible cataract formation. Emission of ultraviolet radiation from halogen lamps is thought to be in the range of wavelength responsible for inducing skin cancer.

Mechanical injury is caused by physical impact or irritation. Most mechanical stresses, however, are subtle and can cause accumulative injuries and disorders over time.

Noise trauma can be caused by acute loud noise or by the cumulative effects of various intensities, frequencies, and durations of noise. Acoustic trauma impairs hearing.

3. Identify various cellular accumulations occurring in response to injury and the subsequent manifestations of cellular damage.
Study pages 78-82; refer to Figures 3-7 through 3-9 and Table 3-2.

Cellular accumulations occur whenever normal substances are produced in excess, normal and abnormal substances are ineffectively catabolized, or harmful exogenous materials accumulate intracellularly. (See box on page 15 of *Workbook*.)

4. Identify the major types of cellular necrosis and cite examples of the tissues involved in each type. Compare necrosis with apoptosis.
Study pages 82-83; refer to Figure 3-10.

Necrosis is local cell death and involves the process of cellular self-digestion known as autodigestion or autolysis. As necrosis progresses, most organelles are disrupted and karyolysis, nuclear dissolution from the action of hydrolytic enzymes, becomes evident. There are four major types of necrosis: coagulative, liquefactive, caseous, and fatty. Gangrenous necrosis is not a distinctive type of cell death but refers to large areas of tissue death.

Coagulative necrosis occurs primarily in the kidneys, heart, and adrenal glands and usually results from hypoxia caused by severe ischemia. Protein denaturation causes coagulation.

Liquefactive necrosis is common following ischemic injury to neurons and glial cells in the brain. Because brain cells are rich in digestive hydrolytic enzymes and lipids, the brain cells are digested by their own hydrolases. The brain tissue becomes soft, liquefies, and is walled off from healthy tissue to form cysts. Bacterial infections are causes of liquefactive necrosis.

Caseous necrosis is commonly seen in tuberculous pulmonary infection and is a combination of coagulative and liquefactive necrosis. The necrotic debris is not digested completely by hydrolases, so tissues appear soft and granular and resemble clumped cheese. A granulomatous inflammatory wall may enclose the central areas of caseous necrosis.

Cellular Accumulations

Accumulation	Causes	Injury
H_2O	Extracellular H_2O shifts into cell, reduced ATP and ATPase, sodium accumulates in cell	Cellular swelling, vacuolation, hydropic degeneration
Lipids, Carbohydrates	Imbalance in production, utilization, or mobilization of lipid or carbohydrates	Vacuolation, displaced nucleus and organelles, leads to fibrosis and scarring
Glycogen	Genetic disorders, diabetes mellitus	Cytoplasmic vacuolation
Proteins	Enzymes digest cellular organelles, renal disorders, plasma cell tumor	Disrupted function and intracellular communication, displaced cellular organelles
Pigments	Exogenous particle ingestion, UV light stimulates melanin production, malignancy, loss of hormonal feedback, genetic defects, bruising and hemorrhage increases hemosiderin, liver dysfunction	Membrane injury, disrupted cellular metabolism
Calcium	Altered membrane permeability, influx of extracellular calcium, excretion of H^+ leading to more OH^- which precipitates Ca^{++}, endocrine disturbances	Hardening of cellular structure, interferes with function
Urate	Absence of enzymes	Crystal deposition, inflammation

The **fatty necrosis** found in the breast, pancreas, and other abdominal structures is a specific cellular dissolution caused by lipases. Lipases break down triglycerides and release free fatty acids which then combine with calcium, magnesium, and sodium ions to create soaps, or saponification. The necrotic tissue appears opaque and chalk white.

Gangrenous necrosis refers to death of tissue, usually in considerable mass and putrefaction. It results from severe hypoxic injury subsequent to arteriosclerosis or blockage of major arteries followed by bacterial invasion. Dry gangrene is usually due to a coagulative necrosis, while wet gangrene develops when neutrophils invade the site and cause liquefactive necrosis. Gas gangrene, a special type of gangrene, is due to bacterial infection of injured tissue by species of *Clostridium*. These anaerobic bacteria produce hydrolytic enzymes and toxins that destroy connective tissue and cellular membrane; bubbles of gas likely form in muscle cells.

Apoptosis is an important, distinct type of cell death that differs from necrosis. It is an active process of cellular self-destruction in both normal and pathologic tissue changes. Apoptosis likely plays a role in deletion of cells during embryonic development and in endocrine-dependent tissues that are undergoing atrophic change. It may occur spontaneously in malignant tumors and in normal, rapidly proliferating cells treated with cancer chemotherapeutic agents and ionizing radiation. Unlike necrosis, apoptosis affects scattered, single cells and results in shrinkage of a cell, whereas in necrosis, cells swell and lyse.

5. Compare the different theories of aging.
Study pages 83-88; refer to Figure 3-11 and Tables 3-3 and 3-4.

Much of the confusion about aging arises from the difficulty of distinguishing between normal aging and changes that are secondary to disease. Health and longevity are affected by a number of factors such as heredity, culture, race, and nutrition. Mechanisms of aging likely involve (1) cellular changes produced by genetic and environmental factors, (2) changes in cellular regulatory or control mechanisms, and (3) degenerative extravascular and vascular alterations. Each mechanistic theory provides clues to the processes involved in aging.

Genetic and Environmental Factors—Cells may be programmed at birth or injured during life by factors such as ionizing radiation that cause mitotic division and replication errors. This could lead to either cellular atrophy or death. Regardless of damaging environmental factors, it is proposed that each cell may have a finite number of times it can replicate; there exists a limited number of cellular doublings. In this model, an intrinsic program within the human genome progressively slows or terminates mitosis.

Cellular Control Mechanistic Alterations—The neuroendocrine theory of aging states that hormonal and neural agents relay a genetic program for aging to peripheral tissues. Mechanisms may increase hormonal degradation or decrease hormonal synthesis or secretion.

The immune system likely is involved in aging since immune function declines with age. This decline may be related to certain diseases such as cancer or may occur in response to any increase in autoantibodies that attack body tissues.

Degenerative Extracellular Changes—Aging affects extracellular matrix by increasing collagen cross-linking. This process decreases cell permeability to nutrients and renders collagen less functional.

Free radicals serve as central agents in the changes observed with aging. Free radicals are parts of molecules or molecules that have had an electron stripped from their structure. Diffusible free radicals damage or alter the original structure or function of other molecules by attaching to these other molecules. This theory has been linked to the idea of oxygen toxicity since oxidation of carbohydrate, fat, protein, and other elements in the body results in the formation of free oxygen radicals.

6. Characterize somatic death and its manifestations.
Study page 88.

Somatic death is death of the entire organism. Unlike the changes that follow cellular death in a viable body, somatic death is diffuse and does not involve components of the inflammatory response, a vascular response to injury. The most notable manifestations of somatic death are that there is complete cessation of respiration and circulation, the surface of the skin usually becomes pale and yellowish, and body temperature falls gradually until, after 24 hours, body temperature equals that of the environment.

Within six hours after death, depletion of ATP interferes with ATP-dependent detachment of the contractile proteins, and muscle stiffening or rigor mortis develops. Within 12 to 14 hours, rigor mortis usually affects the entire body. Rigor mortis gradually diminishes as the body becomes flaccid due to the release of enzymes and lytic dissolution.

Practice Examination

1. A cellular adaptation observable in uterine cervical epithelium is:

   a. atrophy.
   b. hyperplasia.
   c. hypertrophy.
   d. dysplasia.
   e. metaplasia.

2. What are the consequences when a cell is forced into anaerobic glycolysis? (*More than one answer may be correct.*)

   a. insufficient glucose production
   b. excessive pyruvic acid retention
   c. increased lactic acid
   d. inadequate ATP production
   e. excessive CO_2 production

Match the descriptor with the term.

3. ____ reduced oxygen tension	a. anoxia
4. ____ accumulates in mitochondria	b. melanin
	c. lipids
	d. hypoxia
	e. calcium

5. What is the probable cause of cellular swelling in the early stages of cell injury?

   a. fat inclusion
   b. loss of genetic integrity
   c. hydrolytic enzyme activation
   d. Na-K pump fails to remove intracellular Na^+.
   e. None of the above is correct.

Match the process with its cause.

6. ____ lipid peroxidation	a. carbon monoxide
7. ____ neurotransmitter interference	b. oxygen-deprived free radicals
8. ____ asphyxiation	c. ethanol
9. ____ depressed fatty acid oxidation	d. lead
10. ____ depressed protein synthesis	e. detached ribosomes
	f. increased lactate
	g. lysosomal edema

11. Dystrophic calcification:

   a. occurs in dying or dead tissues.
   b. is the result of too much calcium in the blood.
   c. is observed in chronic lesions.
   d. Both a and c are correct.
   e. a, b, and c are correct.

12. Cellular swelling is:

    a. irreversible.
    b. evident early in all types of cellular injury.
    c. manifested by decreased intracellular sodium.
    d. None of the above is correct.
    e. Both b and c are correct.

13. Which is not reversible?

    a. karyolysis
    b. fatty infiltration
    c. hydropic degeneration
    d. All of the above are reversible.

14. Aging:

    a. is easy to distinguish from pathology.
    b. does not have a genetic relationship.
    c. is more advanced in primitive societies.
    d. None of the above is correct.
    e. a, b, and c are correct.

15. In aging, cross-linking implies that:

    a. the life span and number of times a cell can replicate are programmed.
    b. the number of cell doublings is limited.
    c. there is oxygen toxicity.
    d. cell permeability decreases.
    e. Both a and b are correct.

Match the manifestation with the condition.

16. ____ necrosis caused by *Clostridia*	a. liquefactive
17. ____ rigidity of muscles after somatic death	b. rigor mortis
18. ____ increased cell numbers	c. gas gangrene
19. ____ necrosis resulting from lysosomal release	d. hyperplasia
20. ____ replacement of one cell type with another, more suitable type	e. metaplasia
	f. cloudy swelling
	g. coagulation

Match the circumstance with the condition.

21. ____ decreased cell size
22. ____ pancreatic necrosis
23. ____ coagulative and liquefactive necrosis
24. ____ tissue death
25. ____ normal and pathologic cellular self-destruction

a. fatty necrosis
b. gangrene
c. atrophy
d. caseous necrosis
e. apoptosis
f. algor mortis
g. hypertrophy

CHAPTER

4

Fluids and Electrolytes, Acids and Bases

Foundational Objectives

a. Describe the different compartments for body fluids and identify the fluid distribution changes occurring with age. Review pages 94-97; refer to Figure 4-1 and Tables 4-1 through 4-3.

b. Describe the factors that affect water movement. Review pages 94-97; refer to Figure 4-2.

c. Identify the distribution of electrolytes in body compartments. Refer to Table 4-4.

> **Memory Check!**
>
> - $\text{mEq/L} = \dfrac{\text{milligrams of ion per liter of solution} \times \text{number of charges of one ion}}{\text{atomic weight of ion}}$
> - mEq/L expresses the concentration of chemicals dissolved in body fluids; they relate to chemical activity.

d. Identify the role of ADH, aldosterone, and natriuretic hormone in water and electrolyte balance. Review pages 98-99.

e. Identify body mechanisms to buffer excessive hydrogen ion/acid and explain the mechanics of the most important buffer. Distinguish between short-term and long-term adjustments. Review pages 108-110; refer to Figure 4-6 and Tables 4-9 and 4-10.

> **Memory Check!**
>
> - Pulmonary acid/base regulation of blood involves CO_2 and is rapid.
>
> $CO_2 + H_2O \leftrightarrow H_2CO_3 \leftrightarrow H^+ + HCO_3^-$
>
>   An increase in CO_2 tension liberates hydrogen ions; thus, the pH decreases. A decrease in CO_2 tension results in fewer hydrogen ions; thus, the pH increases.
> - Renal acid/base regulation of blood involves HCO_3^- conservation and H^+ and NH_3 excretion and is slow. This process essentially secretes H^+ into the urine and returns HCO_3^- to the blood plasma.

Objectives

After review of this chapter, the learner will be able to:

1. **Identify the mechanisms causing edema.**
Study pages 97-98; refer to Figure 4-3.

Edema is the accumulation of fluid within interstitial spaces. It may be excess or sequestered fluid.

Common Causes of Edema

- High capillary pressure, high hydrostatic pressure, venous obstruction or arteriolar dilation
- Low blood protein or plasma-filtered oncotic pressure, albumin loss from kidney disease or burns, protein malnutrition
- Lymphatic blockage, filtered proteins from the blood failing to reenter the capillaries thus drawing water from capillaries, cancer therapy with removal of lymph nodes and vessels (mastectomy)
- Increased capillary permeability to histamine, inflammation

Edema may be localized or generalized. Localized edema appears confined to traumatized tissues or within organ systems. Generalized edema exhibits a uniform distribution of fluid in the interstitial spaces.

Fluid movement can be explained by the following formula:

Q = (BHP + IFOP) - (IFHP + BOP)
[from vessel] [to vessel]

Q = fluid movement, BHP = blood hydrostatic pressure, IFOP = interstitial fluid osmotic pressure, IFHP = interstitial fluid hydrostatic pressure, and BOP = blood osmotic pressure.

Memory Check!

- Water moves from high concentration to low concentration and to dilute the solute.

2. **Define isotonic, hypertonic, and hypotonic water and solute alterations.**
Study pages 99-103; refer to Table 4-5.

Isotonic Imbalances—Extracellular fluid loss or gain is accompanied by proportional changes of electrolytes in these alterations. Losses are seen in hemorrhage or excessive sweating. Gains occur in administration of intravenous normal saline or renal retention of sodium and water. Cells do not shrink or swell in isotonic fluids.

Hypertonic Imbalances—Water loss or solute gain occurs in these changes. These alterations are seen in administration of hypertonic saline solutions, hyperaldosteronism, Cushing syndrome, diabetes, diarrhea, or insufficient water intake. Cells shrink in hypertonic fluid.

Hypotonic Imbalances—Water gain or solute loss occurs in these changes. These alterations may be caused by vomiting, diarrhea, burns, diuretics, excessive sweating, or renal failure to excrete water. Cells swell in hypotonic fluid.

3. **Identify the major consequences of abnormal levels of sodium, potassium, calcium, phosphate, and magnesium. Define the terms associated with excess or deficit of each electrolyte.**
Study pages 99-108; refer to Figures 4-4 and 4-5 and Tables 4-6 through 4-8.

(See box on page 22 of *Workbook.*)

4. **Differentiate between metabolic/respiratory acidosis and metabolic/respiratory alkalosis.**
Study pages 110-116; refer to Figures 4-8 through 4-11 and Table 4-11.

Important values include the following: pH = 7.35-7.45, K^+ = 5 mEq/L, Na^+ = 142 mEq/L, Cl^- = 104 mEq/L, HCO_3^- = 24 mEq/L, pCO_2 = 35-45 mm Hg, and CO_2 = 28 mEq/L.

Essentially, acidosis causes nervous system depression, and alkalosis causes nervous system irritability. The manifestations vary with the degree of alteration. (See box on page 23 of *Workbook.*)

Clinical Manifestations of Excess and Deficit States of Major Electrolytes

Excess	Deficit
Sodium	
Hypernatremia **> 147 mEq/L**	**Hyponatremia** **< 135 mEq/L**
Cellular shrinking due to hypertonic extracellular fluid, may cause central nervous system irritability, tachycardia, dry and flushed skin, hypertension, thirst, elevated temperature, rapid pulse, weight loss, oliguria, anuria	Cellular swelling, may cause cerebral edema, headache, stupor, coma, peripheral edema, polyuria, absence of thirst, decreased body temperature, rapid pulse, hypotension, nausea, vomiting
Potassium	
Hyperkalemia **> 5.5 mEq/L**	**Hypokalemia** **< 3.5 mEq/L**
Depressed conductivity in heart, muscle cramping, paresthesias, nausea, diarrhea, associated with metabolic acidosis	Cardiac irritability, dysrhythmias, vomiting, paralytic ileus, thirst, associated with metabolic alkalosis, inability to concentrate urine
Calcium	
Hypercalcemia **> 12 mg/dl**	**Hypocalcemia** **< 8.5 mg/dl**
Decreased neuromuscular excitability, muscle weakness, central nervous system depression, stupor to coma, increased risk of bone fracture, vomiting, constipation, kidney stones	Increased neuromuscular excitability, skeletal muscle cramps, tetany, laryngospasm, asphyxiation, death
Phosphate	
Hyperphosphatemia **> 4.5 mg/dl**	**Hypophosphatemia** **< 2.0 mg/dl**
See Hypocalcemia	Anorexia, weakness, osteomalacia, muscle weakness, tremors, seizures, coma, anemia, bleeding disorders, leukocytic alterations
Magnesium	
Hypermagnesemia **> 2.5 mEq/L**	**Hypomagnesemia** **< 1.5 mEq/L**
Skeletal muscle depression, muscle weakness, hypotension, bradycardia, respiratory depression	Hypocalcemia and hypokalemia, neuromuscular irritability, tetany, convulsions, tachycardia, hypertension

Comparison of Common Acid-Base Disturbances

Disturbance	Primary Disturbance	Correction/ Compensation	Usual Causes
Metabolic acidosis ($HCO_3^- < 24$ mEq/L)	Excess endogenous acid depletes bicarbonate or bicarbonate is lost by kidneys	Hyperventilation lowers pCO_2, kidneys excrete more hydrogen ions and retain more bicarbonate	Renal failure, ketosis, aspirin poisoning, over-production of lactic acid
Respiratory acidosis ($pCO_2 > 45$ mm Hg)	Inefficient excretion of carbon dioxide by lungs	Additional bicarbonate retention and H^+ excretion by kidneys	Chronic pulmonary disease, drug depression of respiratory center
Metabolic alkalosis ($HCO_3^- > 26$ mEq/L)	Excess plasma bicarbonate	Hypoventilation raises pCO_2 to acidify blood, kidneys increase H^+ retention and excrete HCO_3^-	Loss of gastric juice, chloride depletion, excess corticosteroid hormones, ingestion of excessive bicarbonate or other antacids
Respiratory alkalosis ($pCO_2 < 35$ mm Hg)	Hyperventilation lowers pCO_2	Increased excretion of bicarbonate and retention of H^+ by kidneys	Severe anxiety with hyperventilation, central nervous system disease, hypoxia, pulmonary imbalances

5. Describe what is meant by the "anion gap" and explain the significance of an abnormal anion gap in metabolic acidosis.
Study page 111.

The blood and cellular electrolytes must maintain osmotic neutrality; i.e., the number of cations must equal the number of anions present. Routine measurement of serum electrolytes usually involves only Na^+ and K^+ cations and the anions of Cl^- and HCO_3^- as total CO_2. There are about 12 mEq/L of other anions present in the blood that are not routinely measured; i.e., phosphates, sulfates, and protein anions. Therefore, assuming that no abnormal anions are present, an individual's serum sodium and potassium should equal the chloride + bicarbonate + 12 mEq/L of unmeasured, normal anions. If this is true, then the individual would have a normal **anion gap**. This may be expressed by the following formula:

$Na^+ + K^+ = Cl^- + HCO_3^- + 12$ mEq/L of unmeasured anions

In metabolic acidosis, a normal anion gap is related to bicarbonate loss and retention of chloride to maintain an ionic balance. This is described as hyperchloremic metabolic acidosis.

The significance of an abnormally large anion gap is that an abnormal anion is present in the blood from lactic acid, ketone bodies, salicylates, etc. When this is the case, the individual will have a low bicarbonate but there is not a corresponding increase in chloride. The anion gap will be greater than 12 mEq/L. If the anion gap is normal but the Cl^- has increased and the HCO_3^- is low, the metabolic acidosis may be due to diarrhea, ammonium chloride ingestion, or renal dysfunction.

Practice Examination

1. The total water loss per day in the adult is approximately:

   a. 0.8 liter.
   b. 1.2 liter.
   c. 1.8 liter.
   d. 2.2 liter.
   e. 2.8 liter.

2. Of the 60% of the body weight made up of water, about two-thirds is:

   a. extracellular water.
   b. intracellular water.
   c. intravascular water.
   d. interstitial water.
   e. None of the above is correct.

3. Sodium is responsible for:

   a. ICF osmotic balance.
   b. ECF osmotic balance.
   c. TBW osmolality.
   d. osmotic equilibrium.

4. A milliequivalent is a unit of:

   a. mass.
   b. physical activity.
   c. chemical activity.
   d. osmotic concentration.

5. Which statement is true?

   a. The number of ions and anions in the body must be equal.
   b. Intravascular molecules of protein are without charge.
   c. The sodium ions must be united with chloride ions.
   d. The positive and negative charges in blood plasma must be equal to each other.

6. Aldosterone controls ECF volume by:

   a. carbohydrate, fat, and protein catabolism.
   b. sodium reabsorption.
   c. potassium reabsorption.
   d. water reabsorption.
   e. Both b and d are correct.

7. The release of ADH is not stimulated by:

   a. stress.
   b. hyponatremia.
   c. hypernatremia.
   d. an increase in plasma osmolality.
   e. a decrease in plasma volume.

Match the term with its definition.

8. ____ hydrostatic pressure
9. ____ oncotic pressure

a. water-pulling effect of plasma proteins
b. pressure of blood within the capillaries
c. mechanism to move fluid to lymph glands
d. movement of fluid through semipermeable membrane

10. Laboratory studies of an adult reveal the following:
Plasma sodium = 110 mEq/L
Plasma chloride = 85 mEq/L
Plasma potassium = 4.8 mEq/L
Plasma calcium = 5.2 mEq/L
Plasma bicarbonate = 26 mEq/L

The most likely alteration is:

a. base bicarbonate deficit (metabolic acidosis).
b. hypokalemia.
c. hyponatremia.
d. base bicarbonate excess (metabolic alkalosis).
e. calcium deficit.

11. An individual suffers from weakness, dizziness, irritability, and intestinal cramps. Laboratory studies reveal the following:
Plasma sodium = 138 mEq/L
Plasma potassium = 6.8 mEq/L
Blood pH = 7.38
Plasma bicarbonate = 25 mEq/L
An EKG with tall, peaked T wave but otherwise normal

The individual is suffering from:

a. hypernatremia.
b. hyponatremia.
c. hypercalcemia.
d. hyperkalemia.
e. hypokalemia.

12. An acid is:

a. an anion.
b. a cation.
c. a substance/chemical that combines with a hydrogen ion to lower pH.
d. a substance/chemical that donates a hydrogen ion or a proton.

13. Strong acids (more than one answer may be correct):

a. include phosphoric acid.
b. contribute many H^+ to the solution.
c. have a pH of 7.
d. have a pH of 14.
e. are eliminated by the renal tubules.
f. are good buffers.

14. The blood pH is maintained near 7.4 by systems. The sequence from the fastest acting to the slowest acting system is:

a. lungs, kidney, blood buffers.
b. blood buffers, lungs, kidneys.
c. blood buffers, kidneys, lungs.
d. lungs, blood buffers, kidneys.

15. The pH of saliva is about 7 and the pH of gastric juice is about 2. How many times more concentrated is the hydrogen ion in gastric juice than in saliva?

a. 5
b. 50
c. 100
d. 10,000
e. 100,000

16. Which would not shift the blood pH toward alkalosis?

a. hydrogen ion secretion into urine
b. exhalation of carbon dioxide
c. bicarbonate ion secretion into urine
d. All of the above would shift the blood pH toward alkalosis.
e. None of the above would do so.

17. A young female became quite agitated and apprehensive and eventually lost consciousness. At the hospital emergency room, the following laboratory values were obtained:
Plasma sodium = 137 mEq/L
Plasma potassium = 5.0 mEq/L
Blood pH = 7.53
Serum CO_2 = 22 mm Hg
Plasma bicarbonate = 24 mEq/L

Her immediate diagnosis was:

a. hypokalemia.
b. metabolic acidosis.
c. metabolic alkalosis.
d. respiratory acidosis.
e. respiratory alkalosis.

18. As HCO_3^- shifts from the red blood cell to the blood plasma, it is expected that the plasma:

a. Na^+ increases.
b. Cl^- shifts into the red blood cell.
c. K^+ increases.
d. pH decreases.

Match the acid-base imbalance with the probable cause.

19. ____ respiratory acidosis
20. ____ respiratory alkalosis
21. ____ metabolic alkalosis

a. severe anxiety
b. diabetes
c. chronic diarrhea
d. emphysema
e. excessive baking soda ingestion

Match the acid-base imbalance with the compensatory mechanism.

22. ____ respiratory acidosis
23. ____ respiratory alkalosis
24. ____ metabolic acidosis

a. kidneys retain H^+ and excrete HCO_3^-
b. kidneys excrete H^+ and retain HCO_3^-
c. respirations increase, more CO_2 is eliminated
d. respirations decrease, more CO_2 is retained

25. An elevated anion gap is associated with an accumulation of:

    a. chloride anions.
    b. lactate anion.
    c. Both a and b are correct.
    d. Neither a nor b is correct.

CHAPTER 5

Immunity

Objectives

After review of this chapter, the learner will be able to:

1. **Distinguish between natural and acquired immunity, between primary and secondary responses, and between humoral and cell-mediated immunity.**
   Review pages 122-126; refer to Figures 5-3 through 5-6 and Table 5-1.

2. **Distinguish among the HLA complex, the Rh system, and the ABO system.**
   Review pages 127-128; refer to Figures 5-7 and 5-8.

3. **Describe the role of the B cell in humoral immunity.**
   Review pages 128-136; refer to Figures 5-9 and 5-13.

4. **Identify the structure and an important role for each of the five classes of immunoglobulins.**
   Review page 134; refer to Figures 5-10 through 5-12 and Table 5-2.

5. **Describe the secretory immune system.**
   Review pages 134-136; refer to Figure 5-14.

6. **Describe the role of the T cell in cellular immunity.**
   Review pages 136-138; refer to Figure 5-15 and Table 5-3.

7. **Characterize the interactions within the immune response; describe the cytokines.**
   Review pages 138-143; refer to Figures 5-16 through 5-18 and Table 5-4.

Practice Examination

Match the term with its definition.

1. ____ phagocytosis
2. ____ specific immunity
3. ____ macrophage
4. ____ nonspecific immunity
5. ____ antigen

a. immunoglobulins, lymphokines

b. lymphocyte that attacks antibodies directly

c. ingestion and destruction

d. phagocytic, agranular leukocyte of the immune system

e. resists a large variety of antigens

f. macromolecular pattern for antibody production

g. protein produced by T cells

h. exclusively thymus-dependent

6. Antigenicity depends on:

a. chemical structure.
b. foreignness.
c. complexity.
d. Both b and c are correct.
e. a, b, and c are correct.

7. The HLA complex:

a. has both A and B antibodies.
b. antigens are found on the surfaces of most cells except erythrocytes.
c. is an antigen system found on erythrocytes.
d. None of the above is correct.

8. When antigen binds to its appropriate antibody:

a. agglutination may occur.
b. phagocytosis may occur.
c. antigen neutralization may occur.
d. All of the above are correct.
e. None of the above is correct.

9. Antibodies are produced by:

a. B cells.
b. T cells.
c. helper cells.
d. plasma cells.
e. memory cells.

10. An immunoglobulin contains:

    a. two heavy and two light polypeptide chains.
    b. four heavy and four light polypeptide chains.
    c. two heavy and four light polypeptide chains.
    d. four heavy and two light polypeptide chains.

11. The antibody class having the highest concentration in the blood is:

    a. IgA.
    b. IgD.
    c. IgE.
    d. IgG.
    e. IgM.

12. Which antibody is matched with its appropriate role?

    a. IgA/allergic reactions
    b. IgD/found in respiratory secretions
    c. IgE/found in gastric secretions
    d. IgG/first to challenge the antigen
    e. IgM/first to challenge the antigen

13. The primary immune response involves:

    a. a rapid plasma cell response with peak antibody by three days.
    b. macrophage production of antibodies.
    c. T cell production of antibodies.
    d. a latent period followed by peak antibody production.

14. Which cells are phagocytic?

    a. B cells
    b. T cells
    c. T suppressors
    d. T killers
    e. macrophages

15. When a child develops measles and acquires an immunity to subsequent infections, the immunity is:

    a. acquired.
    b. active.
    c. natural.
    d. Both a and b are correct.

Match the term with its descriptor.

16. ____ antibody combining site
17. ____ epitopes
18. ____ monoclonal antibodies
19. ____ mucous membrane
20. ____ memory cell

a. antigenic determinants

b. useful for diagnosis

c. first line of defense

d. relies on the specificity between antibody and antigen

e. secretes antibodies

f. long-term immunity

g. produced after initial contact with an antigen

h. predominant antibody of secondary response

Match the descriptor with the lymphocytic activity.

21. ____ capable of forming clones
22. ____ produce lymphokines
23. ____ helper and suppressor cells
24. ____ antibody formation
25. ____ cell-mediated response

a. T cell involvement

b. B cell involvement

c. both T cell and B cell involvement

CHAPTER 6

Inflammation

Objectives

After review of this chapter, the learner will be able to:

1. **Describe inflammation and contrast it to immunity.**
   Review pages 147-148; refer to Figures 6-1 through 6-3.

2. **Indicate the causes of mast cell degranulation and the effects of histamine.**
   Review pages 149-150; refer to Figures 6-4 and 6-5.

3. **State the effects of the synthetic products of the mast cell.**
   Review page 150.

4. **Identify the plasma protein systems and their interactions in inflammation.**
   Review pages 151-158; refer to Figures 6-6 through 6-13.

5. **Identify a role for neutrophils, monocytes, macrophages, and eosinophils in the inflammatory process.**
   Review pages 158-162; refer to Figures 6-14 through 6-18.

6. **State the roles for inflammatory cytokines; note their relationships within the immune system.**
   Review pages 162-164; refer to Figure 6-19 and Table 6-1.

7. **Name and describe the systemic and local signs of inflammation.**
   Review pages 164-167; refer to Figures 6-20 and 6-21 and Table 6-2.

8. **Differentiate between the repair and regeneration processes; identify the adverse factors affecting wound healing.**
   Review pages 167-172; refer to Figures 6-21 and 6-22.

Practice Examination

1. Inflammation:

   a. destroys injurious agents.
   b. confines injurious agents.
   c. stimulates and enhances immunity.
   d. promotes healing.
   e. All of the above are correct.

2. Inflammatory microcirculation changes involve all of the following except:

   a. vasodilation.
   b. requires days to develop.
   c. increased vascular permeability.
   d. exudation of leukocytes to injury site.

3. A phagocyte's role begins with an inflammatory response. The sequence for phagocytosis is:

   a. margination or pavementing, recognition of the target, adherence or binding, fusion with lysosomes inside the phagocyte.
   b. diapedesis, margination or pavementing, phagosome formation, recognition of the target, fusion with lysosomes inside the phagocyte.
   c. recognition of the target, margination or pavementing, destruction of the target by lysosomal enzymes.
   d. margination, diapedesis, recognition, adherence, ingestion, fusion with lysosomes inside the phagocyte, destruction of the target.

4. Chemotactic factors for phagocytes include all of the following except:

   a. complement components.
   b. streptolysins.
   c. plasminogen activator.
   d. prostaglandins.
   e. mast cell degranulation products.

5. Which is not a local manifestation of inflammation?

   a. swelling
   b. pain
   c. heat
   d. leukocytosis
   e. redness

6. Complement is:

   a. a series of proteins in the blood.
   b. an antibody.
   c. a hormone.
   d. a lymphokine.

7. Diapedesis is a process in which:

   a. neutrophils migrate from the bloodstream to an injured tissue site.
   b. phagocytes stick to capillary and venule walls.
   c. bacteria are "coated" with an opsonin.
   d. there is oxygen-dependent killing of cells.

8. Interferon:

   a. interferes with the ability of bacteria to cause disease.
   b. prevents viruses from infecting healthy host cells.
   c. inhibits macrophage migration from inflamed sites.
   d. increases the phagocytic activity of macrophages.
   e. increases the number of circulating neutrophils.

9. The complement system can be activated by:

   a. the binding of complement 1 to a complement binding site of an antibody.
   b. components of other plasma protein systems.
   c. the binding of complement 3 to bacteria.
   d. Both a and c are correct.
   e. a, b, and c are correct.

10. Which is not a systemic manifestation of inflammation?

    a. leukocytosis
    b. fever
    c. increased acute-phase reactants
    d. exudation

11. The inflammatory response:

    a. prevents blood from entering the injured tissue.
    b. elevates body temperature to prevent spread of infection.
    c. prevents formation of abscesses.
    d. minimizes injury and promotes healing.

12. Scar tissue is:

    a. nonfunctional collagenous and fibrotic tissue.
    b. functional tissue that follows wound healing.
    c. regenerated tissue formed in the area of injury.
    d. fibrinogen which has entrapped phagocytes and neurons.

13. Repair involves processes that:

    a. fill in the wound.
    b. cover or seal the wound.
    c. shrink the wound.
    d. Both a and b are correct.
    e. a, b, and c are correct.

14. Swelling during acute inflammation is caused by:

    a. collagenase.
    b. the fluid and cellular exudation.
    c. lymphocytic margination.
    d. neutrophilic margination.
    e. anaerobic glycolysis.

15. Which is not released from mast cells during degranulation?

    a. chemotactic factors
    b. histamine
    c. complement
    d. vasoactive amines

16. Chronic inflammation is characterized by:

    a. hypertrophy.
    b. metaplasia.
    c. neutrophilic infiltration.
    d. lymphocytic and macrophagic infiltration.
    e. All of the above are correct.

17. Which is synthesized by mast cells?

    a. histamine
    b. serotonin
    c. neutrophil chemotactic factor
    d. leukotrienes
    c. eosinophil chemotactic factor

18. Primary intention healing:

    a. involves collagen synthesis.
    b. requires little wound contraction.
    c. requires little wound epithelialization.
    d. Both b and c are correct.
    e. a, b, and c are correct.

19. Interleukins:

    a. provide messages between leukocytes.
    b. are produced in response to tissue injury.
    c. stimulate cells to produce antiviral substances.
    d. increase antibody production and populations of T cells.
    e. All of the above are correct.

20. Eosinophils:

    a. are agranulocytes.
    b. control the vascular effects of serotonin and histamine by lysosomal mediators.
    c. have a lysosomal protein that can dissolve the surface membranes of parasites.
    d. All of the above are correct.
    e. Both b and c are correct.

Match the term with its definition or characteristic.

21. ____ resolution
22. ____ bradykinin
23. ____ granulation tissue
24. ____ fibroblasts
25. ____ scar

a. increases the phagocytic activity of macrophages
b. original structure and physiologic function
c. inhibits macrophage migration from the inflamed area
d. increases vascular permeability
e. new capillaries, fibroblasts, and macrophages
f. avascular
g. synthesize and secrete collagen
h. proliferate antigen-specific clones of B and T cells

CHAPTER 7

Hypersensitivities, Infection, and Immunodeficiencies

Foundational Objectives

a. Chart the development and activities of specific immunity. Review pages 124-125.

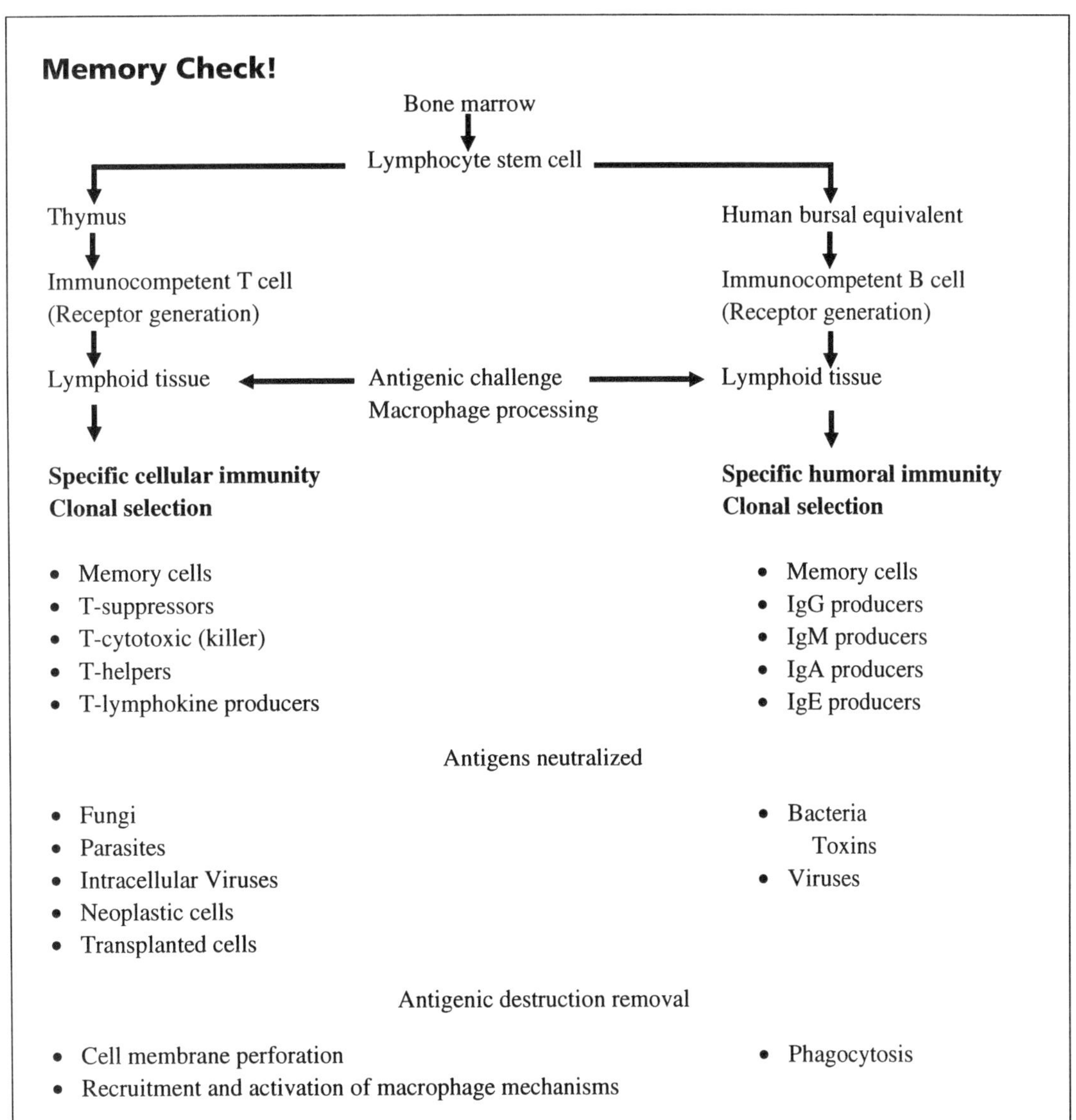

b. Diagram the interrelationships between CMI and HI. Review page 126; refer to Figures 5-16 through 5-18.

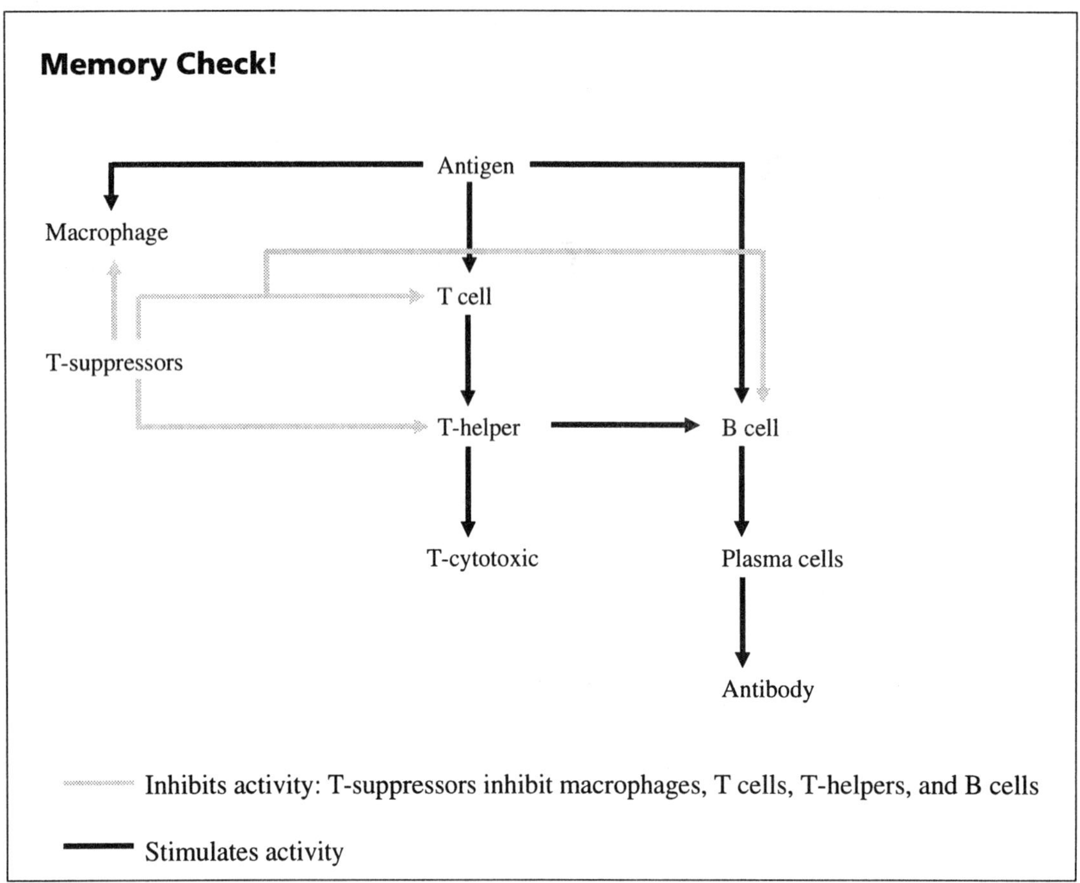

c. Diagram a scheme for complement's role in amplifying the immune response. Relate opsonization, inflammation, and cytolysis to the components of complement. Review pages 151-152; refer to Figures 6-6 and 6-7.

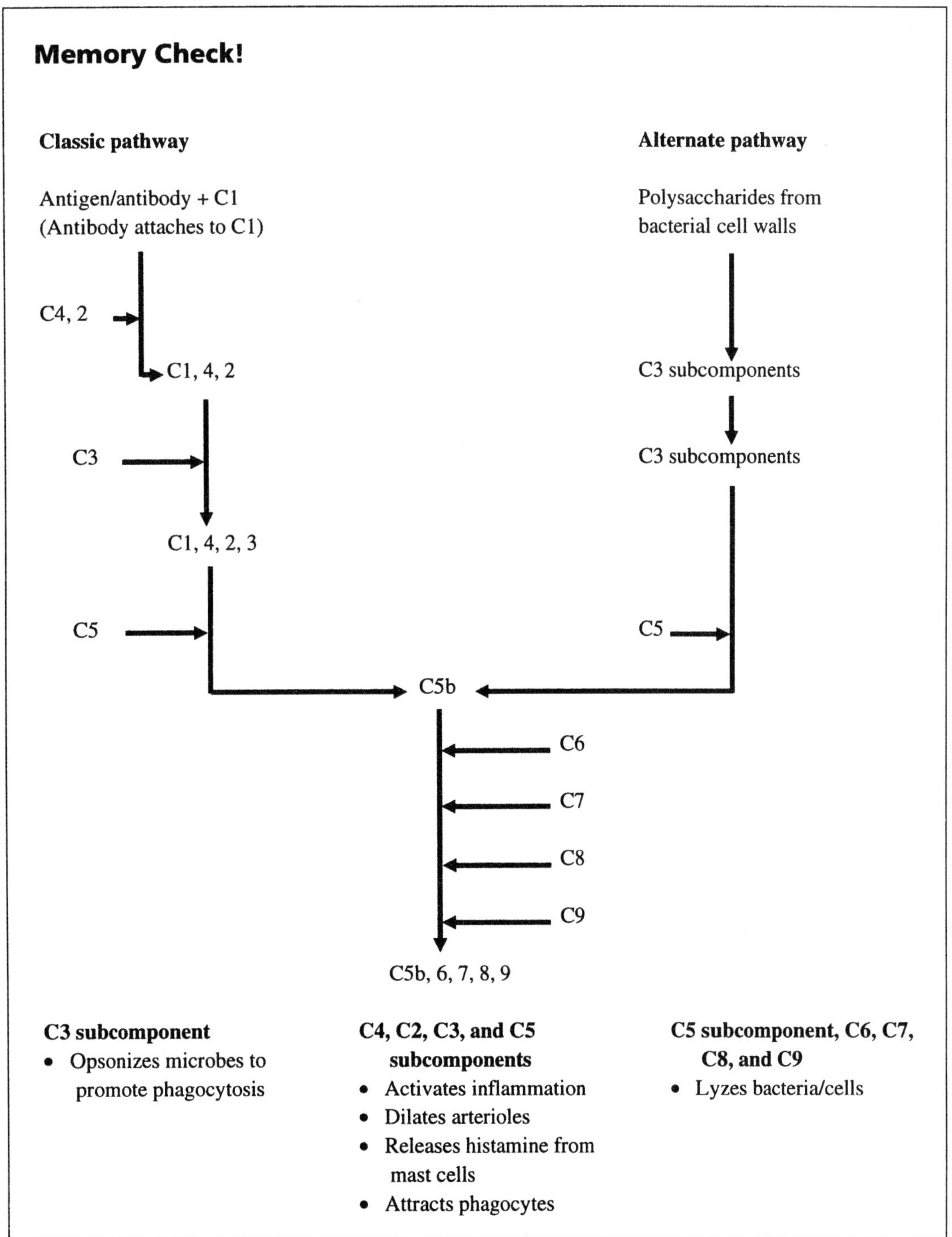

d. Diagram the interaction between lymphocytes and phagocytes. Review pages 139-141.

Memory Check!

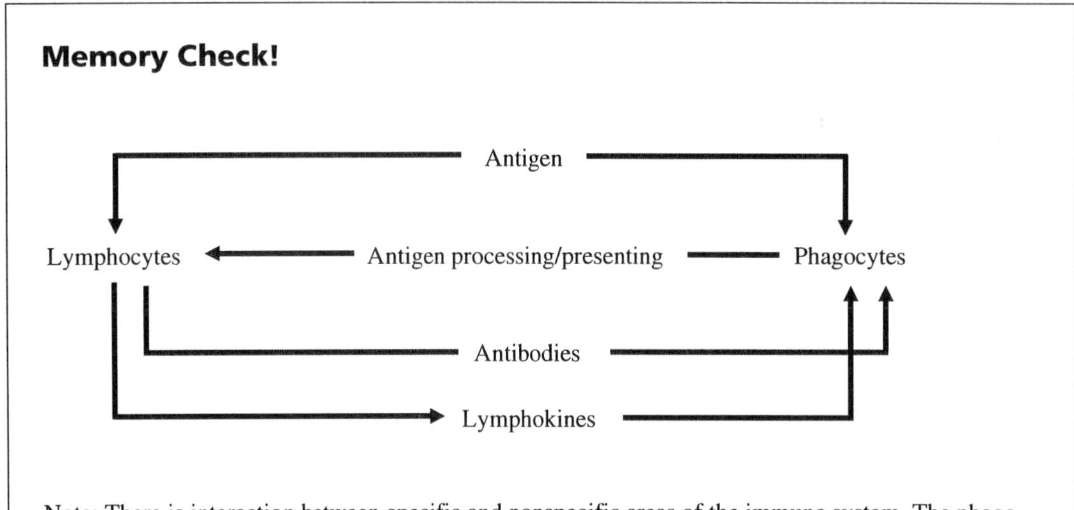

Note: There is interaction between specific and nonspecific areas of the immune system. The phagocytes cannot specifically recognize antigens but process and present them to the lymphocytes. Lymphocytes specifically recognize and produce antibodies or lymphokines which help the phagocytes combat the antigen.

Objectives

After review of this chapter, the learner will be able to:

1. **Compare the four hypersensitivities.**
   Study pages 177-185; refer to Figures 7-1 through 7-7 and Tables 7-1 and 7-3 through 7-5.

   (See box on page 41 of *Workbook.*)

2. **Describe the likely causes of autoimmune and alloimmune diseases; cite examples.**
   Study pages 185-187; refer to Table 7-2.

Self-antigens are usually tolerated by the host's own immune system. This immunologic tolerance develops in humans during the embryonic period. Autoreactive lymphocytes are either eliminated or suppressed. **Autoimmunity** is a breakdown of tolerance in which the body's immune system begins to recognize self-antigens as foreign. The mechanisms of breakdown of tolerance are varied and often unknown. Mechanisms implicated in the development of autoimmunity include alterations of self-antigenic markers by infectious diseases and genetic factors associated with the products of the HLA locus or the histocompatibility-complex-linked immune response genes.

Alloimmunity occurs when an individual's immune system reacts against antigens of the tissues of other members of the same species. Two examples of this reactivity are transient neonatal diseases and transplant rejection and transfusion reactions. Since a fetus has mother and father antigens, fetal paternal antigens different from maternal antigens can cross the placenta and elicit an immune response in the mother. Maternally produced antibody may be transported into the fetal circulation to produce alloimmune disease in the fetus. Examples of diseases that can affect the fetus, neonate, or child include Graves disease, myasthenia gravis, systemic lupus erythematosus, immune thrombocytopenic purpura, and erythroblastosis fetalis.

Transplantation of organs is commonly complicated by an immune response against donor antigens. The primary mechanism of the rejection of transplanted organs is a Type IV, cell-mediated reaction. HLA antigens are the principle targets of the rejection reaction.

Transplant rejection is classified as hyperacute, acute, or chronic depending on the amount of time that elapses between transplantation and rejection. Hyperacute rejection usually occurs in recipients having preexisting IgG or IgM antibody to antigens in the graft. As circulation to the graft is rees-

Comparison of Hypersensitivity Disorders

Hypersensitivity	Immunity Response Time	Effectors	Examples
Type I IgE-mediated Anaphylactic	Humoral Immediate	*Antigen* reacts with IgE bound to *mast cells, histamine* release, histamine effects	Allergic rhinitis, asthma, urticaria, food allergies, anaphylactic shock
Type II Cytotoxic Tissue-specific	Humoral Immediate	*IgG or IgM* reacts with *antigen* on cell's membrane, *complement* is activated, lysis or phagocytosis by macrophage of cell, cell-mediated cytolysis, antibody binding to receptors	Immediate drug reaction, hemolytic anemia, Graves disease
Type III Immune complex	Humoral Immediate	*IgG or IgM* unites with *antigen* to form a complex that is deposited in vessel walls or tissues, neutrophil attraction, *complement* activation, *lysosomal enzymes* injure tissue	Serum sickness, Arthus reaction, celiac disease, allergic alveolitis, glomerulonephritis, systemic lupus erythematosus
Type IV Cell-mediated	Cellular Delayed	Reaction of sensitized *T lymphocytes* with *antigen* leads to *lymphokine* release, recruitment of *macrophages* and *lysosomal* release	Contact dermatitis, graft rejection, tuberculin reaction, rheumatoid arthritis, autoimmune thyroiditis

tablished, antibody binds to the grafted tissue and activates the inflammatory response. This response initiates the coagulation or blood-clotting cascade, which results in cessation of blood flow into the graft.

Acute rejection is a cell-mediated immune response that occurs approximately two weeks after the transplantation. The recipient develops an immune response against unmatched HLA antigens and shows an infiltration of lymphocytes and macrophages characteristic of Type IV hypersensitivity reaction.

Chronic rejection may occur after months or years of normal function. It is characterized by slow, progressive organ failure. Chronic rejection may be caused by inflammatory damage to endothelial cells lining blood vessels. It is likely a result of a weak immunologic reaction against minor histocompatibility antigens on the grafted tissue.

3. **Describe the relationships between humans and infectious agents.**
   Study pages 187-191; refer to Figure 7-9 and Tables 7-8 and 7-10.

Many microbes grow and flourish in our bodies. Symbiosis, mutualism, commensalism, and pathogenicity are relationships between hosts and microorganisms. **Symbiosis** benefits the human without harming the microbe. **Mutualism** benefits both host and microbe. **Commensalism** benefits the microorganism without harming the human host. **Pathogenicity** benefits the microbe while harming the human host.

Pathogens injure cells and tissue because they circumvent the defensive barriers, the inflammatory system, and the immune system of the host. Pathogenic microbes directly damage cells, interfere with cellular metabolism, and render the cell dysfunctional because of their increased numbers.

A bacterial pathogen's **virulence** or ability to cause disease is increased by enzymes and either exotoxins or endotoxins. Some bacteria produce thick capsules of carbohydrate or protein that are antiphagocytic. Viral pathogens bypass many defense mechanisms because they develop intracellularly, thus avoiding inflammatory or immune responses.

The first line of human host defense against infectious organisms is the intact skin and mucous membranes. The digestive, respiratory, and genitourinary tracts form a closed barrier between the internal organs and external environment. The second and third lines of defense are the inflammatory response and immune system including the lymphatic system. The lymphatic system provides a network for internal defensive products to circulate throughout the body.

4. Describe the mechanisms of infection and cellular injury of bacteria, viruses, and fungi.

Study pages 191-197; refer to Figures 7-10 through 7-13 and Tables 7-11 and 7-12.

Bacteria are prokaryotes lacking a discrete nucleus; they are relatively small. Their survival and growth depend on the effectiveness of the host's defense mechanisms and on the bacterium's ability to resist these defenses. Some bacteria have coatings that protect them from phagocytosis. These coatings include polysaccharide coverings for the pneumococcus, the waxy capsule surrounding the tubercle bacillus, and the M protein cell wall of the streptococcus.

Other bacteria survive and proliferate in the body by producing hemolysins, leukocidins, coagulases, exotoxins, and endotoxins that injure cells and tissues. **Exotoxins** are metabolic proteins released into the environment primarily from gram-positive bacteria during bacterial growth. These proteins have highly specific effects on host cells. **Endotoxins** are lipopolysaccharides contained in the cell walls of gram-negative bacteria that are released from cell walls during lysis or destruction of the bacteria. Their effects are generalized. Endotoxins can be released from the bacterial membrane during treatment with antibiotics. Therefore, antibiotics cannot prevent the toxic effects of endotoxins. Once in the host's blood, endotoxins cause the release of vasoactive peptides that produce vasodilation. This, in turn, reduces blood pressure, decreases oxygen delivery, and can result in cardiovascular shock.

Viruses are intracellular parasites that take over the genetic and metabolic machinery of host cells and use them for their own survival and replication. Viruses contain genetic information in either DNA or RNA. This genetic material is protected by a protein coat that must be removed in the cytoplasm of the host cell if the virus is to replicate. Viruses are incapable of independent reproduction; replication depends totally on their ability to infect a **permissive** host cell—a cell unable to resist viral invasion and replication. Infection with a virus requires its binding to a **specific receptor** on the plasma membrane of the host cell. Viral replication depends on absorption, penetration, uncoating, replication, assembly, and release of new virions.

Once inside the host cell, virions have many harmful effects, including the following: (1) cell protein synthesis cessation, (2) disruption of lysosomal membranes resulting in release of enzymes that can kill the host cell, (3) fusion of host cells, (4) alteration of antigenic properties causing the immune system to attack the host cell as if it were foreign, and (5) transformation of host cell into cancerous cells. Cells damaged by viruses may enable secondary bacterial infections to develop.

Fungi are relatively large organisms with thick walls that grow as either single-celled yeasts or multicelled molds. Molds are aerobic, and yeasts are facultative anaerobes. Pathogenic fungi release mycotoxins and enzymes that damage connective tissues.

Diseases caused by fungi are called **mycoses**. Most fungi grow as parasites on or near skin or mucous membranes and usually produce mild and superficial disease. Injury to tissue can lead to secondary bacterial infection.

Fungi causing deep infection enter the body through inhalation or through open wounds. Deep infections are most common in association with other diseases or as opportunistic infections in immunosuppressed individuals. Some fungi are part of the normal body flora and become pathogenic when antibiotics kill bacteria that normally compete for nutrients and preclude fungal growth. For example, yeasts in vagina may undergo rapid proliferation when vaginal bacteria are killed by antibiotics.

5. **Characterize immunodeficiencies; describe examples of congenital or primary diseases.**
   Study pages 200-203; refer to Figure 7-15 and Table 7-14.

Immune deficiencies occur because of impaired function of one or more components of the immune or inflammatory response. B cells, T cells, phagocytic cells, or complement may be involved. The clinical manifestation of immune deficiency is a tendency to develop unusual or recurrent severe infections. Deficiencies in T cell immune responses are suspected when recurrent infections are caused by certain viruses, fungi, and yeasts or certain atypical organisms. B cell deficiencies are suspected if the individual has recurrent infections with encapsulated bacteria or viruses against which humoral immunity is normally effective.

It may be unsafe to administer conventional immunizing agents or blood products to many immunologically compromised individuals because of the risk that the immunizing agent will cause an uncontrolled infection. Uncontrolled infection is particularly a problem when attenuated vaccines that contain live, but weakened, microorganisms are used. Vaccinia virus used for immunization against smallpox is an example of such a vaccine. Although the virus is attenuated enough to be destroyed by a normal immune system, it can survive, multiply, and cause severe disease in an immunodeficient recipient.

Individuals with immune deficiencies are also at risk for graft-versus-host disease. This occurs if T cells in transfused blood are mature and capable of the cell-mediated destruction of tissues in the graft recipient. The grafted T cells are controlled by normal immune systems and no tissue destruction occurs. If the recipient's immune system is deficient, the grafted T cells will attack the recipient's tissue.

Congenital or primary immune deficiency occurs if lymphocyte development is disturbed in the fetus or embryo or if there is a genetic anomaly. Some diseases are primarily caused by a defect in one or the other of the cell lines, although both T and B cell lines may be partially deficient.

Severe combined immune deficiencies (SCID) occur when a common stem cell for all white blood cells is absent. Therefore, T cells, B cells, and phagocytic cells never develop. Most children with SCID caused by reticular dysgenesis, the most severe SCID form, die in utero or very soon after birth. Many individuals with SCID are deficient only in a stem cell for lymphocyte development rather than for all white blood cells, as in reticular dysgenesis, and therefore have normal numbers of all other white cells. T and B lymphocytes are few or totally absent in the circulation, the spleen, and the lymph nodes. The thymus is usually underdeveloped. IgM and IgA immunoglobulin levels are absent or greatly reduced; however, IgG levels may be almost normal because of the presence of maternal antibodies. Other forms of SCID are caused by autosomal recessive enzymatic defects that result in the accumulation of toxic metabolites to rapidly dividing lymphocytes.

DiGeorge syndrome is the complete lack or, more commonly, partial lack of the thymus. This thymus deficiency causes lymphopenia and greatly decreased T cell numbers and function. **Bruton agammaglobulinemia** is caused by failure of B cell precursors to become mature B cells because of the lack of normal bursal-equivalent tissue. There are few or no circulating B cells, though T cell number and function are normal.

Some immune deficiencies involve a defect that results in depressed development of a small portion of the immune system. An example is **Wiskott-Aldrich syndrome**, an X-linked recessive disorder, in which IgM antibody production is greatly depressed. Therefore, antibody responses against polysaccharide antigens from bacterial cell walls are deficient.

Another common defect in which a particular class of antibody is affected is selective IgA deficiency. Individuals with selective **IgA deficiency** are able to produce other classes of immunoglobulin but fail to produce IgA. Individuals with IgA deficiency frequently present with chronic intestinal candidiasis. IgA may normally prevent the uptake of allergens from the environment. Therefore, IgA deficiency may lead to increased allergen uptake and a more intense challenge to the immune system because of prolonged exposure to environmental antigens.

6. Cite causes and consequences of acquired or secondary immune deficiencies.
Study pages 203-204.

Acquired or secondary immune and inflammatory deficiency develops after birth and is not related to genetic defects. **Nutritional deficits** in calorie or protein intake can lead to deficiencies in T cell function and numbers. The humoral immune response is less affected by starvation, although complement activity, neutrophilic chemotaxis, and bacterial killing by neutrophils are frequently depressed. Enzyme cofactors, such as zinc and vitamins, may result in severe depressions of both B and T cell function.

Iatrogenic disorders are caused by some form of medical treatment. Cancer chemotherapeutic agents suppress blood cell formation in the bone marrow. Immunosuppressive corticosteroids for treatment of individuals with transplants or autoimmune diseases depress B and T cell formation. The consequence of these therapies for cancer and immunosuppression is manifested as a progressive increase in infections with opportunistic microorganisms.

Trauma in burn victims makes these individuals more susceptible to severe bacterial infections because of decreased neutrophil function and complement levels. Burn victims also have increased suppressor cell function which may increase antigen-specific suppression.

A relationship between **emotional stress** and depressed immune function seems to exist. Many lymphoid organs are innervated and can be affected by nerve stimulation. Also, lymphocytes have receptors for many hormones such as neurotransmitters and can respond to changing levels of these chemicals with increased or decreased function.

7. Describe acquired immune deficiency syndrome, AIDS.
Study pages 204-209; refer to Figures 7-16 through 7-19.

AIDS is caused by a virus currently named human immunodeficiency virus, or HIV. The virus was isolated by researchers at the National Institutes of Health as the human T-lymphotropic virus type III, or HLV-III, and earlier by the Pasteur Institute as the lymphadenopathy/AIDS virus, or LAV. At least one other AIDS virus (HIV-2) has been identified.

HIV is a retrovirus carrying genetic information in RNA rather than DNA. Retroviruses infect cells by binding a target cell through a surface receptor and inserting their RNA into the target cell. A viral enzyme, reverse transcriptase, converts the viral RNA to DNA and inserts that DNA into the infected cell's genetic material. Viral proliferation may occur, resulting in the lysis and death of the infected cell. If, however, the cell remains relatively dormant rather than active, the viral genetic material integrated into the infected cell's DNA may remain latent for years, if not for the life of the individual.

CD4 is an antigen on the surface of cells that acts as a receptor for the HIV. The virus primarily infects CD4-positive T-helper lymphocytes, but it may also infect and lyze various other cells that express the CD4 antigen.

At the time of diagnosis, the individual may manifest one of four different conditions: serologically negative, serologically positive but asymptomatic, early stages of HIV disease, or AIDS. The currently accepted Centers for Disease Control definition of AIDS relies on both laboratory tests and clinical symptoms. The most common laboratory test is for antibodies against HIV. Without a positive test for antibodies, individuals can be diagnosed as having AIDS if they have a lymphoma of the brain and are less than 60 years of age or if they have lymphoid interstitial pneumonitis and are less than 13 years of age. If they are seropositive, the diagnosis of AIDS is made in association with a variety of clinical symptoms. These include disseminated coccidioidomycosis or histoplasmosis, extrapulmonary tuberculosis, persistent isosporiasis, recurrent salmonella septicemia, recurrent bacterial infections, HIV encephalopathy, HIV wasting syndrome, lymphoma of the brain at any age, non-Hodgkin lymphoma, and uterine cervical cancer. Other clinical symptoms of AIDS include persistent lymphadenopathy, weight loss, recurrent fevers, neurologic abnormalities with dementia in late stages, recurrent pulmonary infiltrates, and the development of opportunistic infections such as *Pneumocystis carinii* pneumonia and other atypical malignancies such as Kaposi sarcoma.

The major immunologic finding in AIDS is the striking decrease of T-helper cells or CD4-positive cells. Suppressor cells which have the CD8 antigen are usually normal or slightly elevated. This results in a reversal of the normal helper-to-suppressor T cell ratio, which is about 1.9. Most individuals with AIDS have ratios much lower than 0.9 and frequently near 0. In contrast, B cell numbers are usually normal.

The presence of circulating antibody against the AIDS virus apparently indicates infection by the virus. Antibody appears soon after infection through blood products, usually within four to seven weeks. After sexual exposure, the individual can be infected yet seronegative for 6 to 14 months. In the late stages of the disease, some individuals become seronegative because of a deficient immune system. The period between infection and the appearance of antibody is referred to as the window period. Although the patient may not have antibody, he or she may be viremic and infectious to others within two weeks of being infected.

Treatment for AIDS can involve restoration of immune function or prevention of viral replication. Restoration of immune function has been attempted with bone marrow transplants, transfusions of white blood cells from healthy donors, and the injection of interleuken-2 interferon. These attempts have shown little or no success because the virus quickly infects the donor cells. Several agents have been tried to prevent viral replication. Some of these agents are designed to block reverse transcriptase activity, and some have been successful against other viruses or parasites such as acyclovir against herpes simplex virus. Azidothymidine, AZT, and its less toxic analogue cyanothymidine, CNT, have shown remarkable effects in extremely advanced AIDS cases with recurrent *P. carinii* infections.

Drug therapy for AIDS is difficult because the AIDS retrovirus incorporates into the genetic material of the host and may never be removed by antiviral therapy. Therefore, drug administration may have to continue for the lifetime of the individual.

The development of an effective AIDS vaccine has been slowed by several major difficulties. The AIDS virus is genetically and antigenically variable. Thus, a vaccine created against one variant may not provide protection against another variant. This is a real problem, since as many as 30 to 40 different genetic variants have been isolated from the same individual during the progression of the disease. Many of these may coexist in the individual. Although individuals with AIDS have high levels of circulating antibodies against the virus, these antibodies do not appear to be protective. The AIDS virus is transmitted from cell to cell and may initially enter the body in an infected cell that is not susceptible to circulating antibody. Also, HIV-infected cells tend to fuse with other cells, so infection can spread to uninfected cells without viral particles being produced.

Finally, the only good model for AIDS experimentation is the chimpanzee, which is a protected animal species and relatively unavailable for medical research. Thus, efficacy and toxicity of possible vaccines cannot easily be evaluated.

Practice Examination

Match the condition with the immunologic mechanism.

1. ____ Graves disease
2. ____ serum sickness
3. ____ allergic rhinitis
4. ____ systemic lupus erythematosus
5. ____ contact dermatitis
6. ____ hemolytic anemia
7. ____ tuberculin reaction

a. IgE-mediated
b. cytotoxic/tissue-specific
c. immune complex
d. cell-mediated

8. Immunologic response(s) recognized as disease is/are:

   a. immediate hypersensitivity.
   b. delayed hypersensitivities.
   c. Both a and b are correct.
   d. Neither a nor b is correct.

9. Which is not characteristic of hypersensitivity?

   a. specificity
   b. immunologic mechanisms
   c. inappropriate or injurious response
   d. prior contact unnecessary to elicit a response

10. When the body produces antibodies against its own tissue, it is a/an:

    a. hypersensitivity.
    b. antibody reaction.
    c. cell-mediated immunity.
    d. autoimmune disease.
    e. opsonization.

11. Which hypersensitivity is caused by poison ivy?

    a. Type I
    b. Type II
    c. Type III
    d. Type IV

12. The mechanism of hypersensitivity for drugs is:

    a. Type I.
    b. Type II.
    c. Type III.
    d. Type IV.
    e. a, b, and c are correct.

13. Which is not an autoimmune disease?

    a. multiple sclerosis
    b. pernicious anemia
    c. transfusion reaction
    d. ulcerative colitis
    e. Goodpasture disease

14. Damage in SLE is due to the formation of antigen/antibody complexes mediated by:

    a. IgE.
    b. mast cells.
    c. the cell-mediated immune system.
    d. the humoral immune system and complement.
    e. lymphokines.

15. The classical complement cascade begins with:

    a. antigen/antibody complexes binding to a component of the complement system.
    b. opsonization.
    c. chemotaxis.
    d. cytolysis.

16. An alloimmune disorder is:

    a. erythroblastosis fetalis.
    b. insulin-dependent diabetes.
    c. myxedema.
    d. All of the above are correct.
    e. None of the above is correct.

17. Immunodeficiencies occur because of impaired function of:

    a. B and T cells.
    b. phagocytic cells.
    c. complement.
    d. All of the above are correct.
    e. Both a and c are correct.

18. An X-linked recessive disorder of immunodeficiency involves a deficit of:

    a. IgA.
    b. IgD.
    c. IgE.
    d. IgG.
    e. IgM.

19. Deficiencies in B cell immune responses are suspected when unusual or recurrent severe infections are caused by:

    a. fungi.
    b. yeasts.
    c. encapsulated bacteria.
    d. Both a and b are correct.
    e. a, b, and c are correct.

20. DiGeorge syndrome is a primary immunodeficiency caused by:

    a. failure of B cells to mature.
    b. congenital lack of thymic tissue.
    c. failure of the formed elements of blood to develop.
    d. selective deficiency of IgG.
    e. selective deficiency of IgA.

21. Acquired or secondary immunodeficiencies:

    a. develop after birth.
    b. may be caused by viral infections.
    c. may develop following immunosuppressive therapy.
    d. Both a and c are correct.
    e. a, b, and c are correct.

22. Rejection of a kidney transplant occurred after two weeks. The reaction was because of:

    a. immune response against recipient HLA antigen.
    b. immune response against donor HLA antigens.
    c. a Type IV hypersensitivity.
    d. Both a and b are correct.
    e. Both b and c are correct.

23. Zinc and vitamin deficits can depress:

    a. only B cell function.
    b. only T cell function.
    c. only complement activity.
    d. both B and T cell function.

24. A positive HIV antibody test signifies that the:

    a. individual is infected with HIV and likely so for life.
    b. asymptomatic individual will absolutely progress to AIDS.
    c. individual isn't viremic.
    d. sexually active individual was infected last weekend.

25. Which is incorrect regarding AIDS?

    a. The T_4/T_8 ratio will be less than 1:1.
    b. The patient will be anti-HIV.
    c. The patient will likely develop opportunistic infections and cancer.
    d. The patient will have increased numbers of CD4 cells or T-helper cells.

CHAPTER 8

Stress and Disease

Foundational Objectives

a. Define stress. Review page 216.

> **Memory Check!**
>
> - Stress arises when a person interacts or transacts with situations in certain ways. People are not disturbed by situations as they exist but by the ways they individually appraise and react to situations. Stress is a condition in which a demand exceeds a person's coping abilities. Stress reactions may include disturbance of cognition, emotion, and behavior that can adversely affect well-being.

b. Describe Selye's original general adaptation syndrome; cite its stages. Review page 216; refer to Figure 8-1.

> **Memory Check!**
>
> - While attempting to discover a new sex hormone, Selye injected crude ovarian extracts into rats. Repeatedly, he found the following triad of structural changes: (1) enlargement of the cortex of the adrenal gland, (2) atrophy of the thymus gland and other lymphoid structures, and (3) development of bleeding ulcers of the stomach and duodenal lining. Selye discovered that this triad of manifestations was not specific for his ovarian extracts but also occurred after he exposed the rats to other noxious stimuli such as cold, surgical injury, and restraint. Selye concluded that this triad or syndrome of manifestations represented a nonspecific response to noxious stimuli. Because many diverse agents caused the same syndrome, Selye suggested that it be called the general adaptation syndrome (GAS).
>
> - Selye later defined three successive stages in the development of the GAS: (1) the alarm stage, (2) the stage of resistance or adaptation, and (3) the stage of exhaustion. The nonspecific physiologic response identified by Selye consists of interaction among the sympathetic branch of the autonomic nervous system and two glands, the pituitary gland and the adrenal gland. The alarm phase of the GAS begins when a stressor triggers the actions of the pituitary gland and the sympathetic nervous system. The resistance or adaptation phase begins with the actions of cortisol, norepinephrine, and epinephrine. Exhaustion occurs if stress continues and adaptation is not successful. The ultimate signs of exhaustion are impairment of the immune response, heart failure, and kidney failure leading to death.

c. Identify current concepts that modify Selye's work; define homeostasis and cite an example. Review pages 216-218.

Memory Check!

- Studies show that activation of the adrenal cortex occurs in humans in response to psychologic stressors. Several factors, including degrees of discomfort/unpleasantness or suddenness of the stress, may account for the presence or absence of the physiologic stress response. In experiments in which psychologic reactions were minimized, physical stressors did not appear to stimulate the pituitary or adrenal cortex in a nonspecific fashion. To support Selye's concept of nonspecificity, evidence is needed that increased adrenal cortical or medullary activity can promote adaptations to both cold and heat. In fact, no single hormone responds to all stressful stimuli in an absolutely nonspecific fashion.

- Selye considered homeostasis the sum of the process by which the body maintains itself at a relatively constant composition. He expanded Cannon's definition to mean that the body's need determines body responses and that adaptive responses are necessary to maintain body stability. Research has since demonstrated that homeostasis does not mean "constant composition" but rather a dynamic steady state representing the net effect of all the turnover or synthesis and breakdown of all bodily substances.

- Stressors cause a series of reactions that alter the dynamic steady state. This alteration may be either short- or long-term. For example, the normal concentration of glucose in the blood is about 80 mg/100 ml. The concentration of glucose rises with acute stress and then slowly returns to normal as stress subsides. If blood glucose remains high in the absence of a known stressor, it is diagnosed as a sign of disease, probably diabetes mellitus.

d. Summarize the major interactions of the nervous, endocrine, and immune systems in the stress response. Review pages 218-223; refer to Figure 8-2 and Tables 8-1 through 8-3.

Memory Check!

- Corticotropin-releasing factor (CRF) may be a primary mediator of many stress-induced alterations to immune functions because of its role as an initiator of biologic brain responses to stress. It activates the hypothalamic-pituitary-adrenal (HPA) axis and the autonomic nervous system (ANS). However, direct suppressive effects of CRF have also been reported on two immune cell types processing CRF receptors, namely the monocyte-macrophage and CD4 (T-helper) lymphocyte. The production of CRF is initiated by a high level of IL-1. Production of IL-1 by activated macrophages and monocytes is inhibited by circulating glucocorticoids. The stimulation of CRF production in the hypothalamus by IL-1 demonstrates immune-induced regulation of the CNS and the cytokines (TNF and IFN). The T cell growth factor IL-2 can increase pituitary ACTH as well.

(Continued)

Memory Check! (cont'd)

The following flow chart summarizes interaction of the three systems:

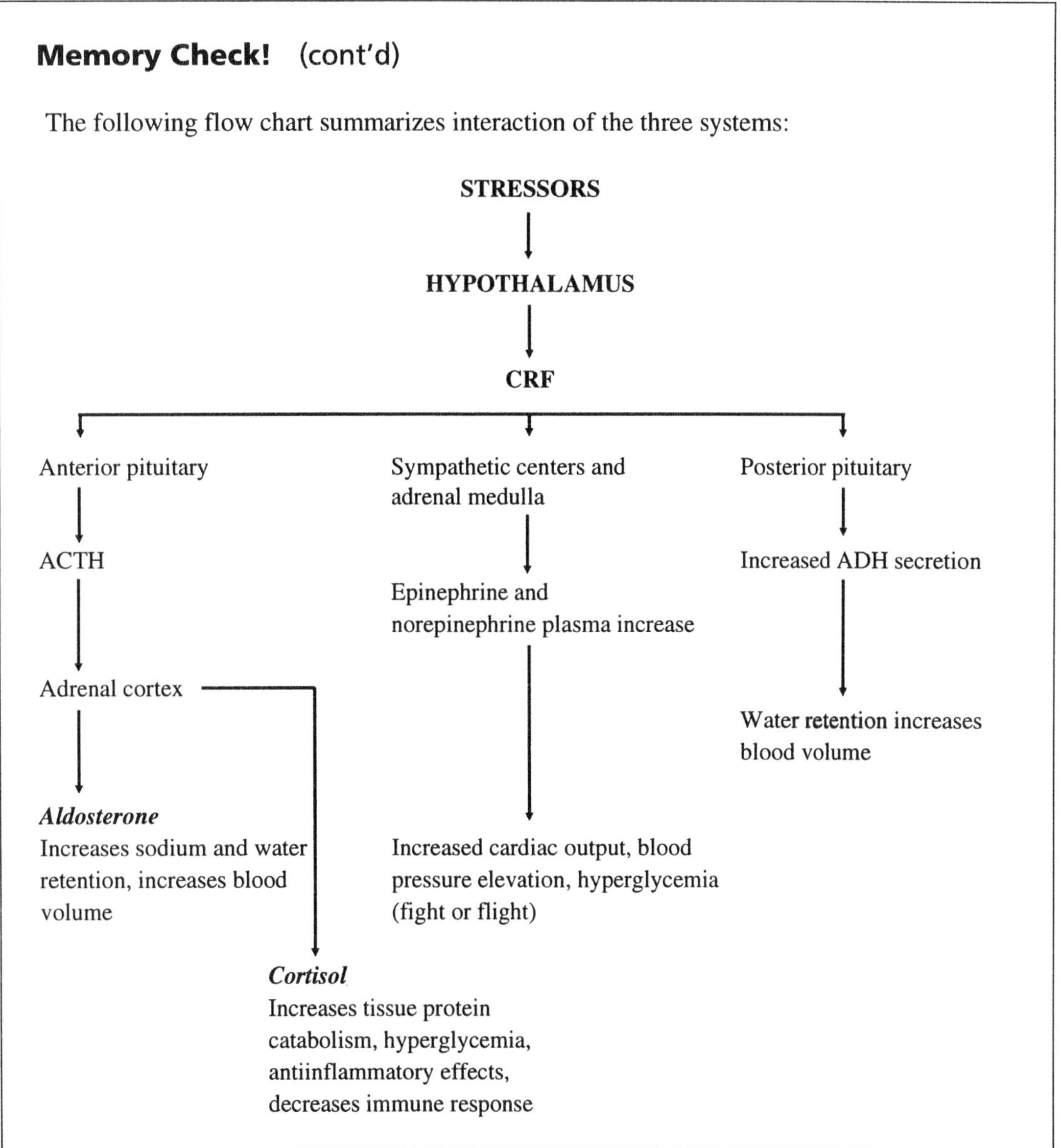

Objectives

After review of this chapter, the learner will be able to:

1. **Describe stress and coping.**
   Study pages 223-225; refer to Figure 8-3.

Stress is not an independent entity but a system of interdependent processes that are moderated by the nature, intensity, and duration of the stressor. The perception, appraisal, and coping efficacy of the affected individual mediate the psychologic and physiologic responses to stress. Coping is managing stressful demands that exceed the individual's resources.

Periods of depression and emotional upheaval with ineffective coping place the affected individual at risk for immunological deficits. Adverse life events that have the most negative effect on immunity have been characterized as those events that are uncontrollable and undesirable and that overtax the individual's ability to cope. Those individuals unable to cope may develop immune dysfunction. Factors that may influence stress susceptibility or resilience include age, socioeconomic status, gender, social support status, personality, self-esteem, genetics, life events, past experiences, and current health status.

Problem-focused and social support coping processes have a beneficial influence during stressful experiences. An individual experiencing distress may draw upon internal and external resources to meet the demands. Social support groups can improve psychologic coping and immune function by increasing natural killer cell activity.

2. Cite examples of stress-related diseases.
Refer to Table 8-4.

Stress-related Diseases

System	Disease or Condition
Cardiovascular	Coronary artery disease, hypertension, stroke, arrhythmia
Muscles	Tension headaches, backache
Connective tissues	Rheumatoid arthritis
Pulmonary	Asthma, hay fever
Immune	Immunosuppression, deficiency, autoimmunity
Gastrointestinal	Ulcer, irritable bowel syndrome, diarrhea, nausea and vomiting, ulcerative colitis
Integumentary	Eczema, neurodermatitis, acne
Endocrine	Diabetes mellitus, amenorrhea
Central nervous	Fatigue and lethargy, type A behavior, overeating, depression, insomnia

Note: The above is an abbreviated grouping of tissues and systems and some stress-related diseases.

Practice Examination

Match the substance with its activity.

1. ____ IL-1
2. ____ IL-2
3. ____ somatotropin
4. ____ testosterone
5. ____ endorphin

a. secreted by the anterior pituitary

b. stimulates the perception of pain

c. produced by macrophages, stimulates release of CRF

d. chronic stress suppresses

e. decreased by psychologic stimuli

f. release of CRF potentiates B and T cell activity

g. may inhibit CRF secretion

h. released from mast cells, vasoactive

6. Which is not a characteristic of Selye's stress syndrome?

   a. adrenal atrophy
   b. shrinkage of the thymus
   c. bleeding gastrointestinal ulcers
   d. shrinkage of lymphatic organs

7. Which characterizes the alarm stage?

   a. increased lymphocytes
   b. increased sympathetic activity
   c. increased parasympathetic activity
   d. increased eosinophils

8. Glucocorticoids would be highest during the stage of:

   a. exhaustion.
   b. alarm.
   c. resistance.

9. Which is a correct sequence for Selye's hypothesis for stress?

   a. increased ACTH secretion, alarm
   b. increased ACTH in the blood, hypertrophy of the adrenal cortex
   c. stimulation of the sympathetic centers, alarm
   d. increased secretion of epinephrine, increased ACTH in the blood

10. CRF is released by the:

    a. adrenal medulla.
    b. adrenal cortex.
    c. anterior pituitary.
    d. hypothalamus.

11. Stress may be defined as any factor that:

    a. stimulates the posterior pituitary.
    b. stimulates the anterior pituitary.
    c. stimulates the hypothalamus to release CRF.
    d. stimulates the hypothalamus to release ADH.

12. Which statement is not true?

    a. Stressors are the same for all individuals.
    b. Stressors are extreme stimuli.
    c. The emotions of fear, anxiety, and grief can act as stressors.
    d. Stressors differ in different individuals and in one individual at different times.

13. What determines which stimuli are stressors for an individual?

    a. heredity
    b. past experience
    c. diet
    d. All of the above are correct.

14. Which statement is not true?

    a. Generally, psychological stress is independent of the physiological stress.
    b. Physiological stress is usually accompanied by some degree of psychological stress.
    c. Identical psychological stressors do not induce identical physiological responses.
    d. For any one individual, adaptive responses are selective and counteract specific body changes.

15. The production of cortisol in response to stress can be initiated by:

    a. hypothalamus, anterior pituitary, adrenal cortex.
    b. hypothalamus, posterior pituitary, adrenal cortex.
    c. hypothalamus, sympathetic nerve fibers, adrenal cortex.
    d. hypothalamus, sympathetic nerve fibers, adrenal medulla.

16. Cortisol:

    a. increases protein catabolism.
    b. decreases blood sugar.
    c. increases immune response.
    d. increases allergic reactions.

17. Which would not occur in response to stress?

    a. increased systolic blood pressure
    b. increased epinephrine
    c. constriction of the pupils
    d. increased adrenocorticoids

18. Which would not be useful to assess stress?

    a. total blood cholesterol
    b. eosinophil count
    c. lymphocyte count
    d. adrenocorticoid levels

19. In response to stress, the adrenal cortex secretes:

    a. norepinephrine.
    b. norepinephrine and cortisol.
    c. cortisol and aldosterone.
    d. norepinephrine and aldosterone.

20. Severe stress results in all of the following except:

    a. an overactive immune system.
    b. increased heart rate.
    c. a rise in epinephrine levels.
    d. changes in breathing patterns.

Match the term with its definition.

21. ____ corticoids
22. ____ stressors
23. ____ stress response
24. ____ exhaustion stage
25. ____ alarm stage

a. sympathetic activity returns to normal
b. glucocorticoids return to normal
c. secreted by adrenal cortex in response to stress
d. Selye's changes seen in stress
e. stimulates the release of CRF
f. high resistance to stressor
g. bodily changes initiated by stress
h. impaired immune response
i. triggers sympathetic nervous system

CHAPTER 9

Biology of Cancer

Foundational Objectives

a. Describe the phases of cellular mitosis and cytokinesis. Review pages 23-24.

Memory Check!

- The reproduction or division of somatic cells involves two sequential phases: mitosis, or nuclear, division and cytokinesis, or cytoplasmic, division. These phases occur in close succession, with cytokinesis beginning toward the end of mitosis. Before a cell can divide, it must double its mass and duplicate all of its contents. Most of the preparation for division occurs during the growth phase or interphase. The alternation between mitosis and interphase in all tissues having cellular turnover is known as the cell cycle.
- There are four designated phases of the cell cycle. They are (1) the S phase (synthesis), in which DNA is synthesized in the cell nucleus; (2) the G_2 phase, in which RNA and protein synthesis occurs; (3) the M phase (mitosis), which includes both nuclear and cytoplasmic division; and (4) the G_1 phase, which is the period between the M phase and the start of DNA synthesis. Interphase, consisting of the G_1, S, and G_2 phases, is the longest phase of the cell cycle.
- The M phase of the cell cycle, mitosis and cytokinesis, begins with prophase or the first appearance of chromosomes. Each chromosome has two identical halves called chromatids which lie side by side and are attached together at a site called a centromere. The nuclear membrane disappears in this phase. Spindle fibers are microtubules formed in the cytoplasm that radiate from two centrioles located at opposite poles of the cell.
- During metaphase, the next phase of mitosis and cytokinesis, the spindle fibers pull the centromeres till they are aligned in the middle of the spindle or at the equatorial plate.
- Anaphase begins when the centromeres separate and the genetically identical chromatids are pulled apart. The chromatids are pulled, centromeres first, toward opposite sides of the cell. When the identical chromatids are separated, each is considered to be a chromosome. Thus, the cell has 92 chromosomes during this stage. By the end of anaphase, there are 46 chromosomes at each side of the identical cell. Each of the two groups of 46 chromosomes should be identical to the original 46 chromosomes present at the start of the cell cycle.
- During telophase, a new nuclear membrane is formed around each group of 46 chromosomes, the spindle fibers disappear, and the chromosomes begin to uncoil. Cytokinesis causes the cytoplasm to divide into roughly equal parts during this phase. At the end of telophase, two identical diploid cells, called daughter cells, have been formed from the original cell.
- The difference between slowly and rapidly dividing cells is the length of time spent in the G_1 phase of the cell cycle. Some cells that divide very slowly can remain in the G_1 phase for years. Once the S phase begins, progression through mitosis requires a relatively constant amount of time. Once a cell has progressed out of the G_1 phase, it must complete the S, G_2, and M phases.

b. Identify mechanisms that control cell division. Review page 24; refer to Table 1-5.

Memory Check!

- Protein growth factors govern the proliferation of different cell types in conjunction with genes involved in the social control or relationship of cells within tissues. It is likely that some genes code for growth factors, some for growth factor receptors, some for intracellular regulatory proteins involved in cell adhesion, and some for proteins that help relay signals for cell division to the cell nucleus.
- Cells require highly specific proteins to stimulate cell division. These growth factors are present in the serum in very low concentrations. For example, platelet-derived growth factor stimulates the production of connective tissue cells. Another important growth factor is interleukin, which stimulates proliferation of T cells. Cells responding to a particular growth factor have specific receptors for the specific growth factor in their plasma membrane. Some growth factors also are regulators of cellular differentiation.

Objectives

After review of this chapter, the learner will be able to:

1. **Define neoplasia or cancer.**
   Study pages 231-232; refer to Figures 9-1 and 9-2 and Table 9-1.

Cancerous cells are defined by two heritable properties, autonomy and anaplasia. **Autonomy** is the cancer cell's independence from normal cellular controls. **Anaplasia** is the loss of differentiation or specialization. The cancer cell has lost its ability to function normally and to control its growth and division.

Transformation is the process by which a normal cell becomes a cancer cell. Genes known as protooncogenes that were normally turned off during levels of differentiation can be mutated, transformed, or reactivated by carcinogenic agents to become **neoplastic** cells.

Cancer is considered a disorder of growth and differentiation because neoplasms resemble undifferentiated tissue. The less the tumor resembles normal tissue, the more undifferentiated or anaplastic the tumor becomes. As malignant cells grow and divide, they lose their mature characteristics and no longer resemble their tissue of origin.

2. **Cite the method for naming and classifying tumors; provide examples.**
   Refer to Table 9-2.

Tumors are named according to the tissue of origin with the suffix "oma" added. Cancers having an epithelial tissue origin are identified as carcinomas while those with a connective tissue origin are sarcomas. Lymphomas arise from lymphatic tissue, gliomas arise from glial cells of the central nervous system, and leukemias arise from the bone marrow. (See box at top of page 58 of *Workbook.*)

3. **Identify some cellular changes that occur in cancerous cells and their functional significance.**
   Study pages 234-238; refer to Figures 9-3 and 9-4 and Tables 9-4 and 9-5.

(See box at bottom of page 58 of *Workbook.*)

Common Benign and Malignant Tumors

Tissue	Benign Tumor	Malignant Tumor
Connective tissue		
Adult fibrous	Fibroma	Fibrosarcoma
Cartilage	Chondroma	Chondrosarcoma
Bone	Osteoma	Osteosarcoma
Fat	Lipoma	Liposarcoma
Muscle		
Smooth muscle	Leiomyoma	Leiomyosarcoma
Striated muscle	Rhabdomyoma	Rhabdomyosarcoma
Blood tissue		
Lymph vessels	Lymphangioma	Lymphangiosarcoma
Blood vessels	Hemangioma	Hemangiosarcoma
Lymphoid tissue	Infectious mononucleosis	Lymphosarcoma (Lymphoma)
Bone marrow	Infectious mononucleosis	Leukemia
Neural tissue		
Nerve sheath	Neurilemmoma	Neurogenic sarcoma
Glial tissue	Gliosis	Glioma
Epithelium		
Squamous epithelium	Papilloma	Squamous carcinoma
Glandular epithelium	Adenoma	Adenocarcinoma

Cancerous Cell Changes and Their Significance

Change	Significance
Surface loss or alteration of glycoprotein or glycolipid	Receptor alterations change response to growth factors, abnormal cellular proliferation, impaired cell-to-cell recognition
Reduced fibronectin	Changes cellular organization, decreases adhesion, increases migration
Altered membranes	Increases metabolite transport
Increased plasminogen activator	Increased extracellular proteolysis
Disorganized actin filaments	Cells maintain "rounded-up" nature which is characteristic of mitotic cells
Fewer anchoring junctions	Encourages proliferation of transformed cells, cells metastasize and grow in new environment
Altered gap junctions	Decreases intercellular communication, causes loss of density-dependent inhibition of growth

4. Postulate a model for the causes of carcinogenesis.
Study pages 238-245; refer to Figures 9-5 through 9-9 and Table 9-1.

Why does a normal cell lose control and become abnormal? There likely are several reasons. First, there are environmental agents. A chemical or other environmental agent that produces cancer increases the frequency of mutations in somatic cells.

Viruses are another cause of cancer. These tiny packages of nucleic acids, either DNA or RNA, are capable of infecting cells and converting them to transformed cells. Oncogenes are genes that can transform a normal cell into a cancerous cell when they are activated by oncogenic viruses. Oncogenes develop from normal genes that regulate growth and development. These genes may undergo some change that either causes them to produce an abnormal product or disrupts their control so that they are expressed inappropriately.

Some cancers are not caused by oncogenes but rather by genes called tumor suppressor genes that have mutated. These genes produce proteins that normally oppose the action of an oncogene or inhibit cell division. Carcinogenesis inactivates tumor suppressor genes and activates oncogenes.

The multistep process of cancer seems to involve the loss of the cell's ability to terminally differentiate and control growth. In addition, the neoplastic cell must travel to distant tissues, invade, and colonize these tissues. Tumors appear to be derived from a single stem cell. Tumor development requires several independent accidents to occur together in one cell. If a single mutation were responsible, the chance of developing cancer in any given year would be independent of age. However, the cancerous change increases at a rapid rate with increasing age, so a multistep process is likely.

In most cancers, the cells of the initial mutant clone undergo further mutation that enables them to divide more rapidly before they terminally differentiate. Because of rapid division, the cancer cells begin to outnumber the normal cells as well as those having the primary mutation.

(See box below.)

5. Describe the initiation-promotion-progression theory of carcinogenesis.
Study pages 245-247; refer to Figures 9-10 and 9-11 and Table 9-7.

Initiation is an irreversible cellular step requiring exposure to a carcinogen. The affected cell has its DNA irreversibly altered or mutated. However, the initiated cell may not be considered cancerous until a promoting agent acts on that cell to produce an altered cell. **Promotion** accelerates the process by which the initiated cells become cancerous. Initiation and promotion mechanisms have not been experimentally shown for all cancers. However, the

Causes of Neoplasia

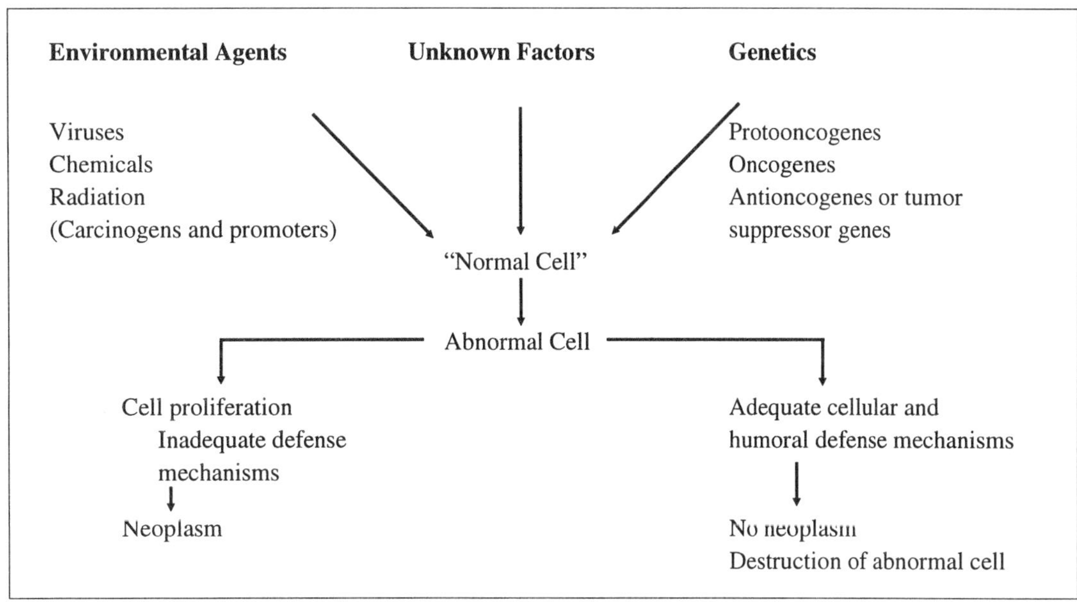

process can be applied to chemical agents found in coal tar or cigarette smoke, ionizing and nonionizing radiation, viruses, and hormones.

Initiators cause interruptions in the DNA chain, errors in DNA repair, or an elimination of a base pair or sugar. Promoters may affect cell proliferation by altering cell-to-cell communication, by the production of oxygen radicals, or by interfering with the process of differentiation, usually after division has occurred.

6. **Characterize common carcinogens as chemical, physical, or viral.**
   Study pages 247-253; refer to Figure 9-12 and Table 9-9.

Chemical carcinogens include naturally occurring products, drugs, metals, and industrial carcinogens.

Cancers of the oral cavity, lungs, and bladder are associated with exposure to cigarette smoking. Nitrosamines and other nitrosocompounds develop from chemical interactions between nitrites and other secondary amines. Numerous drugs and nicotine may supply the amines for the process of converting nitrites to nitrosamine. Nitrites are present in foods as additives. These agents may be contributors to gastric carcinomas.

Heavy consumption of alcohol is associated with cancer of the mouth, pharynx, esophagus, larynx, and liver. Alcohol apparently enhances the effect of carcinogens such as nicotine by increasing their solubility. Aflatoxin, a mold, has been linked to liver cancer in humans.

Asbestos is associated with cancer of the lung. The fibers function as promoters for other carcinogens such as cigarette smoke.

Carcinoma of the breast, endometrium, ovary, and prostate are associated with hormones. These neoplasms occur because of hormone responses.

Ionizing radiation is a **physical carcinogen** that causes cellular mutations. Damage to DNA may be direct or indirect. Radiation can directly damage macromolecules and nucleic acids. Indirect damage occurs when a secondary electron interacts with a water molecule, giving rise to a free radical, which then damages DNA. Evidence links adult leukemia to exposure to large doses of irradiation. The frequency of breast cancer and thyroid cancer increases with irradiation during childhood. Radiographs of the fetus in utero increase chances of developing childhood cancer.

Ultraviolet radiation from the sun is a major cause of skin cancer. UV light causes the release of tumor necrosis factor in the epidermis, which may reduce immune surveillance against skin cancer.

Viruses implicated in human cancers are called oncogenic viruses. Viruses alter the genome of the infected cell which then alters the progeny of the host cell. Oncogenic viruses are either deoxyribonucleic acid (DNA) or ribonucleic acid (RNA). The DNA viruses are incorporated into the genes of the host and are then transmitted to subsequent generations. The DNA viruses are implicated in cancers of the cervix and liver and some lymphomas.

The RNA viruses involve a synthesis of DNA from an RNA template using an enzyme called reverse transcriptase. In this mechanism, genes are expanded and new DNA sequences are integrated into the host's DNA. The RNA viruses are implicated in the development of certain types of adult T cell leukemia-lymphoma.

7. **Describe the theory of tumor immune surveillance as a defense against neoplasia; identify tumor antigens.**
   Study pages 254-256; refer to Figure 9-13 and Table 9-10.

Cell-mediated cytotoxicity by immunologic cells such as lymphocytes has evolved as a protection against "foreign" structures found on emerging cancer cells. The identification of tumor antigens, the increased risk of some cancers in immune-suppressed individuals, the identification of tumor reactive antibodies in some individuals with cancer, and the demonstration of tumor-specific T cell-mediated cellular immunity—all confirm immune surveillance for neoplastic cells.

Human cancer cells express numerous "foreign" molecules on their surfaces that can be recognized by the immune system as **tumor-specific antigens** (TSAs). Because cancer is a disease of unregulated cell growth and differentiation, the differences between the molecules expressed on the surfaces of normal and cancer cells may be minor. Thus, the recognition of a molecule as a TSA results from a complex interaction between the tumor and the host's immune system. Serologically defined human TSAs include viral antigens, oncofetal antigens, oncogene products, and "mutant" proteins and carbohydrates. The **viral antigens** are products expressed by virally transformed cells. Viral antigens are common to all tumors induced by the same virus.

The **oncofetal antigens** are expressed by cells during certain stages of embryonic development but are absent or expressed at very low concentrations by normal adult cells. **Alphafetoprotein** (a-FP) and **carcinoembryonic antigens** are common examples of these antigens. Individuals with hepatic, pancreatic, and malignant tumors of epithelial cells have high levels of a-FP in their serum. Pancreas and breast cancer patients have detectable CEA antibody titers. Malignancies of hematopoietic tissues express a unique form of oncofetal antigens. The common acute lymphoblastic leukemia-associated antigen referred to as CALLA is a valuable marker of lymphoblastic leukemia (ALL).

A large number of **oncogene-related antigens** are associated with individual tumors; a complex activation of certain oncogenes is required for transformation of normal cells. A number of oncogene-related antigens are expressed by lung cancers and are associated with cellular growth and differentiation.

Carbohydrate TSAs are expressed by melanomas and other neuroectodermal cancers. Expression of blood group A antigen on lung cancers has a poor prognosis.

The major histocompatibility class II antigen, HLA-DR, is not usually expressed by normal epithelial cells. However, HLA-DR as a **protein TSA** is expressed to varying degrees by melanomas, gastric carcinomas, larynx carcinomas, lung carcinomas, colorectal carcinomas, and breast carcinomas. An example of an enzyme marker is prostate-specific antigen (PSA) found in prostate tumors.

8. Indicate the limitations of immune surveillance as a defense against cancer.
Study pages 257-258; refer to Figure 9-14.

Host immunologic potential and the characteristics of growing cancer cells constantly change. Therefore, many cancers can bypass the host's immune surveillance system and escape destruction. Tumors escape immunologic rejection by (1) antigenic modulation, (2) secretion of immunosuppressive substances, (3) escape and sneaking through, (4) blocking factor, (5) immunostimulation, and (6) TSA-reactive suppressor T lymphocytes.

Essentially, tumor growth or rejection depends on complex interactions between cancer cells and the host's immune system. Transformation processes may select for cancer cells that escape the host's immune surveillance system. It is likely that many carcinogenic agents cause immune suppression; this makes individuals more susceptible to the growth of neoplasia or cancers.

Practice Examination

Match the term with its definition.

1. ____ neoplasia
2. ____ anaplasia
3. ____ transformation

a. variation in size, shape, and arrangement of cells

b. differentiation of dividing cells into cellular types not ordinarily found in a given area

c. abnormal, proliferating cells possessing a higher degree of autonomy

d. increase in absolute number of cells

e. lack of cellular differentiation or specialization, primitive cells

f. normal cell becomes cancerous

4. Which characterizes cancer cells?

   a. poorly differentiated
   b. metastasis
   c. impaired cell-to-cell recognition
   d. poor cellular cohesiveness
   e. All of the above are correct.

5. Which statement is false regarding neoplasms?

   a. Malignant neoplasms secrete plasminogen-activating factor.
   b. Malignant neoplasms exhibit abnormal cellular arrangement.
   c. Malignant neoplasms have increased cell-to-cell adhesion.
   d. Malignant neoplasms lack cellular differentiation.

6. The group of individuals most susceptible to cancer often:

   a. are immunodeficient.
   b. are anemic.
   c. have hypercalcemia.
   d. have chronic joint disturbance.
   e. have neurologic dysfunction.

7. Metastasis is:

   a. an alteration in normal cellular growth.
   b. growth of benign or malignant neoplastic cells.
   c. mutational.
   d. the ability to establish a secondary neoplasm at a new site.

8. Carcinoma in situ is:

   a. preinvasive.
   b. a glandular or epithelial neoplasm.
   c. a teratoma.
   d. carcinoma that has broken through the basement membrane.
   e. Both a and b are correct.

Match the cellular change with its functional significance.

9. ____ fewer anchoring junctions
10. ____ reduced fibronectin
11. ____ loss of surface glycolipid
12. ____ increased gap junctions

a. increased metabolite transport
b. proliferation of transformed cell encouraged
c. altered response to growth factors
d. loss of density-dependent inhibition of growth
e. "rounded-up" cells
f. increased migration, decreased adhesion
g. increased extracellular proteolysis

13. Which are carcinogens or promoters?

a. viruses
b. chemicals
c. radiation
d. Both b and c are correct.
e. a, b, and c are correct.

14. Tumor suppressor genes are:

a. genes having the ability to transform a normal cell into a cancerous cell.
b. normal genes that regulate growth and development.
c. genes that produce proteins that inhibit cellular division.
d. Both b and c are correct.

15. In a theory of carcinogenesis, promotion:

a. precedes initiation.
b. accelerates the process by which initiated cells become cancerous.
c. interrupts DNA chain sequence.
d. may alter cell-to-cell communication.
e. Both b and d are correct.

16. Carcinogens for lung cancer include:

a. saccharin.
b. tobacco smoke condensates.
c. nitrates and food additives.
d. aflatoxin.
e. All of the above are correct.

17. Oncogenic viruses are:

a. DNA viruses.
b. RNA viruses.
c. capable of incorporation into host genes.
d. capable of establishing new DNA sequences.
e. All of the above are correct.

18. Ionizing radiation:

a. injures the DNA of a cell as DNA interacts with an electron.
b. causes cellular mutations.
c. damages DNA because of interaction of DNA with a free radical.
d. Both a and b are correct.
e. a, b, and c are correct.

19. Which serum TSA is an example of an oncofetal antigen?

a. carcinoembryonic antigen
b. prostate-specific antigen
c. HLA-DR antigen
d. Both a and b are correct.
e. None of the above is correct.

20. The postulate in the immune surveillance theory is:

a. cancerous cells do not express "nonself" antigens.
b. neoplastic "nonself" antigens are tolerated.
c. TSAs are very similar to those of normal cells.
d. neoplastic cells express antigens recognized as "nonself" which are then rejected.
e. Both b and c are correct.

21. Neoplasms may "escape" immunological rejection by:

a. producing blocking antibodies.
b. stimulating suppressor cells.
c. secreting immunosuppressive substances.
d. Both a and c are correct.
e. a, b, and c are correct.

Match the cancer with the carcinogen.

22. ____ liver cancer
23. ____ uterine cervical cancer
24. ____ lung cancer
25. ____ melanoma

a. asbestos
b. estrogen
c. aflatoxin
d. human papillomavirus
e. ionizing radiation
f. ultraviolet radiation

CHAPTER

10

Tumor Spread in Adults and Cancer in Children

Foundational Objective

a. Describe mechanisms that confine cells and tissues to a specific anatomical site. Review pages 25-27.

Memory Check!

- All cells are within a network of extracellular macromolecules known as the extracellular matrix. The extracellular matrix holds cells and tissues together and provides an organized framework in which cells can interact with each other.
- To confine themselves and form tissues, cells must have intercellular recognition and adhesion. Specialized cells likely form a tissue in one of two ways. The first way is mitosis of one or more founder cells. Founder cells, basic precursor cells, are prevented from "wandering away" by macromolecules in the extracellular matrix and by adherence to one another at specialized junctions on their plasma membranes. The second way specialized cells form tissues involves their migration to and subsequent accumulation at the site of tissue formation. Migrant cells are thought to arrive at the specific site of tissue formation through chemotaxis or contact guidance. Cells at the migrant cells' destination secrete a chemical known as chemotactic factor, which attracts specific migrant cells. Contact guidance is movement along a pathway or "pavement" within the extracellular matrix. In order to stay together in groups, cells must recognize each other and remain distinct from the cells of surrounding tissues.
- Cells in direct physical contact with neighboring cells are often linked together at specialized regions of their plasma membranes. These regions are known as cell junctions. Cell junctions hold cells together and allow small molecules to pass from cell to cell. This coordinates the activities of cells that form tissues. There are three main types of cell junctions: (1) desmosomes, (2) tight junctions, and (3) gap junctions. Desmosomes hold cells together by forming either continuous bands of epithelial sheets or buttonlike points of contact. Desmosomes also provide a system of braces to maintain structural stability. Tight junctions act as a barrier to diffusion, prevent movement of substances through transport proteins of the plasma membrane, and prevent the leakage of small molecules between the plasma membranes of adjacent cells. Gap junctions are clusters of protein channels that allow small ions and molecules to pass directly from the inside of one cell to the inside of another. Cells connected by gap junctions are considered ionically and metabolically joined. Gap junctions coordinate the activities of adjacent cells. For example, these junctions synchronize contractions of heart muscle cells through ionic coupling. The junctions permit action potentials to spread rapidly from cell to cell in neural tissues.

Objectives

After review of this chapter, the learner will be able to:

1. Describe prerequisites for metastasis to occur.
Study page 265; refer to Figure 10-1.

Invasion or local spread is a prerequisite for metastasis and is the first step in the metastatic process. In early stages, local invasion may occur by direct tumor extension. Eventually, cells or clumps of cells become detached from the primary tumor and invade the surrounding interstitial spaces. Possible important factors in local invasion include (1) cellular multiplication, (2) mechanical pressure, (3) release of lytic enzymes, (4) decreased cell-to-cell adhesion, and (5) increased motility of individual tumor cells. These mechanisms are not mutually exclusive, and it is likely that in a given neoplasm any combination of the five may be involved.

The rate of cellular multiplication depends on the cell generation time, the number of cells that are dividing, and the cell loss from the tumor. Malignant cells can divide rapidly, but the tumor may not grow because cells are rapidly dying.

Mechanical pressure generates pressure that forces cellular sheets or fingerlike projections along the lines of least mechanical resistance; spread is enhanced. Growing mass blocks local blood vessels and leads to local tissue death. This reduces mechanical resistance and further aids the spread.

Many tumors have higher levels of protease and collagenases, plasminogen activators, and lysosomal enzymes than corresponding normal tissue. These lytic enzymes destroy normal tissue, which increases tumor invasion.

Cancer cells do not adhere to one another as well as normal cells. This trait has partially been attributed to fibronectin. Cancer cells may either make a defective type of fibronectin or break down fibronectin as they make it. Low levels or loss of this anchoring molecule may help cancer cells "slip" between normal cells and allow more invasion.

Cell movement is essential for tumor cells to invade and travel. The neoplastic cell must detach and infiltrate into adjacent tissue, migrate through the vascular wall into the circulation, and then migrate out of the vascular wall into a secondary site. Tumor cells may actually move by means of their own chemotactic factors known as "autocrine motility factors." In these mechanisms, the tumor cell would secrete a factor that binds to a specific receptor on the cell surface to stimulate motility. Thus, the neoplastic cell acquires independent and continuous stimulation for its motile and invasive behavior.

2. Describe the proposed sequence of events during tumor cell invasion of extracellular matrix.
Study pages 265-266; refer to Figures 10-2 and 10-3.

Once the tumor cell is in the blood circulation, a three-step theory likely describes the events during tumor cell invasion of the extracellular matrix. These steps involve tumor cell attachment to the basement membrane of vascular matrix, degradation or dissolution of the matrix, and locomotion or movement into the interstitial matrix. **Laminin** is a complex glycoprotein and a major constituent of all basement membranes. Since membrane vesicles of tumor cells are rich in **laminin receptors**, the first step is complete when binding occurs between the vascular basement membrane laminin and its receptors. Once anchored, the tumor cell either secretes **collagenase** or induces host cells to produce proteolytic enzymes. Degradation of the matrix constitutes the second step. Such enzymes may degrade both the attachment proteins and the structural collagenous proteins of the vascular basement membrane matrix. The third step is tumor cell locomotion. Fingerlike projections, called pseudopodia, extend from the tumor cell and attach to blood vessel walls that cross the basement membrane. Thus, the tumor cells leave the vasculature and enter the interstitial stroma. The direction of locomotion site is likely influenced by chemotactic factors.

3. Describe the avenues for metastatic spread.
Study pages 266-268.

Three routes for metastasis exist: direct or continuous extension, lymphatic spread, and bloodstream dissemination. These routes are not mutually exclusive. Tumor dissemination through one route often facilitates metastasis through others because tumor cells move through numerous microscopic anatomic connections.

Direct tumor extension is thought to be initiated by a complex sequence of events. These events are initiated by loss of intracellular adhesion, enabling cells to "slip" past one another. Movement of cells through tissue barriers is further influenced by protease and autocrine motility factors.

The process of metastasis involves invasion and penetration of tumor cells into and from blood vessels or via lymphatics or both. The most common route for distant metastases is **lymphatic spread**. Tumors generally lack a well-formed lymphatic network; rather, lymphatic channels occur at the periphery of the tumor and not within the tumor mass. Tumor cells entering the lymphatic vessels from interstitial sites are carried to regional lymph nodes that initially may prevent the further spread of tumor cells into the lymphatics. A cancer cell that becomes lodged in lymph nodes may die as a result of local inflammatory reaction or, because of an incompatible local environment, grow into a discernable lump, remain dormant for unknown reasons, or detach and enter the efferent lymphatics. If tumor cell emboli are released into efferent lymphatic vessels, lymphatic metastasis occurs. The shedding of emboli may be caused by changes in vessel pressure, by turbulent alterations in lymphatic flow, or by manipulation of the tumor during diagnostic tests or surgery. Tumor cells eventually move into the venous drainage because of numerous venolymphatic communications.

Hematogenous spread requires tumor cells to penetrate and detach from blood vessels and spread to distant organs. To establish a metastatic site, tumor cells must "escape" host defenses, survive mechanical trauma in the bloodstream, and lodge in the vascular bed of the target organ. Tumor cells circulate and attach directly to the endothelial surface of the basement membrane. The formation of a leukocyte-fibrin-platelet complex around tumor cells is thought to protect tumor cells within these complexes from host defenses and to assist successful attachment to the vascular epithelium. After invading the vascular wall, these neoplastic cells leave the vascular bed, enter the interstitial stroma, and invade the parenchyma of the target organ.

4. Describe angiogenesis; identify factors that may determine metastatic sites.
Study pages 268-269; refer to Table 10-1.

Tumors likely cannot grow more than a few millimeters in diameter without developing new blood vessels. This new vascular network development is called **angiogenesis**. Development of blood vessels is the result of diffusible substances secreted by the tumor. These secreted substances are known as **tumor-angiogenesis factors** (TAF). Also, **thrombospondin**—a protein that inhibits growth of new blood vessels—production drops suddenly in cancer cells.

The ability of metastatic cells to grow and develop requires not only the development of a vascular network but evasion of host defenses and a compatible new environment. The metastatic potential of many common carcinomas is related to the size of the primary tumor. Larger tumors may overwhelm host defenses, thus favoring survival of disseminated malignant cells.

Distant metastatic sites may or may not be the first capillary bed encountered by the circulating cells. Instead, preferential growth in specific organs is observed. This feature is called "organ tropism." This tropism may result from local growth factors or hormones present in the target organ, preferential adherence by tumor receptors to the surface of certain target organs, or the presence of chemotactic factors diffusing from the target organ, which cause circulating tumor cells to extravasate from the vessels and accumulate in the target organ. Evidence exists that organ tropism is genetically determined.

5. Describe the clinical manifestations of cancer.
Study pages 269-271; refer to Figure 10-4 and Table 10-2.

Usually little or no **pain** is associated with the early stages of malignant disease, but pain will affect 60 to 80 percent of individuals terminally ill with cancer. The pain may or may not be directly related to the malignancy but might be the result of inflammation and infection. A very common cause of pain is bone metastasis; it is caused by periosteal irritation, medullary pressure, or pathologic fractures. Abdominal pain is often caused by stretching, obstructions, or surgical adhesions of the hollow visceral organs. An enlarged liver from hepatic malignancies results in a dull pain or fullness over the right upper quadrant of the abdomen. Any tumor having very little space to grow without compressing blood vessels and nerve endings against bone will elicit pain. Tissue destruction from infection and necrosis can cause pain.

Fatigue is the most frequently reported symptom of cancer and cancer treatment. Likely causes of fatigue include sleep disturbance, biochemical changes, psychological factors, altered nutritional status, and level of activity.

Decreased muscle contractibility and function are observed in individuals with cancer. Muscle loss may result from cancer treatment or from circulating tumor necrosis factor and IL-1.

Cachexia is a severe wasting, emaciation, and decreased quality of life seen in malignancy. Anorexia, or loss of appetite, contributes to the syndrome of cachexia. Reductions in sensitivities to sweet, sour, and salty tastes make ordinary seasoned foods seem bland. Also, aversions to food likely develop because of poor use of glucose and increased mobilization of protein. Elevated glucose and amino acid levels in the blood stimulate the satiety center, resulting in reduced appetite.

Anemia is commonly associated with malignancy. The majority of individuals with cancer usually have a mild anemia, although 20 percent may have hemoglobin concentrations which are depressed to below 9 g/dl. Chronic bleeding, severe malnutrition, medical therapies, or malignancy in blood-forming organs may cause anemia.

Direct tumor invasion into the bone marrow causes decreased leukocyte counts and decreased numbers of platelets. Chemotherapy and radiotherapy of areas of the bone marrow cause **leukopenia** and **thrombocytopenia**.

Infection is the most significant cause of complications and death in individuals with malignant disease. Individuals with cancer are very susceptible to infection because of reductions in immunologic functions, debility from advanced disease, and immunosuppression from radiotherapy and chemotherapy. Surgery can create favorable residual sites for infection. The incidence of hospital-related or nosocomial infections for cancer patients is increased because of indwelling medical devices, compromised wound care, and the introduction of microorganisms from visitors and other patients.

6. **Compare the modalities for the treatment of neoplasms; identify the advantages of immune therapy.**
   Study pages 271-273; refer to Tables 10-3 through 10-5.

Cancer is treated by chemotherapy, radiotherapy, surgery, immunotherapy, and combinations of these modalities. The mechanism by which **chemotherapy** acts to eradicate tumor cells depends largely on its effect on the cell cycle. To be effective, chemotherapy must eliminate enough neoplastic cells so that the body's own defenses can eradicate the remaining cells.

To eradicate neoplastic cells without producing excessive toxicity and to avoid damage to normal structures is the challenge of **radiation therapy**. Ionizing radiation damages important macromolecules, especially DNA. Rapidly renewing and dividing cells are generally more radiosensitive than other cells.

Surgical therapy is useful when the neoplasm is accessible and has not yet spread beyond the limits of surgical excision. If there is any chance of regional lymph node involvement and there is no evidence of distant disease, the lymph nodes also should be removed. Palliative surgery, alleviation without cure, may be used to relieve or avoid symptoms of malignancy. Surgery is also indicated for benign tumors and those that could become malignant.

Immunotherapy is promising in the treatment of cancer. A specific method, like immunotherapy, may eliminate transformed cells without damaging normal tissues. Also, immune memory cells are long-lived and capable of providing extended protection against the emergence of recurrent primary tumor cells and metastatic cancer cells.

Immunotherapies for the treatment of cancer are known as **biological response modifiers** (BRMs). These BRMs can have a direct cytotoxic effect on cancer cells, initiate or augment the host's tumor-immune rejection response, or modify cancer cells' susceptibility to the lytic or tumor-arresting effects of the immune system. The BRMs include immunomodulating agents, interferons, thymosins, antigens, effector cells, lymphokines, cytokines, and monoclonal antibodies.

7. **Compare childhood neoplasms with adult neoplasms.**
   Study pages 273-277; refer to Tables 10-6 through 10-8.

(See box on page 69 of *Workbook.*)

Comparison of Usual Childhood and Adult Cancers

Characteristic	Childhood Cancers	Adult Cancers
Incidence	< 1% of all cancers	> 99% of all cancers
Environmental causation	Weak relationship to environmental exposures and lifestyle	Strong relationship to environmental exposures and lifestyle
Latency (from initiation to diagnosis)	Short	Long
Sites involved	Tissue	Organs
Cells involved	Nonepithelial: sarcomas, embryonal, leukemia, lymphoma	Epithelial: carcinomas
Prevention	Few strategies to prevent	80% may be preventable
Early detection	Generally accidental	Possible by early detection screening tests/exams
Stage at diagnosis	80% have metastasized	Local or regional spread
Treatment/side effects	Less difficulty with acute toxicity but more significant long-term consequences	More difficulty with acute toxicity but fewer long-term consequences
Response to treatment	Very responsive to chemotherapy	Less responsive to chemotherapy
Prognosis	> 60% cure	< 60% cure

Practice Examination

1. Tumor spread depends on:

   a. growth rate of tumor and its degree of differentiation.
   b. unknown factors.
   c. the presence or absence of anatomical barriers.
   d. Both a and c are correct.
   e. a, b, and c are correct.

2. Which is the correct sequence during the process of metastasis?

   a. vascularization, adherence of neoplastic cells, invasion into lymph and vascular systems
   b. transport, vascularization, adherence of neoplastic cells
   c. local invasion, invasion into lymph and vascular systems, transport
   d. vascularization, extravasation, transport

3. In order for metastasis to occur, local invasive factors include all of the following except:

   a. cellular multiplication.
   b. mechanical pressure.
   c. lytic enzyme release.
   d. increased cellular adhesion.
   e. increased individual tumor cells.

4. Known routes for metastasis of malignant cells include:

   a. continuous extension.
   b. lymphatic spread.
   c. bloodstream dissemination.
   d. Both b and c are correct.
   e. a, b, and c are correct.

5. Frequent sites for metastatic cells include all of the following except:

   a. lung.
   b. liver.
   c. brain.
   d. bone.
   e. heart.

6. A malignant cell that becomes lodged in a lymph node may:

   a. die.
   b. divide.
   c. become dormant.
   d. enter efferent lymphatics.
   e. All of the above are correct.

7. The process by which tumors develop new vascular networks is:

   a. heparinization.
   b. angiogenesis.
   c. anaplasia.
   d. autonomy.
   e. differentiation.

8. Organ tropism involves:

   a. local growth factors.
   b. chemotactic factors.
   c. tumor receptors.
   d. genetic determinants.
   e. All of the above are correct.

9. Likely causes for the fatigue observed in individuals with cancer include:

   a. biochemical changes because of treatment.
   b. muscle loss.
   c. psychological factors.
   d. All of the above are correct.
   e. Both a and c are correct.

10. Neoplasms may cause all of the following except:

    a. obstruction of passageways.
    b. hormonal imbalances.
    c. viral infections.
    d. nutrient depletion.

11. Metastatic behavior may be due to:

    a. altered cytoplasm.
    b. altered ribosomes.
    c. altered genetic code.
    d. chromosomal breakage.

12. The pain experienced with cancer:

    a. affects the individual in the early stages of malignancy.
    b. occurs in bone metastasis.
    c. results from tissue necrosis.
    d. Both b and c are correct.
    e. a, b, and c are correct.

13. The anorexia or loss of appetite seen in the syndrome of cancer cachexia may occur because of:

    a. altered blood serum levels of glucose and amino acids.
    b. hyperinsulinism.
    c. late satiety.
    d. hypoproteinemia.

14. The anemia associated with malignancy can be:

    a. due to depletion of hemoglobin building blocks.
    b. severe in the majority of cases.
    c. caused by destruction of bone marrow.
    d. All of the above are correct.
    e. Both a and c are correct.

15. Chemotherapy for cancer:

    a. prevents transcription.
    b. damages cells undergoing mitosis.
    c. Both a and b are correct.
    d. Neither a nor b is correct.

16. Immunotherapy for cancer:

    a. is a nonspecific treatment.
    b. injures both transformed and normal cells.
    c. suppresses tumor-immune response.
    d. is augmented by memory cells.
    e. None of the above is correct.

17. BRMs:

    a. directly kill cancer cells.
    b. augment the tumor-immune rejection response.
    c. modify the cancer cell's susceptibility to lysis.
    d. All of the above are correct.
    e. None of the above is correct.

18. Childhood cancers:

    a. most often involve nonepithelial tissue.
    b. most often involve epithelial tissue.
    c. have a strong relationship to environmental exposure.
    d. are less responsive to chemotherapy than adult cancers.
    e. None of the above is correct.

19. Adult cancers have:

    a. a better cure rate than childhood cancers.
    b. a short latency period.
    c. mostly metastasized at time of diagnosis.
    d. organ involvement more often than tissue involvement.
    e. None of the above is correct.

20. Which is not involved in metastasis?

    a. initial establishment
    b. interference
    c. invasion
    d. dissemination
    e. proliferation

Match the cancer treatment with its characteristic.

21. ____ radiation
22. ____ monoclonal antibodies
23. ____ immunomodulating agents
24. ____ surgery
25. ____ mitomycin

a. cross-linking of DNA strands
b. T cell transfer
c. specific antibodies for tumor antigen
d. cancerous cells attacked in cell cycle
e. stimulation of immune system
f. tumor removal
g. direct ionization

PART *Two*

BODY SYSTEMS AND DISEASES

CHAPTER 11

Structure and Function of the Neurologic System

Objectives

After review of this chapter, the learner will be able to:

1. **Identify the structural and functional subdivisions of the nervous system.**
   Review page 286.

2. **Compare the functions of neurons and neuroglia; identify the parts of neurons.**
   Review pages 286-287; refer to Figures 11-1 through 11-3 and Table 11-1.

3. **Describe the circumstances under which nervous tissue can regenerate.**
   Review pages 287-289; refer to Figure 11-4.

4. **Describe transmission of impulses by neurotransmitters.**
   Review pages 289-291; refer to Table 11-2.

5. **Identify the three main divisions of the brain; characterize their associated structures and functions.**
   Review pages 291-296; refer to Figures 11-6 through 11-8 and Table 11-3.

6. **Identify the significance of decussation of motor fibers.**
   Review page 296; refer to Figure 11-9.

7. **Describe the location and structure of the spinal cord; define a reflex arc.**
   Review pages 296-297; refer to Figures 11-10 through 11-14.

8. **Identify the structures responsible for maintaining and protecting the central nervous system.**
   Review pages 297-301; refer to Figures 11-15 through 11-17 and Table 11-4.

9. **Identify the route of blood circulation within the central nervous system; note the significance of the circle of Willis.**
   Review pages 301-306; refer to Figures 11-18 through 11-22 and Table 11-5.

10. **Describe the structure of a spinal nerve; locate plexuses.**
    Review pages 306-308; refer to Figure 11-23.

11. **Name the cranial nerves and state functions of each.**
    Refer to Table 11-6.

12. **Identify the subdivisions of the autonomic nervous system, their origins, and general functions.**
    Review pages 308-315; refer to Figures 11-24 through 11-26 and 11-28.

13. **Identify the type of neurotransmitter secreted by preganglionic and postganglionic fibers in the autonomic nervous system.**
    Review pages 309-310; refer to Figure 11-27 and Table 11-7.

Practice Examination

1. One function of the somatic nervous system that is not performed by the autonomic nervous system is:

   a. conduction of impulses to involuntary muscles and glands.
   b. conduction of impulses to the central nervous system.
   c. conduction of impulses to skeletal muscles.
   d. conduction of impulses between the brain and spinal cord.

2. A neuron with a single dendrite at one end of the cell body and a single axon at the other end of the cell body would be classified as:

   a. unipolar.
   b. multipolar.
   c. monopolar.
   d. bipolar.

3. Neurons that carry impulses away from the CNS are called:

   a. afferent neurons.
   b. sensory neurons.
   c. efferent neurons.
   d. association neurons.

Match the structure with its function or description.

4. ____ Schwann cell
5. ____ dendrite

a. the outer, nucleated layer of a certain cell type
b. produces myelin sheath
c. carries impulses away from perikaryon
d. a covering over neuron fibers
e. conducts impulses to cell body

6. Neurons are specialized for the conduction of impulses, whereas neuroglia:

   a. support nerve tissue.
   b. serve as motor end plates.
   c. synthesize acetylcholine and cholinesterase.
   d. All of the above are correct.

7. There is one-way conduction at a synapse because:

   a. only postsynaptic neurons contain synaptic vesicles.
   b. acetylcholine prevents nerve impulses from traveling in both directions.
   c. only the presynaptic neuron contains neurotransmitters.
   d. only dendrites release neurotransmitters.

8. Which contains the thalamus and hypothalamus?

   a. diencephalon
   b. cerebrum
   c. medulla oblongata
   d. brain stem

9. The reticular activating system:

   a. programs for fine repetitive motor movements.
   b. maintains wakefulness.
   c. maintains constant internal environments.
   d. affects the positioning of the head to improve hearing.

10. Which phrases best describe the spinal cord? (*More than one answer may be correct.*)

   a. descends inferior to the lumbar vertebrae
   b. conducts motor impulses from the brain
   c. descends to the fourth lumbar vertebra
   d. conducts sensory impulses to the brain

Match the component of a reflex arc with its descriptor.

11. ____ sensory neuron
12. ____ effector

a. carries impulses to the CNS
b. carries impulses to a responding organ
c. responds to motor impulse
d. stimulated by one neuron and passes impulse on to another neuron
e. responds directly to changes in environment

13. Which is not a protective covering of the CNS?

   a. cauda equine
   b. dura mater
   c. arachnoid
   d. cranial bone

14. The composition of cerebrospinal fluid is:

   a. the same as blood.
   b. distilled H_2O with dissolved salts.
   c. a plasmalike liquid with glucose, salts, and proteins.
   d. a heavy mucous solution with dissolved salts, glucose, and urea.

Match the function with the cranial nerve.

15. ____ tasting
16. ____ balance maintenance

a. facial
b. olfactory
c. vestibulocochlear
d. hypoglossal
e. optic

17. An autonomic ganglion can be described as:

    a. the site of synapses between visceral efferent neurons.
    b. a site where spinal reflexes occur.
    c. a point of synapse between parasympathetic and sympathetic neurons.
    d. the place where unconscious sensations occur.

18 The sympathetic division of the autonomic nervous system:

    a. mobilizes energy in times of need.
    b. is innervated by cell bodies from T1 through L2.
    c. is innervated by cell bodies located in the cranial nerve nuclei.
    d. Both a and b are correct.
    e. Both a and c are correct.

19. The parasympathetic division of the autonomic nervous system:

    a. conserves and stores energy.
    b. has relatively short postganglionic neurons.
    c. Both a and b are correct.
    d. has paravertebral ganglia.

Match the characteristic with the division of the autonomic nervous system.

20. ____ more extensive use of norepinephrine as a transmitter substance	a. sympathetic
	b. parasympathetic
21. ____ effects more widespread and generalized	
22. ____ elicits rest-response	

Classify the effect of sympathetic nerve stimulation on the structure.

23. ____ breathing passageways	a. increases diameter
24. ____ intestines	b. decreases diameter
25. ____ liver	c. increases activity
	d. decreases activity

CHAPTER

12

Pain, Temperature, Sleep, and Sensory Function

Foundational Objectives

a. Identify receptors, pathways, and perceptors for pain. Review pages 320-323; refer to Figure 12-1 and Table 12-2.

Memory Check!

- Pain receptors, also known as nociceptors, are small unmyelinated and lightly myelinated nerve endings of afferent neurons found in nearly every tissue in the body. These neurons respond to chemical, thermal, and mechanical stimuli. Sensory nerves transmit the stimuli from pain receptors into the dorsal horn of the spinal cord. The impulses ascend by either the neospinothalamic tract or the paleospinothalamic tract. The paleospinothalamic tract carries information to the reticular formation, the pons, the limbic system, and the midbrain. The neospinothalamic tract carries information to the midbrain, the postcentral gyrus where pain is perceived, and the cortex where precision and discrimination occur.

b. Describe thermoregulation. Review pages 326-327; refer to Table 12-5.

Memory Check!

- The control of body temperature is a function of centers located in the hypothalamus. Thermoreceptors provide the hypothalamus with information about peripheral and core temperatures. If the temperature is low, the body initiates heat conservation measures by a series of hormonal mechanisms. Heat production begins with hypothalamic release of TSH-RH which stimulates release of TSH from the anterior pituitary. The TSH causes release of thyroxine from the thyroid gland. This hormone causes release of epinephrine from the adrenal medulla. Epinephrine causes vasoconstriction, glycolysis, and increased metabolic rates which increase heat production. Warmer peripheral and core temperatures reverse the process. Decreasing the sympathetic pathway produces vasodilation, decreased muscle tone, and increased perspiration.

c. Identify the normal sleep stages; describe nervous system control of sleep. Review page 330.

Memory Check!

- Normal sleep has two phases that can be documented by electroencephalography (EEG): rapid eye movement (REM) sleep and non-REM, or slow wave, sleep. Non-REM sleep is initiated by the withdrawal of neurotransmitters from the reticular formation and by the inhibition of arousal mechanisms. During non-REM sleep, respiration is controlled by metabolic processes. The basal metabolic rate, temperature, heart rate, blood pressure, and muscle tone all decrease. Knee-jerk reflexes are absent. Pupils are constricted. During various stages, cerebral blood flow to the brain decreases, growth hormone is released, and levels of corticosteroids and catecholamines are depressed.
- REM sleep occurs about every 90 minutes beginning after one or two hours of non-REM sleep. The EEG pattern of REM sleep is similar to the normal awake pattern. Alternating periods of REM and non-REM sleep occur throughout the night, with lengthening intervals of REM sleep and fewer intervals of the deeper stages of non-REM sleep toward morning. REM sleep is characterized by rapid eye movement; loss of tone of antigravity muscles; loss of temperature regulation; alteration in heart rate, blood pressure, and respiration; penile erection in men and clitoral engorgement in women; and a high rate of memorable dreams. Steroids are released in short bursts and cerebral blood flow is increased. The reticular formation is primarily responsible for generating REM sleep. Projections from the reticular formation and other areas of the mesencephalon and brain stem produce non-REM sleep.

d. Describe the eye and its structure. Review pages 331-333; refer to Figures 12-6 through 12-8.

Memory Check!

- The wall of the eye is formed of three layers: sclera, choroid, and retina. It becomes transparent at the cornea in the central anterior region, which allows light to enter the eye. The choroid is the pigmented middle layer that prevents light from scattering inside the eye. The iris, part of the choroid, has a round opening, the pupil, through which light passes.
- The innermost layer of the eye, the retina, contains the rods and cones. These photoreceptors convert light energy into nerve impulses.
- Nerve impulses pass through the optic nerves to the optic chiasm. Nerves from the nasal halves of the retinas cross and join fibers from the temporal halves of the retinas to form the optic tracts. The optic tracts connect to the primary visual cortex in the occipital lobe of the brain. Light entering the eye is focused on the retina by the lens, which is a flexible, biconvex, crystal-like structure. The lens separates the anterior cavity from the vitreous chamber. The aqueous humor of the anterior cavity helps maintain pressure inside the eye and provides nutrients to the lens and the cornea. The vitreous chamber is filled with a gel-like vitreous humor which prevents the eyeball from collapsing inward.
- Six extrinsic eye muscles allow gross eye movements and permit eyes to follow a moving object. The external structures protecting the eye include the eyelids, conjunctiva, and lacrimal apparatus.

e. Describe the parts of the ear. Review pages 336-337; refer to Figures 12-11 and 12-12.

Memory Check!

- The ear is divided into three areas: the external ear, involved only with hearing; the middle ear, involved only with hearing; and the inner ear, involved with hearing and equilibrium.
- The external ear is composed of the pinna, which is visible, and the external auditory canal that leads to the middle ear. Sound waves entering the external auditory canal hit the tympanic membrane and cause it to vibrate. This membrane separates the external ear from the middle ear.
- The middle ear is composed of the tympanic cavity within the temporal bone. Three ossicles transmit the vibration of the tympanic membrane to the inner ear and set the fluids of the inner ear in motion.
- The inner ear is a system of osseous labyrinths filled with perilymph. The bony labyrinth is divided into the cochlea, the vestibule, and the semicircular canals.
- Sound waves that reach the cochlea through vibrations of the tympanic membrane, ossicles, and oval window set the cochlear fluids in motion. Receptor cells on the basilar membrane are stimulated and transmit impulses along the cochlear nerve, a division of the vestibulocochlear nerve, to the auditory cortex of the temporal lobe for sound interpretation.
- The semicircular canals and vestibule of the inner ear contain equilibrium receptors. In the semicircular canals, the dynamic equilibrium receptors respond to changes in direction of movement. The vestibule in the inner ear contains receptors essential to the body's sense of static equilibrium. Both of these impulses are transmitted through the vestibular nerve, a division of the vestibulocochlear nerve, to the cerebellum.

Objectives

After review of this chapter, the learner will be able to:

1. **Compare the theories of pain.**
   Study page 323; refer to Figure 12-2.

Theories proposed to describe the mechanism of pain include the specificity theory, the intensity theory, the pattern theory, and the gate control theory. The **specificity theory** identifies cutaneous sensation as (1) touch, (2) warmth, (3) cold, or (4) pain. Each cutaneous sensation results from stimulation of specific receptor sites on the skin. Impulses are transmitted to discrete areas of the thalamus and cerebral cortex for perception of pain. This theory fails to account for adaptation to pain and the effects of psychosocial factors on pain perception.

The **intensity theory** proposes that pain results from excessive stimulation of sensory receptors. Pain occurs if the stimulus is of sufficient intensity. This theory does not explain the intense stimulation of some sites that produces no pain.

The **pattern theory** suggests that pain perception is the result of the length of time, the amount of tissue involved, and the summation of the afferent impulses. Summation may occur in the spinal cord or in the brain. Although pattern theories do not account for adaptation to pain, they do allow for multiple pain perception factors.

According to the **gate control theory**, nociceptive impulses are transmitted from specialized skin receptors to the spinal cord through large A and small C fibers. These fibers terminate in the dorsal horn of the spinal cord. Cells in the substantia gelatinosa of the dorsal horn function as a gate and permit some impulses to reach the central nervous system for interpretation. Stimulation of larger, faster-transmitting fibers causes the cells in the substantia gelatinosa to "close the gate." A closed gate decreases stimulation of trigger cells, decreases transmission impulses, and diminishes pain perception. Persistent stimulation of the large fibers, however, allows adaptation. When adaptation to impulses from large fibers occurs, the result is a relative increase in small neuron activity. With time, adaptation by larger fibers may thus "open the gate." Slower-transmitting small-fiber input inhibits cells in the substantia gelatinosa and opens the gate. An open gate increases the stimulation of trigger cells, increases transmission of impulses, and enhances pain perception. In addition to gate control through large- and small-fiber stimulation, the central nervous system through efferent pathways may close, partially close, or open the gate. This theory does not explain chronic pain problems such as phantom limb pain.

2. Identify chemicals that modulate pain.
Study page 324; refer to Figure 12-3.

Tissue injury results in the release of prostaglandins and lymphokines that trigger release of neuromodulators. These neuromodulators include **substance P, calcitonin-gene-related peptide, norepinephrine**, and **5-hydroxytryptamine**.

Endorphins are neuropeptides that inhibit transmission of pain impulses in the spinal cord and brain. All endorphins attach to opiate receptors on the plasma membrane of the afferent neuron. The combination of the opiate receptor and endorphin inhibits the release of excitatory neurotransmitters, thereby blocking the transmission of the painful stimulus. Stress, excessive physical exertion, acupuncture, and intercourse are factors that increase the level of circulating endorphins, serotonin, norepinephrine, and other neurotransmitters, thus raising the pain threshold.

3. Differentiate between acute and chronic pain.
Study pages 324-326; refer to Figure 12-4 and Table 12-1.

Acute pain may be somatic, visceral, or referred. **Somatic pain** comes from the skin or close to the surface of the body and is well localized. **Visceral pain** occurs in internal organs, the abdomen, or skeleton. It is poorly localized. It is associated with nausea and vomiting, hypotension, restlessness, and possible shock. Visceral pain often radiates or is referred. **Referred pain** is present in an area removed or distant from its point of origin. The area of referred pain is supplied by the same spinal segment as the actual site of injury. Impulses from many cutaneous and visceral neurons converge on the same ascending neuron, and the brain cannot distinguish between the origin of the two.

Chronic pain is prolonged; it may last longer than six months and may either persist or be intermittent. Causes of chronic pain include decreased levels of endorphins or a predominance of C neuron stimulation. Physiologic responses to chronic pain depend on the persistent or intermittent nature of the pain. **Intermittent pain** produces physiologic response similar to acute pain, whereas **persistent pain** permits physiologic adaptation. Individuals with chronic pain often are depressed, have difficulty sleeping and eating, and may become preoccupied with their pain.

4. Describe the alterations occurring in fever, hyperthermia, and hypothermia.
Study pages 327-330; refer to Figure 12-5 and Table 12-5.

Fever is not the failure of the normal thermoregulatory mechanism. Instead, it is considered "a resetting of the hypothalamic thermostat" to a higher level. The normal thermoregulatory mechanisms are raised so that the thermoregulatory center adjusts heat production, conservation, and loss to maintain the core temperature at a new, higher set-point temperature.

The pathophysiology of fever begins with exogenous pyrogens or endotoxins stimulating the release of interleukin-1 (IL-1), tumor necrosis factor, and interleukin-6 which raise the set-point. As the set-point is raised, the hypothalamus signals an increase in heat production and conservation to raise body temperature to the new level.

As fever breaks, the set-point is returned to normal. The hypothalamus signals a decrease in heat production and an increase in heat reduction.

Fever can be beneficial. Elevated body temperature kills many microorganisms and has adverse effects on the growth and replication of others. Increased temperature causes lysosomal breakdown with autodestruction of cells; this prevents viral replication in infected cells. Heat increases lymphocytic transformation and motility of polymorphonuclear neutrophils, which facilitate the immune response.

Hyperthermia can produce nerve damage, coagulation of cell proteins, and death. At 41° C (106° F), nerve damage produces convulsions in the adult. At 43° C (109° F), death follows. In hyperthermia, there is no resetting of the hypothalamic set-point. Forms of accidental hyperthermia are heat cramps, heat exhaustion, and heatstroke.

Heat cramps are severe, spasmodic cramps in the abdomen and extremities subsequent to prolonged sweating and associated sodium loss. Heat cramps usually appear in individuals who are unaccustomed to heat or who are performing strenuous work in very warm climates. Fever, rapid pulse, and increased blood pressure often accompany the cramps.

Heat exhaustion or collapse results from prolonged high body core or environmental temperatures. These high temperatures cause profound vasodilation and profuse sweating. Over a prolonged period of elevated temperatures, the hypothalamic responses produce dehydration, decreased plasma volumes, hypotension, decreased cardiac output, and tachycardia.

Heatstroke is a potentially lethal consequence of a breakdown in control of an overstressed thermoregulatory center. In cases of very high core temperatures, the regulatory center may cease to function appropriately.

High core temperatures and vascular collapse produce cerebral edema, degeneration of the central nervous system, and renal tubular necrosis. Death results unless immediate, effective treatment is initiated.

Malignant hyperthermia is a potentially lethal complication of an inherited muscle disorder. Malignant hyperthermia causes intracellular calcium levels to rise, producing sustained, uncoordinated muscle contractions. As a result of these contractions, acidosis develops. Cardiac dysrhythmias, hypotension, decreased cardiac output, or cardiac arrest may follow.

Hypothermia slows chemical reactions, increases blood viscosity, slows blood flow, facilitates blood coagulation, and stimulates profound vasoconstriction. Accidental hypothermia is generally the result of sudden immersion in cold water or prolonged exposure to cold environments. The young and the elderly are at risk because of their less effective thermoregulatory mechanisms. Individuals with conditions that diminish their ability to generate heat, such as hypothyroidism, hypopituitarism, malnutrition, Parkinson disease, and rheumatoid arthritis, are also at risk.

The hypothalamic center stimulates shivering in an effort to increase heat production. Thinking becomes sluggish and coordination is decreased. The individual becomes stuporous, heart rate and respiratory rates decline, and cardiac output is diminished. In severe hypothermia, pulse and respirations may be undetectable. Acidosis becomes moderate to severe. Ventricular fibrillation and asystole are common.

Depending on the severity of the hypothermia, rewarming of the peripheral tissues may be the only treatment required. Core rewarming is performed when core temperatures have dropped below 30° C (86° F).

5. Describe sleep disorders; cite examples.
Study pages 330-331.

Sleep disorders are classified by signs and symptoms rather than by their etiology. Sleep disorders can be classified as (1) disorders of initiating sleep, (2) disorders of excessive somnolence, (3) disorders of the sleep-wake schedule, and (4) dysfunctions of sleep, sleep stages, or partial arousals.

Disorders of initiating sleep are classified as **insomnia**, the inability to fall or stay asleep. Insomnia may be transient and related to travel across time zones or due to acute stress. Long-term insomnia is associated with drug or alcohol abuse, chronic pain disorders, or chronic depression.

Two disorders of excessive **somnolence** or excessive daytime sleepiness are **pickwickian syndrome** and **hypersomnia sleep apnea** (HSA) syndrome. Both are associated with periodic breathing and episodes of apnea.

In pickwickian syndrome, the apneic periods are generally due to obesity, decreased chemosensitivity to carbon dioxide and oxygen tensions, or upper airway obstruction occurring while sleeping. HSA syndrome is primarily a result of upper airway obstruction occurring during sleep. The sleep apnea reduces oxygen saturation and eventually produces polycythemia, pulmonary hypertension, right-sided congestive heart failure, liver congestion, cyanosis, and peripheral edema.

Common **disorders of the sleep-wake schedule** include rapid time-zone change or "jet-lag syndrome," an altered sleep schedule with an advance or a delay of three hours or more in sleep time, or a change in total sleep time from day to day. Vigilance of psychomotor performance and arousal are markedly depressed after alterations in the sleep-wake schedule.

Dysfunctions of sleep, **sleep stages**, or **partial arousals** are common in children. They are somnambulism, night terrors, and enuresis. **Somnambulism**, or sleepwalking, appears to resolve itself within several years after the onset of the sleepwalking episodes. During the sleepwalking episode, the child functions at a very low level of arousal and has no memory of the event upon awakening.

Night terrors are characterized by "sudden apparent arousals in which the child expresses intense fear or emotion." However, the child is not awake and is very difficult to arouse. Once awakened, the child has no memory of the night terror event. Neither somnambulism nor night terrors are associated with dreams.

Enuresis, or bedwetting, is disturbing because of social pressure. It is not associated with dreaming. Children eventually do "outgrow" the enuretic episodes.

6. Identify common diseases, their etiology, and manifestations that are associated with the special senses.

Study pages 331-340; refer to Figures 12-9 and 12-10 and Tables 12-6 and 12-7.

Vision

Blepharitis is an inflammation of the eyelids caused by staphylococcal infections or seborrheic dermatitis.

Conjunctivitis is an inflammation of the conjunctiva, or the mucous membrane covering the front part of the eyeball. It may be caused by bacteria, viruses, allergies, or chemical irritations.

Keratitis is an infection of the cornea usually caused by bacteria or viruses. Bacterial infections often cause corneal ulceration and require extensive antibiotic treatment. Type I herpes virus usually infects the cornea and conjunctiva.

Strabismus is the deviation of one eye from the other when the person is looking directly at an object. It is due to a weak or hypertonic muscle in one of the eyes. The deviation may be upward, downward, inward, or outward.

Amblyopia is a vision reduction or dimness for unknown reasons. Amblyopia is associated with diabetes mellitus, renal failure, malaria, and toxic substances such as alcohol and tobacco.

A *scotoma* is a circumscribed defect of the central field of vision. It is most often a sequel to an inflammatory lesion of the optic nerve and is frequently associated with multiple sclerosis.

A *cataract* is a cloudy or opaque ocular lens. The most common form of cataract is degenerative.

Papilledema is edema and inflammation of the optic nerve at its point of entrance into the eyeball. Generally, papilledema is caused by obstruction to the venous return from the retina.

Dark adaptation affects visual acuity. Changes in rhodopsin, a substance found in the rods and responsible for low-light vision, are likely responsible for reduced dark adaptation in older adults. Vitamin A deficiencies can cause the same disorder in individuals of any age.

Glaucoma is characterized by intraocular pressures above the normal range of 12 to 20 mm Hg maintained by the aqueous fluid in homeostasis. Intraocular fluid accumulation blocks the flow of nutrients to optic nerve fibers, leading to their death.

Loss of accommodation in the elderly is termed *presbyopia,* a condition in which the ocular lens becomes larger, firmer, and less elastic. The major symptom is reduced near vision, causing reading material to be held at arm's length.

In *myopia,* or nearsightedness, light rays are focused in front of the retina when the person is looking at a distant object. In *hyperopia,* or farsightedness, light rays are focused behind the retina when the person is looking at a near object. *Astigmatism* is caused by an unequal curvature of the cornea; light rays are bent unevenly and do not come to a single focus on the retina.

Hearing

A *conductive hearing loss* occurs when a change in the outer and/or middle ear impairs sound conduction from the outer to the inner ear. Conditions that commonly cause a conductive hearing loss include impacted cerumen, foreign bodies lodged in the ear canal, neoplasms of the external auditory canal and/or middle ear, eustachian tube dysfunction, otitis media, cholesteatoma, and otosclerosis. Symptoms of conductive hearing loss include diminished hearing and soft speaking voice. The voice is soft because the individual may hear his or her voice conducted by bone ossicles.

A *sensorineural hearing loss* is due to impairment of the organ of Corti and its hearing receptors or its central connections. Conditions that commonly cause sensorineural hearing loss include congenital and hereditary factors, noise exposure, aging, ototoxicity, and systemic diseases. Congenital and neonatal sensorineural hearing loss may be caused by maternal rubella, infant prematurity, traumatic delivery, or erythroblastosis fetalis.

Olfaction

Hyposmia is impaired sense of smell; *anosmia* is complete loss of smell. *Olfactory hallucinations* arise from hyperactivity in cortical neurons and involve the smelling of odors that actually are not present. *Parosmia* is abnormal or perverted sense of smell.

Taste

Hypogeusia is decreased taste sensation; *ageusia* is the absence of taste. These disorders are the result of cranial nerve injuries and can be specific to the area of tongue innervated. *Parageusia* is a perversion of taste in which substances possess an unpleasant flavor. Parageusia is common in individuals receiving chemotherapy for cancer. Parageusia often leads to anorexia.

Touch

Any impairment of reception, transmission, perception, or interpretation of touch alters tactile sensation. Trauma, tumor, infection, metabolic changes, vascular changes, and degenerative disease may cause tactile dysfunction.

Proprioception

Proprioception is the perception and awareness of the position of the body and its parts. It depends on impulses from the inner ear and from receptors in joints and ligaments. *Proprioceptive dysfunction* may be caused by alterations at any level of the nervous system, similar to that observed in tactile dysfunction.

Vestibular nystagmus is the constant, involuntary movement of the eyeball caused when the semicircular canal system is overstimulated. *Vertigo* is the sensation of spinning that occurs with inflammation of the semicircular canals in the ear. *Meniere disease* is a vestibular disorder that can cause proprioceptive dysfunction. The individual with acute Meniere disease may experience loss of proprioception and become unable to stand or walk.

Peripheral neuropathies are probably associated with renal disease and diabetes mellitus. The result is a diminished or absent sense of body position or position of body parts. Gait changes often occur.

Practice Examination

Match the nervous system component with the pain characteristic for which it is responsible.

1. ____ basic perception of pain
2. ____ initiation of pain stimulus
3. ____ discrimination and precision given to painful stimulus

a. nociceptive receptors
b. postcentral gyrus
c. brain stem
d. A fibers
e. cortex

4. Endorphins:

a. increase pain sensations.
b. decrease pain sensations.
c. may increase or decrease pain sensations.
d. have no effect on pain sensations.

5. Referred pain from upper abdominal diseases involves:

a. the sacral region.
b. L2 to L4.
c. T8, L1, and L2.
d. the gluteal regions, posterior thighs, and calves.

6. In the gate control theory of pain:

   a. a "closed gate" increases pain perception.
   b. stimulation of large A fibers "closes the gate."
   c. Both a and b are correct.
   d. Neither a nor b is correct.

7. Which is not a neuromodulator of pain?

   a. prostaglandins
   b. 5-hydroxtryptamine
   c. norepinephrine
   d. lymphokines
   e. heparin

8. Interleukin-1:

   a. raises the hypothalamic set-point.
   b. is an endogenous pyrogen.
   c. is stimulated by exogenous pyrogens.
   d. None of the above is correct.
   e. a, b, and c are correct.

9. Increased serum levels of epinephrine increase body temperature by:

   a. increasing shivering.
   b. increasing muscle tone.
   c. increasing heat production.
   d. decreasing basal metabolic rate.

10. In heatstroke:

    a. core temperature usually doesn't exceed 101° F.
    b. sodium loss follows sweating.
    c. core temperature increases as the regulatory center fails.
    d. Both b and c are correct.

11. Which is involved in fever?

    a. tumor necrosis factor
    b. endotoxins
    c. elevation of the set-point in the hypothalamus
    d. Both a and b are correct.
    e. a, b, and c are correct.

12. In hypothermia:

    a. the viscosity of blood is decreased.
    b. acidosis can develop.
    c. the hypothalamic center prevents shivering.
    d. All of the above are correct.

13. Although non-REM and REM sleep are defined by electrical recordings, they are characterized by physiological events. Which does not occur?

    a. During non-REM sleep, muscle tone decreases.
    b. Non-REM is initiated by withdrawal of neurotransmitters from the reticular formation.
    c. During non-REM, cerebral blood flow to the cortex is decreased.
    d. During non-REM, levels of corticosteroids are increased.

Match the abnormality with the sleep disorder.

14. ____ pickwickian syndrome
15. ____ HSA
16. ____ depressed vigilance
17. ____ insomnia

a. disorder of sleep initiation
b. disorder of somnolence
c. disorder of sleep-wake schedule

18. Sleep apnea:

    a. is lack of breathing during sleep.
    b. results from airway obstruction during sleep.
    c. is associated with "jet-lag syndrome."
    d. All of the above are correct.
    e. Both a and b are correct.

19. Individuals affected by sleep apnea may experience:

    a. polycythemia.
    b. cyanosis.
    c. pulmonary hypertension.
    d. All of the above are correct.

Match the term with its defining characteristic.

20. ____ blepharitis
21. ____ strabismus
22. ____ anosmia
23. ____ hypogeusia
24. ____ vertigo
25. ____ glaucoma

a. inflammation of mucous membrane covering the eyeball
b. infection of the cornea
c. weak muscle in one of the eyes
d. reduction or dimness of vision
e. inflammation of the eyelids
f. high intraocular pressures
g. elevated intraocular pressure
h. inflammation of the semicircular canals
i. decreased taste sensation
j. complete loss of smell

Case Study

Mrs. D. is a 45-year-old female who sought care for chronic insomnia of 15 months' duration. She stated that she awakes 15 to 20 times a night and rarely sleeps more than four hours. Various hypnotics had been unsuccessful.

Her history revealed that about 18 months earlier some important stressful life changes occurred. Her only child, a daughter, left for an out-of-state university. A lifelong friend, who was a confidante, moved to another community. Her husband, a successful dentist, had become more involved in various men's organizations than in the past. A sedating antidepressant was prescribed and a second appointment was made for ten days later.

On the second appointment, which lasted one hour, she noted her sleep patterns had improved. She was able to articulate that she felt unneeded, incompetent, and old.

As a caregiver, how do you assess Mrs. D.'s case?

CHAPTER

13

Concepts of Neurologic Dysfunction

Foundational Objectives

a. Describe the RAS as a modulator of consciousness. Review page 291; refer to Figure 11-5.

Memory Check!

- The reticular activating system (RAS) maintains wakefulness. It ascends from the lower brain stem and projects throughout the cerebral cortex. The ability to respond to stimuli or arousal depends on an intact RAS in the brain stem and the ability to respond to the environment. Cognition relies on an intact cerebral cortex. Therefore, consciousness or responsiveness requires functioning along the reticular formation in the brain stem to the cerebral cortex.

b. Identify the structural and functional components of the brain. Review pages 291-296; refer to Figures 11-6 through 11-8.

Memory Check!

- The central nervous system (CNS) consists of the brain and spinal cord encased within the meninges and bathed in cerebrospinal fluid (CSF). The brain is divided into several areas, including the cerebrum, midbrain, cerebellum, pons, and medulla oblongata. The midbrain, the medulla, and the pons comprise the brain stem.
- The outer covering of the cerebrum is the cortex. The entire cerebrum is divided into two halves or hemispheres connected by a neural bridge, the corpus callosum, that coordinates activities between hemispheres. The cortex is concerned with thinking and sensory perception. Emotional responses and control of body temperature, water and food intake, and sex drive have their origin in the midbrain area. The cerebellum primarily integrates muscular movements to produce coordination in walking, talking, and other complex muscular activities. The medulla oblongata controls vital functions such as respiration, heart rate, and blood pressure, although these are modified by higher brain centers.
- Within the cerebral hemispheres are subdivisions, or lobes. The frontal lobe is located in the anterior portion of each hemisphere. The temporal lobe is located in the lower middle region of each hemisphere. The parietal lobe is the upper, rear portion. The occipital lobe is the lower, rear portion of each hemisphere.
- The basal ganglia are a collection of cell bodies in several areas in the gray matter of the brain including the caudate nucleus, globus pallidus, putamen, and substantia nigra. The function of the basal ganglia is thought to involve the planning and programming of movement.

c. Identify the parts of the CNS that control voluntary muscle movement. Review pages 295-296; refer to Figure 11-9.

Memory Check!

- The cerebral cortex plays a major role in controlling precise, voluntary muscular movements. Motor output to skeletal muscles travels down the spinal cord in two types of descending tracts, the pyramidal tracts and the extrapyramidal tracts. The pyramidal tracts originate in the motor cortex and terminate in the brain stem. They cross to the opposite side at the medulla-spinal cord junction. The pyramidal tracts convey impulses causing precise, voluntary movements of skeletal muscles. The extrapyramidal tracts arise from the cortex and project to innervate the motor neurons; they don't cross to the opposite side. Extrapyramidal tracts convey nerve impulses that program fine repetitive motor movements.

Objectives

After review of this chapter, the learner will be able to:

1. **Define terms describing levels of consciousness.**
   Refer to Table 13-3.

Consciousness is alertness with orientation to person, place, and time. **Confusion** is an inability to think. First, there is **disorientation** to time, then to place, and eventually to person. The attention span is shortened. **Lethargy** may exhibit orientation to person, place, and time. However, slow vocalization and decreased motor skills are present. **Obtundation** is awakening in response to stimulation. Continuous stimulation is needed for arousal. **Stupor** is vocalization only in response to vigorous stimuli. Markedly decreased spontaneous movement is seen. **Coma** displays no vocalization and no arousal to any stimulus.

2. **Identify sites and causes for alterations in arousal.**
   Study page 347; refer to Tables 13-1 and 13-2.

Possible causes of an **altered level of arousal** may be separated into three major groups: structural, metabolic, and psychogenic. Structural causes are divided according to whether the original pathologic condition is above (supratentorial) or below (infratentorial) the tentorial plate.

Supratentorial processes produce a decreased level of consciousness because of compression or displacement of the diencephalon or brain stem. **Infratentorial processes** produce a reduction in arousal by diseases that destroy the brain stem.

Disorders outside the brain, such as neoplasms, bleeding from trauma, and pus, can produce arousal dysfunction. Bleeding, infarcts, emboli, and neoplasms within the brain also can contribute to altered levels of arousal.

A wide spectrum of disorders or agents may produce a **metabolically** induced alteration in arousal. Hypoxia, electrolyte disturbances, hypoglycemia, drugs, and toxins alter arousal.

Psychogenic unresponsiveness may develop in general psychiatric disorders. Despite apparent unconsciousness, the person is actually physiologically awake.

3. **Summarize the changes in levels of consciousness, pupillary response, muscle tone, and respiratory activity as the diencephalon through the medulla is affected.**
   Study pages 347-351; refer to Figures 13-1 through 13-6 and Tables 13-3 through 13-5.

   (See box on page 91 of *Workbook*.)

4. **Distinguish between cerebral death and brain death.**
   Study page 351.

Cerebral death, or irreversible coma, is death of the cerebral hemispheres, exclusive of the brain stem and cerebellum. The individual is permanently unable to respond in any significant way to

Rostral-Caudal Progression of Nonresponsiveness

Area Involved	Level of Consciousness	Pupils	Muscle Tone	Breathing Pattern
Diencephalon (thalamus/ hypothalamus)	Decreased concentration, agitation, dullness, lethargy, obtundation	Respond to light briskly; Full-range eye movements only on "doll's eyes"—none in direction of rotation or after injection of hot or cold water in ear canal (caloric posturing)	Some purposeful movement in response to pain, combative movement Decorticate—flexion in upper extremities and extension in lower extremities	Yawning and sighing to Cheyne-Stokes
Midbrain	Stupor to coma	Midposition fixed (MPF)	Decerebrate—arms rigid, palms turned away from body	Neurogenic hyperventilation
Pons	Coma	MPF	Decerebrate	Apneustic—prolonged inspiration and expiration
Medulla	Coma	MPF	Flaccid	Atactic—uncoordinated and irregular

the environment. The brain may continue to maintain internal homeostasis.

Brain death occurs when irreversible brain damage is so extensive that the brain can no longer maintain the body's internal respiratory and cerebral vascular functions. There is destruction of the brain stem and cerebellum.

5. **Define seizure and cite conditions associated with seizure disorders.**
   Study pages 355-357; refer to Tables 13-6 through 13-8.

A **seizure** is a sudden, explosive disorderly discharge of cerebral neurons and is characterized by a sudden, transient alteration in brain function, usually involving motor, sensory, autonomic, or psychic clinical manifestations and an alteration in level of arousal. The alteration in level of arousal is temporary. Among the causes of seizure activity are:

metabolic defects	motor syndromes
congenital malformation	infection
genetic predisposition	brain tumor
perinatal injury	vascular disease
postnatal trauma	fever

An **epileptogenic focus** may be a group of neurons that have lost their afferent stimulation. The plasma membranes of these neuronal cells appear to be hypersensitive. This makes them more easily activated by hyperthermia, hypoxia, hypoglycemia, hyponatremia, repeated sensory stimulation, and certain sleep phases. The neural excitation spreads to the subcortical, thalamic, and brain stem areas to initiate the tonic phase of muscle contraction, which is followed by increased muscle tone and loss of consciousness.

The clonic phase of alternating contraction and relaxation of muscles begins as inhibitory neurons in the cortex, anterior thalamus, and basal ganglia begin to inhibit the cortical excitation. This inhibition interrupts seizure discharge and produces an intermittent pattern of muscle contractions; the contractions gradually decrease and finally cease.

Common Epileptic Seizure Types

Disorder	Areas Involved	Change in Consciousness	Impaired Capacities/ Symptoms
Partial			
Jacksonian	Simple unilateral	No change in consciousness generally	Disturbance in motor capacity
Psychomotor	Complex unilateral	Loss of consciousness, automatism	Dyscognitive states, loss of awareness
Generalized			
Generalized tonic-clonic movement (grand mal)	Bilateral	Loss of consciousness with postictal sleeping	Major tonic-clonic movement; muscular contraction followed by relaxation or a longer phase of contraction
Absence (petit mal)	Bilateral	Transient losses of consciousness	Blank spells, akinetic seizures, myoclonic jerks

6. **Differentiate between partial and generalized seizures.**
   Refer to Tables 13-7 and 13-8.

7. **Define descriptive terms of cognitive deficits.**
   Refer to Table 13-9.

Selective attention deficit refers to the inability to select appropriately from available, competing environmental stimuli for conscious processing.

Anterograde memory is an inability to form new memories.

A **remote memory deficit** manifests as an inability to recognize sensory input as sounds, sight, or touch or to retrieve past memories.

A **concept-formation deficit** is the inability to analyze the relationships between objects and their properties; individuals cannot generalize or categorize.

A **vigilance deficit** is the inability to concentrate over time or to maintain sustained attention.

A **reasoning deficit** is the inability to understand relationships or to abstract.

Executive function deficit prevents programming, verification, and correction.

Generally, the primary pathophysiological mechanism that operates in cognitive system disorders is due directly to ischemia and hypoxia or indirectly to compression, toxins, and chemicals.

8. **Identify terms used to describe specific cognition disorders.**
   Study pages 357-362; refer to Figure 13-7 and Tables 13-10 through 13-13.

Agnosia is a defect of recognition of the form and nature of objects. Although it most commonly is associated with cerebrovascular accidents, it may arise from any pathologic process that injures specific areas of the brain.

Dysphasia is impairment of comprehension or production of language. Comprehension or use of symbols, in either written or verbal language, is disturbed or lost. **Aphasia** is loss of the comprehension or production of language. Dysphasias usually are associated with cerebrovascular accidents involving the middle cerebral artery or one of its many branches. Dysphasia results from dysfunction in the left cerebral hemisphere and usually involves the frontotemporal region. Dysphasia may be nonfluent; the individual cannot find words for expression and exhibits difficulty in writing. Dysphasia may also be fluent; verbal language is produced, but it is meaningless with inappropriate words.

Acute confusional states result from cerebral dysfunction secondary to drug intoxication or nervous system disease. These states may begin either suddenly or gradually depending on the amount of toxin exposure. The predominant feature of an acute confusional state is impaired or lost vigilance. The individual is unable to concentrate on incoming sensory information or on any one particular mental or motor task.

The **dementias** are characterized by the loss of more than one cognitive or intellectual function. There may be a decrease in orientation, general knowledge and information, vigilance, recent memory, remote memory, concept formation, abstraction, reasoning, and language. Causes of dementia include degeneration, cerebrovascular accidents, compression, toxins, metabolic disorder, biochemical imbalance, demyelinization, and infections. Symptoms of dementia may be grouped according to type of memory deficit: amnestic dementia (loss of recent memory), cognitive dementia (loss of remote memory), or intentional dementia (loss of vigilance and executive function).

9. Characterize the stages of increased intracranial pressure; describe herniation syndrome.
Study pages 363-364; refer to Figures 13-8 and 13-9.

Increased intracranial pressure may result from an increase in intracranial content which occurs with tumor growth, edema, excess cerebrospinal fluid, or hemorrhage. A rise in intracranial pressure from one component requires an equal reduction in volume of other components. The most readily displaced content of the cranial vault is cerebrospinal fluid (CSF).

In Stage 1 of intracranial hypertension, vasoconstriction and external compression of the venous system occur in an attempt to decrease further the intracranial pressure following CSF displacement from the cranial vault.

With continued expansion of the intracranial content, the resulting increase in intracranial pressure may exceed the brain's compensatory capacity to adjust to the increasing pressure. In this state, Stage 2, the pressure begins to compromise neuronal oxygenation. Systemic arterial vasoconstriction occurs to elevate the systemic blood pressure sufficiently to overcome the increased intracranial pressure. Clinical manifestations at this stage are subtle and transient and include confusion, drowsiness, and slight pupillary and breathing changes.

Intracranial pressure begins to approach arterial pressure and the brain tissues begin to experience hypoxia and hypercapnia. Hyperventilation occurs, pupils become sluggish and dilated, pulse pressure widens, and bradycardia develops. Accumulating CO_2 causes local vasodilation and blood volume increases. The brain volume increases, and intracranial pressure continues to rise. This is Stage 3 of intracranial hypertension. Cerebral perfusion pressure falls and cerebral perfusion slows dramatically; the brain tissues experience severe hypoxia and acidosis.

In the last stage of intracranial hypertension, Stage 4, brain tissue shifts or **herniates** from the compartment of greater pressure to the compartment of lesser pressure. The herniated brain tissues increase the volume within the lower pressure compartment, exerting pressure on the brain tissue that normally occupies that compartment. Now, both the herniated and lower tissue's blood supply is impaired. Mean systolic arterial pressure soon equals intracranial pressure, and cerebral blood flow ceases.

Two common types of herniation syndromes exist, supratentorial and infratentorial, based on whether they are located above or below the tentorium.

Supratentorial herniation occurs when brain tissue shifts through the tentorial notch into the posterior fossa and presses on the third cranial nerve. **Infratentorial herniation** occurs as cerebellar tonsils shift inferiorly through the foramen magnum because of increased pressure within the posterior fossa. The clinical manifestations of supratentorial and infratentorial herniation syndromes vary and may be manifested as decreasing levels of consciousness and respiratory abnormalities.

10. Describe the pathogenesis of cerebral edema.
Study pages 364-366; refer to Figure 13-10.

Cerebral edema is an increase of extracellular or intracellular fluid within the brain. It develops after brain insult from trauma, infection, hemorrhage, tumor, ischemia, infarct, or hypoxia. Cerebral edema will distort blood vessels, displace brain tissues, and eventually herniate brain tissue from one brain compartment to another. The four types of cerebral edema are (1) vasogenic edema, (2) cytotoxic (metabolic) edema, (3) ischemic edema, and (4) interstitial edema.

Vasogenic edema is clinically the most important type. It is caused by the increased permeability of the capillary endothelium of the brain after injury to the vascular structure. Plasma proteins leak into the extracellular spaces, drawing water to them, so the water content of the brain parenchyma increases. Vasogenic edema starts in the area of injury and spreads with preferential accumulation in the white matter of the ipsilateral side because the parallel myelinated fibers separate more easily.

In **cytotoxic (metabolic) edema,** toxic factors directly affect the neuronal, glial, and endothelial cells, causing failure of the active transport systems. The cells lose their potassium and gain larger amounts of sodium. Water follows by osmosis into the cells, causing the cells to swell. Cytotoxic edema principally occurs in the gray matter.

Ischemic edema follows cerebral infarction. The initial edema is confined to the intracellular compartment. Later in the process, brain cells begin to undergo necrosis and die. The released lysosomes increase the blood-brain barrier's permeability by lyzing it.

Interstitial edema is caused by movement of cerebrospinal fluid from the ventricles into the extracellular spaces of the brain tissues. The brain fluid volume is mostly increased around the ventricles; increased pressure is within the white matter.

11. Define terms that describe alterations in motor functions.

Study pages 366-376; refer to Tables 13-14, 13-15, and 13-17.

Movements are influenced by the cerebral cortex, the pyramidal system, the extrapyramidal system, and the motor units. Dysfunction in any of these areas may cause motor dysfunction.

Hypotonia is decreased muscle tone shown by passive movement of a muscle against resistance. It likely is due to decreased muscle spindle activity secondary to decreased excitability of neurons. Hypotonia is caused by cerebellar damage or in rare cases by pyramidal tract damage.

Hypertonia is increased muscle tone shown by passive movement of a muscle with resistance. **Spasticity**, a type of hypertonia, results from hyperexcitability of the stretch reflexes and is associated with damage to the motor, premotor, and supplementary motor areas and lateral corticospinal tracts. **Rigidity**, another hypertonia, is produced by tonic reflex activity. The involved muscles are firm and tense; the increase in muscle movement is even and uniform throughout the range of passive movement.

Hyperkinesia is excessive movement, whereas **dyskinesias** are abnormal, involuntary movements.

Hypokinesia, or decreased movement, is a loss of voluntary movement despite consciousness and normal peripheral nerve and muscle function. Types of hypokinesia include paresis/paralysis, akinesia, bradykinesia, and loss of associated movement.

Hemiparesis/hemiplegia is paresis/paralysis of the upper and lower extremity on one side. **Diplegia** is the paralysis of both upper or both lower extremities due to cerebral hemisphere injuries. **Paraparesis/paraplegia** refers to weakness/paralysis of the lower extremities. **Quadriparesis/quadriplegia** refers to paresis/paralysis of all four extremities. Both paraparesis/paraplegia and quadriparesis/quadriplegia may be caused by dysfunction of the spinal cord.

When the pyramidal system is destroyed below the level of the pons, **spinal shock** occurs. It is the complete cessation of spinal cord functions below the lesion. It is characterized by complete flaccid paralysis, absence of reflexes, and marked disturbances in bowel and bladder function.

Lower motor syndrome originating in the anterior horn cells or the motor nuclei of the cranial nerves are called **amyotrophies**. Paralytic poliomyelitis is the prototype of these disorders. In the amyotrophies, muscle strength, muscle tone, and muscle bulk are affected in the muscles innervated by the involved motor neurons.

Several brain stem syndromes involve damage to one or more of the cranial nerve nuclei. These are called **nuclear palsies** and may be caused by vascular occlusion, tumor, aneurysm, tuberculosis, or hemorrhage.

Akinesia is a decrease in associated and voluntary movements. It is related to dysfunction of the extrapyramidal system. Pathogenesis is related to either a deficiency of dopamine or a defect of the postsynaptic dopamine receptors. **Bradykinesia** is slowness of voluntary movements. In **hypokinesia**, the normal, habitually associated movements that provide skill, grace, and balance to voluntary movements are lost. An expressionless face, a statuesque posture, absence of speech inflection, and absence of spontaneous gestures are exhibited as well.

Dystonia is the maintenance of abnormal posture through muscular contractions. **Decorticate posture** is characterized by upper extremities that are flexed at the elbows and held close to the body and lower extremities that are externally rotated and extended. Decorticate posture is thought to occur when the brain stem is not inhibited by the motor function of the cerebral cortex. **Decerebrate posture** refers to increased tone in extensor muscles and trunk muscles with active tonic neck reflexes. The decerebrate posture is caused by severe injury to the brain and brain stem. **Basal ganglion posture** refers to a stooped, hyperflexed posture with a narrow-based, short-stepped gait. **Senile posture** is characterized by an increasingly flexed posture similar to a basal ganglion posture. The posture is associated with frontal lobe dysfunction.

A **spastic gait** is associated with unilateral, pyramidal injury and is manifested by a shuffling gait with the leg extended and held stiff. This gait causes a scraping over the walking surface. A **scissors gait** is associated with bilateral pyramidal injury and spasticity. The legs are abducted, so the legs touch each other. A **cerebellar gait** manifests as a wide-based gait with the feet apart and often turned outward and inward for greater stability. Cerebellar dysfunction accounts for this particular gait. A **basal ganglion gait** is a broad-based gait. Small steps are taken, and there is a decreased arm swing during walking. The individual's head and body are flexed and the arms are semiflexed and abducted, whereas the legs are flexed and rigid in more advanced states. Basal ganglion and frontal lobe dysfunction, respectively, account for these two gaits.

Hypermimesia, a disorder of expression, is most commonly manifested as pathological laughter or crying. Pathological laughter is associated with right hemisphere injury, whereas pathological crying is associated with left hemisphere injury. **Hypomimesia** is manifested as aprosodias, or the loss of emotional language. Aprosodias involve an inability to understand emotion in speech and facial expression. Aprosodias are associated with right hemisphere damage.

Dyspraxia/apraxia is the inability to perform purposeful or skilled motor acts in the absence of paralysis, sensory loss, abnormal posture and tone, abnormal involuntary movement, incoordination, or inattentiveness. Dyspraxias arise when the connecting pathways between the left and right cortical areas are interrupted; conceptualization and execution of a complex motor act is impaired.

12. Differentiate between pyramidal and extrapyramidal motor syndromes and between upper motor neuron and lower motor neuron or motor unit syndromes.
Study pages 369-376; refer to Figures 13-11 through 13-13 and Tables 13-16 and 13-18.

Disturbances in motor function are classified along upper and lower motor neuron structures. Amyotrophic lateral sclerosis can involve both upper and lower neuron structures. Upper motor neuron disorders include cerebral palsies, cerebrovascular accidents, multiple sclerosis, and Parkinson disease. Lower motor neuron disorders include poliomyelitis, muscular dystrophies, myasthenia gravis, and polymyositis.

Pyramidal and Extrapyramidal Motor Syndromes

	Pyramidal Motor Syndrome	Extrapyramidal Motor Syndrome
Unilateral movement	Paralysis	Little or no paralysis
Tendon reflexes	Increased	Normal or slightly increased
Involuntary movements	Absent	Presence of tremor, chorea, or dystonia
Muscle tone	General spasticity in muscles; hypertonia present in flexors of arms and extensors of legs	Possible rigidity or intermittent rigidity

Motor Neuron Syndromes

	Upper Motor Neuron Syndrome	Lower Motor Neuron and Motor Unit Syndromes
Affected muscles	Muscle groups; when movement is possible, relationship among agonists, antagonists, synergists, and fixators is preserved	Individual muscles
Muscle tone	Hypertonia, spasticity	Hypotonia, flaccidity
Tendon reflexes	Hyperreflexia	Hyporeflexia
Atrophy	Slight, due to disuse	Pronounced
Fasciculations	Absent	May be present

Practice Examination

Match the level of consciousness with its characteristic.

1. ____ confusion
2. ____ coma

a. orientation to person, time, and place
b. slow vocalization, decreased oculomotor activity
c. inability to think clearly
d. vocalization in response to pain stimuli
e. no arousal

3. Supratentorial processes reduce arousal by:

a. developing the reticular activating system.
b. encephalitis.
c. destroying the brain stem.
d. Both a and c are correct.
e. None of the above is correct.

4. An individual shows flexion in upper extremities and extension in lower extremities. This is:

a. decorticate posturing.
b. decerebrate posturing.
c. excitation posturing.
d. caloric posturing.

5. Cerebral death:

a. is death of the cerebellum.
b. maintains normal internal homeostasis.
c. no longer maintains respiratory and cardiovascular functions.
d. is death of the brain stem.

6. Precipitating causes of seizure include all of the following except:

   a. meningitis.
   b. stroke.
   c. hyperglycemia.
   d. hyperthermia.
   e. All of the above are correct.

7. Which epileptic seizure is characterized by temporal lobe spikes in the EEG?

   a. autonomic
   b. status epilepticus
   c. absence
   d. Jacksonian
   e. psychomotor

8. Postictal sleeping can be seen in ______ seizures.

   a. partial
   b. unilateral
   c. absence
   d. grand mal
   e. psychomotor

Match the term with its definition.

9. ____ reasoning deficit
10. ____ agnosia
11. ____ vigilance deficit

a. inability to understand relationships
b. inability to verify and correct input
c. inability to concentrate
d. inability to recognize sound
e. inability to abstract

12. Hypotonia is:

    a. spasticity.
    b. caused by cerebellar damage.
    c. rigidity.
    d. abnormal, involuntary movement.
    e. All of the above are correct.

13. Dystonia is:

    a. abnormal posture maintained by muscular contractions.
    b. flexed posture.
    c. stooped, hyperflexed posture.
    d. a spastic gait.

14. An individual with increased intracranial pressure from a head injury shows dilated and sluggish pupils, widened pulse pressure, and bradycardia. Which stage of ICP exists?

    a. Stage 1
    b. Stage 2
    c. Stage 3
    d. Stage 4

15. Infratentorial herniation occurs in:

    a. shifting of the mesencephalon.
    b. shifting of the diencephalon.
    c. shifting of the cerebellum.
    d. Both a and b are correct.
    e. None of the above is correct.

16. In cerebral vasogenic edema:

    a. active transport fails.
    b. there is autodigestion.
    c. plasma proteins leak into extracellular spaces.
    d. cerebrospinal fluid leaves the ventricles.

17. Which statement is not true regarding increasing intracranial pressures?

    a. Accumulating CO_2 causes vasoconstriction.
    b. The brain volume increases.
    c. The blood volume in the vessels increases.
    d. Brain tissue shifts from the compartment of greater pressure to one of lesser pressure.
    e. Both b and c are correct.

18. Intellectual function is impaired in the dementing process. Which intellectual function is not impaired?

    a. recent memory
    b. remote memory
    c. abstraction
    d. language deficits
    e. All of the above functions are impaired.

Match the term with its definition or characteristic.

19. ____ hypertonia
20. ____ rigidity
21. ____ hemiparesis
22. ____ akinesia
23. ____ senile posture
24. ____ dyspraxia
25. ____ lower motor neuron syndrome

a. paralysis of both upper and lower extremities

b. difficult initiation of spontaneous and voluntary movements

c. absence of spontaneous gestures

d. abnormal posture maintained through muscular contractions

e. frontal lobe dysfunction

f. impaired conceptualization and execution of complex acts

g. individual muscles affected

h. involuntary writing movements

i. organically caused impairment of intellectual functions

j. increased muscle tone

k. tonic reflex activity

l. upper and lower extremity paralysis on same side

Case Study

A 12-year-old male complained of strange odors prior to loss of consciousness and a major tonic-clonic seizure. During the seizure, his parents rushed him to the emergency room of a local hospital. On arrival at the hospital, he appeared to be asleep.

Studies at the hospital showed routine laboratory work within normal limits (WNL), lumbar puncture (CSF) was WNL, no evidence of skull fracture on x-ray study was revealed, and an electroencephalograph (EEG) showed no abnormalities.

How would you interpret the episode and findings?

CHAPTER 14

Alterations of Neurologic Function

Foundational Objectives

a. Identify the protective structures of the central nervous system. Review pages 297-300; refer to Figures 11-15 through 11-17 and Table 11-4.

Memory Check!

- The cranium is composed of eight bones that fuse early in childhood. The cranial vault encloses and protects the brain and its associated structures. The floor of the cranial vault is irregular and contains many foramina or openings for cranial nerves, blood vessels, and the spinal cord to exit. The foramen magnum is large enough for the spinal cord to exit. Surrounding the brain and spinal cord are three protective membranes called the meninges: the dura mater, the arachnoid membrane, and the pia mater.
- The dura mater is composed of two layers and has venous sinuses between the layers. The outermost dural layer forms the periosteum of the skull. The inner dural meningeal layer forms the rigid plates that support and separate various brain structures.
- One of these membranous plates, the falx cerebri, transverses between the two cerebral hemispheres and anchors the base of the brain to the ethmoid bone. The tentorium cerebelli is a membrane that surrounds the brain stem and separates the cerebellum from the cerebral structures.
- Below the dura mater lies the arachnoid membrane, which is characterized by its spongy, weblike structure. The space between the dura and arachnoid membrane is the subdural space. Many small bridging veins traverse the subdural space. The subarachnoid space between the arachnoid membrane and the pia mater contains cerebrospinal fluid. The delicate pia mater provides support for blood vessels serving brain tissue. The choroid plexuses, structures that produce cerebrospinal fluid, arise from the pial membrane. The spinal cord is anchored to the vertebrae by extension of the meninges. Between the dura mater and skull is a potential space, the epidural space.
- Cerebrospinal fluid (CSF) is a clear, colorless fluid similar to blood plasma and interstitial fluid. The CNS's soft tissues are cushioned from traumatic jolts and blows because of the CSF's buoyant properties. The choroid plexuses in the lateral, third, and fourth ventricles produce the major portion of CSF.

b. Describe the blood supply to the brain. Review pages 301-306; refer to Figures 11-18 through 11-21 and Table 11-5.

Memory Check!

- The brain receives approximately 20 percent of the cardiac output, or 800 to 1000 ml of blood flow per minute. Carbon dioxide is a potent vasodilator in the CNS and ensures an adequate cerebral blood supply. The brain derives its arterial supply from two systems: the internal carotid arteries and the vertebral arteries.

- The internal carotid arteries originate from the common carotid arteries, enter the cranium through the base of the skull, and pass through the cavernous sinus. After giving off some small branches, they divide into the anterior and middle cerebral arteries. The vertebral arteries originate at the subclavian arteries and pass through the transverse foramina of the cervical vertebrae and enter the cranium through the foramen magnum. They join to form the basilar artery. The basilar artery divides at the level of the midbrain to form paired posterior cerebral arteries. Superficial arteries supply small branches that project into the brain. The circle of Willis is a structure having the ability to provide collateral blood flow. It is formed by many communicating arteries that extend to various brain structures.

- The venous drainage of the brain stem and cerebellum parallels the arterial supply; the venous drainage of the cerebrum does not. The cerebral veins are classified as superficial and deep. The veins drain into venous plexuses and dural sinuses and eventually drain into the internal jugular veins at the base of the skull. The blood-brain barrier selectively inhibits certain substances in the blood from entering the interstitial spaces of the brain or CSF. It is believed that the supporting cells and tight junctions between endothelial cells are involved in the formation of the blood-brain barrier and are responsible for its impermeability.

c. State the functions of the parts and associated structures of the brain. Review pages 291-296; refer to Figures 11-5 through 11-9 and Table 11-3.

Memory Check!

Structural Functions of the Brain

Structure	Function
Brain stem	Performs sensory, motor, and reflex functions; controls cardiac, vasomotor, and respiratory centers; cranial nerve reflex
Cerebellum	Coordinates the activities of groups of muscles, maintains equilibrium, controls posture
Diencephalon	
Thalamus	Conscious recognition of crude pain, temperature, and touch; relays sensory impulses except smell to cerebrum; emotions; arousal mechanism; complex reflex movements
Hypothalamus	Links nervous system to endocrine system; coordinates ANS; controls body temperature, hunger, thirst, and sleep

(Continued)

Memory Check! (cont'd)

Structure	Function
Cerebrum	
Cerebral cortex lobes	
Frontal	Voluntary control of skeletal muscles, unconscious skeletal muscle movement, speaking and writing
Temporal	Interpretation of odor and sound
Parietal	General body sensations
Occipital	Interpretation of sight
All lobes	Memory, emotions, reasoning, and intelligence
Left hemisphere	Language, numerical skills, controls right side of body
Right hemisphere	Musical and artistic awareness, space and pattern perception, insight, controls left side of body

d. Cite some examples of neurotransmitters and neuroreceptors. Review pages 289-291 and 309-310; refer to Figure 11-27 and Tables 11-2 and 11-7.

Memory Check!

Responses of Selected Effector Organs to Automatic Nerve Impulses

Effector	Receptor Type	Adrenergic Response	Cholinergic Response
Eye			
Radial muscle, iris	∂	Contraction	—
Sphincter muscle, iris	β_1	—	Contraction
Heart			
SA node	β_1	Increases heart rate	Decreases heart rate
Ventricles	β_1	Increases contractility	—
Arterioles			
Pulmonary	∂, β_2	Dilation predominates	—
Skeletal muscle	∂, β_2	Dilation predominates	—
Cerebral	∂	Constriction	—
Lung			
Bronchial muscle	β_2	Relaxation	Contraction
Adrenal medulla	—	—	Secretion of epinephrine and norepinephrine

(Continued)

Memory Check! (cont'd)

- Sympathetic preganglionic fibers, parasympathetic preganglionic fibers, and postganglionic fibers release acetylcholine. These fibers are characterized by cholinergic transmission. Most postganglionic sympathetic fibers release norepinephrine (adrenaline) and are considered to function by adrenergic transmission.

- Two types of adrenergic receptors exist, ∂ and β. Cells of effector organs may have only one or both types of these adrenergic receptors. ∂_1 receptors are associated with excitation, while ∂_2 receptors are associated with inhibition. β_1 receptors stimulate cardiac muscle and cause release of renin from the kidney, while β_2 receptors facilitate all other effects attributed to β receptors.

Objectives

After studying this chapter, the learner will be able to:

1. **Differentiate between focal and diffuse brain injury.**
   Study pages 381-386; refer to Figures 14-1 through 14-3 and Tables 14-1 through 14-4.

Traumatic brain injuries are broadly categorized into blunt or closed trauma and open or penetrating trauma. In blunt trauma, the head strikes a hard surface or a rapidly moving object strikes the head. The dura remains intact and brain tissues are not exposed to the environment. Blunt trauma may result in both focal brain injuries and diffuse axonal injuries. When a break in the dura exposes the cranial contents to the environment, open trauma has occurred. Open trauma results in focal brain injuries.

Focal brain injury involves specific, grossly observable brain lesions seen in cortical contusions, epidural hemorrhage, subdural hematoma, and intracerebral hematoma. The force of impact typically produces **contusions**, or bruises, on the brain. The contusion, in turn, produces epidural hemorrhage, subdural hematomas, and intracerebral hematomas. Contusion and bleeding occur because of small tears in blood vessels resulting from these forces. The smaller the area of impact, the greater the severity of injury because the force is concentrated into a smaller area. The focal injury may be coup or contrecoup. **Coup** is the direct impact area. **Contrecoup** lies opposite the line of force; the lesions occur where the brain strikes hard tissue on the opposite side.

The clinical manifestations of a contusion may include immediate loss of consciousness, loss of reflexes, transient cessation of respiration, brief period of bradycardia, and fall in blood pressure. Vital signs may stabilize in a few seconds. Reflexes return next and the person begins to regain consciousness. Returning to full alertness takes variable periods of time from minutes to days. Large contusions and lacerations with hemorrhage may be surgically excised. Otherwise treatment is directed at controlling intracranial pressure and managing symptoms.

Extradural hematomas, also called epidural hematomas or epidural hemorrhages, most often have an artery as the source of bleeding. Extradural hemorrhages may result in herniation through the foramen magnum.

Tearing of the bridging veins is the major cause of rapidly developing and subacutely developing **subdural hematomas**. However, torn cortical veins or venous sinuses and contused tissue may be the source of the bleeding. The subdural space gradually fills with blood, and herniation can result.

In **intracerebral hematomas**, small blood vessels are traumatized by shearing forces. The intracerebral hematoma expands and increases intracranial pressure with compression of brain tissues.

Individuals with classic temporal extradural hematomas lose consciousness at the time of injury; some lucid periods follow. As the hematoma mass accumulates, a headache of increasing severity, vomiting, drowsiness, confusion, seizure, and hemiparesis may develop. Level of consciousness declines rapidly as the temporal lobe herniation begins. Clinical manifestations of temporal lobe herniation also include ipsilateral pupillary dilation and contralateral hemiparesis. Surgical therapy evacuates the hematoma through burr holes followed by ligation of the bleeding vessel(s).

An acute subdural hematoma classically begins with headache, drowsiness, restlessness or agitation, slowed cognition, and confusion. These symptoms worsen over time and progress to loss of consciousness, respiratory pattern changes, and pupillary dilatation. Most persons with chronic subdural hematomas appear to have a progressive dementia accompanied by generalized rigidity. Chronic subdural hematomas require a craniotomy to evacuate the gelatinous blood.

In intracerebral hematomas, as the intracranial pressure rises, clinical manifestations of temporal lobe herniation may appear. Delayed intracerebral hematoma results in the following: sudden, rapidly progressive decreased levels of consciousness with pupillary dilatation, breathing pattern changes, hemiplegia, and bilateral positive Babinski reflexes. Evacuation of a singular intracerebral hematoma is occasionally helpful for subcortical white matter hematomas. Otherwise treatment is directed at reducing the intracranial pressure and allowing the hematoma to reabsorb slowly.

Diffuse brain injury or diffuse axonal injury (DAI) results from the inertial force to the head; it is associated with high levels of acceleration and deceleration. Severity of the diffuse injury correlates with how much shearing force is applied to the brain stem. In DAI, increased intravascular blood within the brain, vasodilation, and increased cerebral blood volume are frequently seen. Several categories of diffuse brain injury exist: mild concussion, classical concussion, mild DAI, moderate DAI, and severe DAI.

Mild concussion involves temporary axonal disturbances. Cerebral cortical dysfunction related to attentional and memory systems results and consciousness is not lost.

Classical cerebral concussion causes reflexes to fail transiently. Confusional states last for hours or days. Loss of consciousness lasts more than six hours.

In **mild DAI**, individuals display decerebrate or decorticate posturing; they may experience prolonged stupor or restlessness. Seventy-eight percent recover in three months.

In **moderate DAI**, widespread physiological impairment exists throughout the cerebral cortex and diencephalon. Actual tearing of some axons in both hemispheres occurs. Basal skull fracture is commonly associated with moderate DAI. Prolonged coma lasting more than 24 hours is present and recovery is often incomplete in surviving individuals. Thirty-eight percent recover in three months.

Severe DAI, formerly called primary brain stem injury or brain stem contusion, involves severe mechanical disruption of many axons in both cerebral hemispheres and those extending to the diencephalon and brain stem. Fifteen percent recover in three months.

DAI is associated with physical, cognitive, psychological/behavioral, and social consequences. Spastic paralysis, peripheral nerve injury, swallowing disorders, dysarthria, visual and hearing impairments, and taste and smell deficits are some of the physical consequences. Common cognitive deficits include disorientation and confusion, short attention span, memory deficits, learning difficulties, dysphasia, poor judgment, and perceptual deficits. Behavioral disorders that emerge include agitation, impulsivity, blunted affect, social withdrawal, and depression.

2. Discuss pathogenesis and manifestations of spinal cord injuries.

Study pages 387-391; refer to Figures 14-4 through 14-7 and Tables 14-5 through 14-7.

Spinal cord injuries mostly occur because of vertebral injuries. Traumatic forces injure the vertebral and/or neural tissues by compressing the tissue, pulling or exerting a traction on the tissue, or shearing tissues so that they slide into one another.

Vertebral injuries occur mostly at the first to second cervical, fourth to seventh cervical, and twelfth thoracic to second lumbar vertebrae. These are the most mobile portions of the vertebral column. The cord occupies most of the vertebral canal in these areas and its size makes it more easily injured. Within a few minutes following injury, microscopic hemorrhages appear in the central gray matter and pia-arachnoid. Edema progresses into the white matter, impairing the microcirculation of the cord with reduced vascular perfusion and development of metabolic changes in spinal cord tissues, including lactate and increasing concentrations of norepinephrine. The elevated norepinephrine levels may produce further ischemia, vascular damage, and necrosis of tissue. Cord swelling increases the individual's degree of dysfunction. In the cervical region cord, swelling may be life-threatening because of impairment of diaphragm function. The traumatized cord is replaced by acellular collagenous tissue usually in three to four weeks. Meninges thicken as part of the scarring process.

Normal activity of the spinal cord cells at and below the level of injury ceases because of the lack of continuous tonic discharges from the brain or brain stem and inhibition of suprasegmental impulses immediately after cord injury. This causes **spinal shock** which is characterized by a complete loss of reflex function in all segments below the level of the lesion. This condition involves all skeletal muscles; bladder, bowel, and sexual function; and autonomic control.

Spinal shock may last for 7 to 20 days following onset; it may persist as long as three months. Indications that spinal shock is terminating include the reappearance of reflex activity, hyperreflexia, spasticity, and reflex emptying of the bladder. Loss of motor function and sensory function depends upon the level and degree of injury. Paraplegia or quadriplegia can result. Return of spinal neuron excitability occurs slowly. Either motor, sensory, reflex, and autonomic functions return to normal or autonomic neural activity in the isolated segment develops.

Autonomic hyperreflexia is a syndrome that may occur at any time after spinal shock resolves. The syndrome is associated with a massive, uncompensated cardiovascular response to stimulation of the sympathetic nervous system. Individuals most likely to be affected have lesions at the T6 level or above. Hyperreflexia involves the stimulation of sensory receptors below the level of the cord injury. The intact autonomic nervous system reflexively responds with an arteriolar spasm that increases blood pressure. Baroreceptors in the cerebral vessels, the carotid sinus, and the aorta sense the hypertension and stimulate the parasympathetic system. The heart rate decreases, but the visceral and peripheral vessels do not dilate because efferent impulses cannot pass through the cord and cardiovascular compensation is incomplete. The most common precipitating cause is a distended bladder or rectum, but any sensory stimulation can elicit autonomic hyperreflexia.

For a suspected or confirmed vertebral fracture or dislocation, the immediate intervention is immobilization of the spine to prevent further injury. Decompression and surgical fixation may be necessary. Corticosteroids are given to decrease secondary cord injury. In cases of autonomic hyperreflexia, intervention must be prompt because cerebrovascular accident is possible. The head of the bed should be elevated and the injurious stimulus should be found and removed. Medications may be used if these measures do not effectively reduce blood pressure.

3. **Cite the causes of low back pain; describe a herniated disk.**
   Study pages 391-396; refer to Figures 14-5, 14-9, and 14-10.

The local processes involved in **low back pain** include tension caused by tumors or disk prolapse, bursitis, synovitis, degenerative joint disease, abnormal bone pressures, spinal immobility, and inflammation caused by osteomyelitis, bony fractures, or ligamentous strains. Pain may be referred from viscera or the posterior peritoneum. General processes resulting in low back pain include bone diseases such as osteoporosis or osteomalacia seen in hyperparathyroidism.

The etiology for **degenerative disk disease** includes biochemical and biomechanical alterations of tissue comprising the intervertebral disk. Fibrocartilage replaces the gelatinous mucoid material of the nucleus pulposus as the disk changes with aging; the narrowing disk results in variable segmental instability. The process seems to stabilize when segmental fibrosis results; often, the incidence of back pain decreases also.

Spondylolysis is a structural defect involving the lamia or neural arch of the vertebra. The most common site is the lumbar spine. Heredity plays a significant role, and spondylolysis is associated with other congenital spinal defects. As a result of torsional and rotational stress, microfractures occur at the affected site and eventually cause dissolution of the pars interarticularis. **Spondylolisthesis** is caused when a vertebra slides forward in relation to an inferior vertebra. **Spinal stenosis** may represent several conditions ranging from entrapment of a single nerve root in the lateral recess to diffuse central stenosis involving many roots.

Most individuals having acute low back pain benefit from bed rest, analgesic medications, exercises, physical therapy, and education. Surgical treatments include diskectomy and spinal fusions. Individuals with chronic low back pain can be treated with antiinflammatory and muscle relaxant medications and exercise programs. Spinal surgery has a limited role in curing chronic low back pain.

Herniation of an intervertebral disk is a protrusion of part of the nucleus pulposus through a tear in the fibrous capsule enclosing the gelatinous center of the disk. Rupture of intervertebral disks is usually caused by trauma, degenerative disease, or both. Lifting with the trunk flexed and sudden straining when the back is in an unstable position are the most common causes; males are more affected than females. Most commonly affected are the lumbosacral disks; disk herniation occasionally occurs in the cervical area. The symptoms may be immediate or occur within a few hours, or they may take months to years to develop. The pain of a herniated disk in the lumbosacral area radiates along the sciatic nerve over the buttock and into the calf or ankle. With the herniation of a lower cervical disk, paresthesia and pain are present in the upper arm, forearm, and hand according to the affected nerve root distribution.

The conservative therapeutic approach comprises traction, bed rest, heat and ice to the affected areas, and an effective analgesic regimen. The surgical approach is indicated if there is weakness and decreased deep tendon reflexes and bladder/bowel reflexes or if the conservative approach is unsuccessful.

4. Compare and contrast cerebrovascular accidents.
Study pages 396-400; refer to Figures 14-11 and 14-12 and Table 14-8.

Cerebrovascular accidents are classified as thrombotic, embolic, or hemorrhagic. The accidents are vascular in origin but are manifested neurologically. **Thrombotic strokes** arise from arterial occlusions caused by thrombi formed in the intracranial vessels or the arteries supplying the brain.

The risk factors for cerebrovascular occlusive disease are:

hypertension
cigarette smoking
elevated blood cholesterol
elevated triglyceride levels
diabetes mellitus
sedentary lifestyle
hypothyroidism
use of oral contraceptives
sickle cell disease
coagulation disorders
polycythemia vera
arteritis
subclavian steal syndrome
chronic hypoxia
dehydration

The development of a cerebral thrombosis is most frequently attributed to atherosclerosis and inflammatory disease processes that damage arterial walls. Atheromatous plaques tend to form at branchings and curves in the cerebral circulation. Degeneration or bleeding into the vessel wall may cause endothelial damage. Platelets and fibrin adhere to the damaged wall and delicate thrombi form. Small thrombi collect over time; gradual

Cerebrovascular Accidents

	Thrombotic	Embolic	Hemorrhagic
Presence of earlier transient ischemia attacks (TIAs)	Frequent	Occasional	Infrequent
Onset	Acute, hours to days	Acute	Acute, progressing, worsening
Associated headache	Occasional, not severe	Often moderately severe	Frequent, severe
Stiff neck	Rare	Rare	Frequent
Loss of consciousness	Occasional, not at onset	Occasional, brief	Frequent
Blood in CSF	Rare	Rare	Frequent

occlusion of the artery occurs. Once the artery is occluded, the thrombus may enlarge lengthwise in the vessel.

Thrombotic strokes may be further subdivided on the basis of clinical manifestations into transient ischemic attacks, strokes-in-evolution, and completed strokes. **Transient ischemic attacks** (TIAs) represent thrombotic particles that cause an intermittent blockage of circulation. In a true transient ischemic attack, all neurologic deficits must completely clear within 24 hours and leave no residual dysfunction. The typical development of thrombotic stroke causes the clinical syndrome known as a **stroke-in-evolution.** An intermittent progression of a neurologic deficit over hours to days is characteristic of thrombotic stroke or slow intracranial hemorrhage. The **completed stroke** has reached its maximum destructiveness in producing deficits, although cerebral edema may not have reached its maximum.

An **embolic stroke** involves fragments that break from a thrombus formed outside the brain. Common sites are in the heart, aorta, common carotid, or thorax. The embolus usually involves small vessels and obstructs a bifurcation or other narrowing to cause ischemia. Conditions associated with an embolic stroke include atrial fibrillation, myocardial infarction, endocarditis, rheumatic heart disease, valvular prostheses, atrial-septal defects, and disorders of the aorta, carotids, or vertebral-basilar circulation. In persons who experience an embolic stroke, usually a second stroke follows at some point because the source of emboli continues to exist. Emboli usually lodge in the distribution of the middle cerebral artery.

Hemorrhagic stroke or intracranial hemorrhage is a frequent cause of cerebrovascular accidents. The most common causes of hemorrhagic stroke are hypertension, ruptured aneurysms or arteriovenous malformation, and hemorrhage associated with bleeding disorders.

Hypertensive hemorrhage is associated with a significant increase in systolic-diastolic pressure over several years and usually occurs within the brain tissue. A mass of blood forms as its volume increases; adjacent brain tissue is displaced and compressed. Rupture or seepage into the ventricular system occurs in many of the cases. The most common sites for hypertensive hemorrhages are in the putamen of the basal ganglia.

Lacunar strokes, or lacunar infarcts, are very small and involve the small arteries predominantly in the basal ganglia, internal capsules, and brain stem. Because of the subcortical location and small area of infarction, these strokes may have limited motor and sensory deficits.

Cerebral infarction results when an area of the brain loses blood supply due to vascular occlusion. In ischemic infarcts, neuronal cell bodies change, myelin sheaths and axis cylinders are interrupted and disintegrate, and there is loss of function.

The symptoms depend on the blood vessel involved. Essentially, if the internal carotid artery branches are involved, there is confusion, inability to plan, aphasia, perception disorders, paralysis, or blindness. If the vertebral artery branches are involved, there is diplopia, ataxia, vertigo, dysphagia, and dysphonia. If a TIA is the cause of the thrombotic lesion, the neurological deficit will usually clear within 24 hours. Other CVA usually have permanent neurological deficits.

In thrombotic strokes, treatment is directed at supportive management to control cerebral edema and increased intracranial pressure. Intervention to restore blood supply may be indicated. Arresting the disease process by controlling risk factors is critical. In embolic strokes, treatment is directed at preventing further embolization by instituting anticoagulation therapy and correcting the primary problem. Rehabilitation is indicated in both thrombotic and embolic stroke. Treatment of an intracranial stroke, regardless of cause, is focused on stopping or reducing the bleeding, controlling the increased intracranial pressure, preventing another hemorrhagic episode, and preventing vasospasm. At times, an attempt is made to evacuate or aspirate the blood.

5. Compare meningitis with encephalitis.

Study pages 400-401 and 402-403; refer to Table 14-9.

(See box on page 108 of *Workbook.*)

6. Characterize CNS abscesses.

Study pages 401-402; refer to Figure 14-13.

Abscesses are localized collections of pus within the parenchyma or functioning cells of the brain and spinal cord. Abscesses occur following open trauma and during neurosurgery; with foci of infection such as the middle ear, mastoid cells, nasal cavity, and nasal sinuses; and through metastatic or hematogenous spread from distant foci. Streptococci, staphylococci, and *Bacteroides* in combination with anaerobes are the most common

Meningitis and Encephalitis

	Bacterial Meningitis	Aseptic Meningitis	Encephalitis
Site	Pia mater, arachnoid, subarachnoid space, CSF, ventricles	Meninges	Meninges, white and gray matter
Infectious agents	*Neisseria, pneumococci haemophilus*	Enteroviral viruses, herpes simplex 1	Arthropod-borne viruses, herpes simplex 1, complications of systemic viral infection
Lesion	Meningeal vessels become hyperemic and permeable	Similar to bacterial	Nerve cell degeneration
Manifestations	Throbbing headache, flexion of legs and thighs, neck stiffens, projectile vomiting, confusion	Mild symptoms compared with bacterial meningitis but similar	Fever, delirium, confusion, coma, seizure, cranial nerve palsies, paresis and paralysis
CSF	Internal pressure, bacteria, elevated protein levels, decreased glucose levels, neutrophils and monocytes	Increased pressure, normal glucose levels, lymphocytes	Same as aseptic meningitis

bacteria that cause abscesses. However, yeast and fungi have also been found in CNS abscess.

Initially, a localized inflammatory process leads to edema, hyperemia, softening, and petechial hemorrhage. After a few days, fibroblasts from capillaries deposit collagen fibers which contain and encapsulate the purulent focus. The infection becomes limited with a center of pus and a wall of granular tissue.

Clinical manifestations of **brain abscesses** include fever, headache, nausea, vomiting, decreasing cognitive abilities, paresis, and seizures. These signs and symptoms develop because of the infection and expanding mass. Clinical manifestations of **spinal cord abscesses** are spinal discomfort, root pain accompanied by spasms of the back muscles and limited vertebral movement due to pain and spasm, weakness due to progressive cord compression, and paralysis.

Aspiration or excision accompanied by antibiotic therapy is the recommended but somewhat controversial treatment for brain abscesses. Intracranial pressure must be managed. Spinal cord abscesses are treated with surgical excision or aspiration because decompression is necessary. Antibiotic and supportive therapy is also required.

7. Identify the neurologic complications of AIDS.

Study pages 403-404.

Approximately 40 to 60 percent of all persons with AIDS develop neurologic complications. The most common neurologic disorder is HIV encephalopathy. Other common neurologic disorders are peripheral neuropathies, vacuolar myelopathy, opportunistic infection of the CNS, and neoplasms.

HIV encephalopathy is characterized by progressive cognitive dysfunction in conjunction with motor and behavioral alterations. HIV encephalopathy is likely the result of direct brain tissue infection by the virus. HIV is mostly found in white matter subcortical areas.

Vacuolar myelopathy involving diffuse degeneration of the spinal cord may occur in persons with AIDS. A progressive spastic paraparesis with ataxia is the predominant clinical manifestation. Leg weakness, upper motor neuron signs, incontinence, and posterior column sensory loss may be present.

Peripheral neuropathy is a sensory neuropathy. Individuals experience painful dysthesias and paresthesias in the extremities. Weakness and decreased or absent distal reflexes may be present.

Some individuals develop an acute **aseptic meningitis** at approximately the time of positive seroconversion. Headache, fever, and meningismus with cranial nerve involvement, especially V and VII, may appear.

Opportunistic viral infections may cause nervous system disease. Persons with cytomegalovirus encephalitis may experience altered cognitive functions, tremor, focal neurologic deficits, and sensory deficits.

Opportunistic nonviral infections are the most common CNS disorders associated with AIDS. Clinical manifestations of CNS toxoplasmosis, a common AIDS disorder, are highly variable and include clumsiness to hemiplegia, aphasia, seizures, ataxia, and cognitive changes.

CNS neoplasms associated with AIDS include CNS lymphoma, systemic non-Hodgkin lymphoma, and metastatic Kaposi sarcoma.

8. Describe Alzheimer disease.
Study pages 404-406; refer to Figures 14-14 and 14-15.

Alzheimer disease is one of the most common causes of severe cognitive dysfunction in older persons. The exact cause of Alzheimer disease is unknown. Several possible theories are notable, including loss of neurotransmitter stimulation by choline acetyltransferase, mutation for encoding amyloid precursor protein, and alteration in apolipoprotein E which binds beta amyloid. Early- and late-onset familial Alzheimer disease (FAD) are linked to genetic defects. Aggregation and precipitation of insoluble amyloid occur with these disorders. Alzheimer disease has also been linked to a lysosomal pathway that yields a neurotoxic substance.

An autoimmune etiology is also being investigated. Familial risk appears to be greatest in families affected by the classic early onset of Alzheimer disease. The risk when a sibling develops Alzheimer disease after age 70 does not differ from that of the general population.

Microscopically, the protein in the neurons becomes distorted and twisted, forming a tangle called a **neurofibrillary tangle**. These abnormal protein fibers accumulate within the neurons. Groups of nerve cells, especially terminal axons, degenerate and coalesce around an amyloid core. These areas appear like plaques and are called **senile plaques**. These plaques disrupt nerve impulse transmission. Senile plaques and neurofibrillary tangles are more concentrated in the cerebral cortex and hippocampus. The greater the number of senile plaques and neurofibrillary tangles, the greater the dysfunction.

Dyspraxias, or the inability to perform coordinated acts, may appear. Motor changes may occur if the posterior frontal lobes are involved. The individual may exhibit rigidity with flexion posturing, propulsion, and retropulsion. There is great variability in age of onset, intensity, and sequence of symptoms and in the location and extent of brain pathology among individuals with the disease.

9. Distinguish between the degenerative diseases of Parkinson, Huntington, multiple sclerosis, and amyotrophic lateral sclerosis (ALS).
Study pages 406-411; refer to Figures 14-16 through 14-19.

(See box on page 110 of *Workbook*.)

10. Describe hydrocephalus.
Study pages 411-412; refer to Table 14-10.

Hydrocephalus refers to various conditions characterized by excess fluid in the cranial vault, subarachnoid space, or both. It occurs because of interference with cerebrospinal fluid flow caused by increased fluid production, obstruction within the ventricular system, or defective reabsorption of the fluid.

Hydrocephalus may develop from infancy through adulthood. Congenital hydrocephalus is rare. **Noncommunicating** or internal hydrocephalus in which the flow from the ventricles is obstructed is seen more frequently in children, and the **communicating** type without obstruction is seen more frequently in adults.

Obstructed cerebrospinal fluid is under pressure and causes atrophy of the cerebral cortex and degeneration of the white matter tracts. There is selective preservation of gray matter.

Acute hydrocephalus manifests signs of rapidly developing increased intracranial pressure. If not promptly treated, the individual quickly becomes comatose. Normal pressure hydrocephalus develops slowly, showing declining memory and cognitive function. In infancy, head enlargement is predominant before cranial suture closure.

Degenerative CNS Diseases

	Parkinson	Huntington	Multiple Sclerosis	ALS
Lesion site	Basal ganglia, degeneration of dopaminergic receptors	Basal ganglia frontal cortex, depletion of GABA	CNS demyelination	Scarring of corticospinal tract in lateral column of spinal cord—upper and lower motor neurons
Etiology	Dopamine insufficiency, trauma, infection, neoplasms, drugs, toxins	Autosomal dominant	Immunogenetic-viral, genetic/ environmental	Viral-immune
Onset	> age 40, peak 60s	40s and 50s	Between 20 and 40 years of age	40s, peaks in early 50s
Manifestations	Resting tremor, muscle stiffness, poverty of movement or akinesia, flexed or forward leaning, possible late-stage dementia	Dementia, delusions, and depression; chorea-type movements beginning in face and arms and finally the entire body	Remissions and exacerbations but progressive paresthesia, diplopia, cerebellar incoordination, urinary dysfunction	Muscle weakness and atrophy, progress to paralysis, normal intellectual and sensory function until death
Treatment	Symptomatic, dopaminergic drugs	No known treatment	Steroids to shorten exacerbations, supportive and rehabilitative management	No known treatment

The diagnosis is based on physical examination, CT scan, and MRI. Hydrocephalus can be treated by surgery to resect cysts, neoplasms, or hematomas. Ventricular bypass into the normal intracranial channel or into an extracranial compartment by a shunt is also used therapeutically.

11. Describe peripheral nervous system disorders; characterize myasthenia gravis.
Study pages 412-414; refer to Table 14-11.

Radiculopathies and **radiculitis** are disorders of the spinal nerve roots. As spinal roots emerge from or enter into the vertebral canal, they may be injured or damaged by compression, inflammation, or direct trauma that stretches or tears the roots.

Plexus injuries involve the nerve plexus distal to the spinal roots but proximal to the the peripheral nerves. Such injuries may be caused by trauma, compression, or infiltration or iatrogenically by positioning during surgery or by intramuscular injections. Clinical manifestations include motor weakness, muscle atrophy, and sensory loss in affected areas. Paralysis can occur with complete plexus lesions.

Where the peripheral nerves themselves are affected, **neuropathy** develops. Sensory neuropathies are mostly caused by leprosy, some industrial solvents, chloramphenicol, and heredity. Motor neuropathies are predominantly caused by Guillain-Barré syndrome, infectious mononucleosis, viral hepatitis, acute porphyria, lead, mercury, and triorthocresylphosphates (TCP).

Sensory alterations are seen in sensory neuropathy. These include paresthesia and dysthesia, as well as decreased or absent primary sensations.

The neurologic dysfunctions observed in **Guillain-Barré syndrome** are associated with earlier respiratory or gastrointestinal infections. The individual may have a symmetrical weakness or paralysis involving the legs, the trunk, and possibly the neck and face. Any paresthesia ascends upward. Individuals then may experience respiratory arrest or cardiovascular collapse.

Myasthenia gravis is a disorder of voluntary or striated muscles characterized by muscle weakness and fatigability because of a defect in nerve impulse transmission at the neuromuscular junction. Between 70 and 80 percent of persons with myasthenia gravis have pathological changes in the thymus; this disorder is an autoimmune disease. Different types of myasthenia gravis exist. **Ocular myasthenia**, which is more common in males, involves muscle weakness confined to the eye muscles. **Generalized myasthenia** involves the proximal musculature throughout the body and exhibits varying rates of progression with possible remissions. **Bulbar myasthenia** involves the muscles innervated by cranial nerves IX through XII and tends to be rapidly progressive or severe.

In myasthenia gravis, postsynaptic acetylcholine receptors on the muscle cell's plasma membrane are no longer recognized as "self." Therefore, IgG antibody is secreted against the acetylcholine receptors. These antibodies fix onto the receptor sites and block the binding of acetylcholine. Eventually, the antibody action causes the destruction of receptor sites and the diminished transmission of the nerve impulse across the neuromuscular junction.

The muscles of the eyes, face, mouth, throat, and neck are usually affected first. Manifestations include diplopia, ptosis, and ocular palsies; facial droop and an expressionless face; difficulty chewing and swallowing; drooling, episodes of choking, and aspirations; and a nasal, low-volume but high-pitched monotonous speech pattern. The muscles of the neck, shoulder girdle, and hip flexor are less frequently affected.

Myasthenic crisis occurs when severe muscle weakness causes extreme quadriparesis or quadriplegia, respiratory insufficiency that can lead to respiratory arrest, and extreme difficulty in swallowing. **Cholinergic crisis** is caused by the muscle hyperactivity secondary to excessive accumulation of acetylcholine at the neuromuscular junctions and excessive parasympathetic activity. As in myasthenic crisis, the individual is in danger of respiratory arrest.

Anticholinesterase drugs, steroids, and immunosuppressant drugs are used to treat myasthenia gravis and myasthenic crisis. Treatment of individuals with cholinergic crisis involves withholding anticholinergic drugs until blood levels fall out of the toxic range while providing ventilatory support.

12. Describe the pathophysiology, manifestations, and treatment of CNS tumors; classify common brain tumors.

Study pages 414-419; refer to Figures 14-20 and 14-21 and Tables 14-12 and 14-13.

Cranial tumors can be either primary or metastatic. **Primary intracerebral tumors** originate from brain substance, neuroglia, neurons, cells of the blood vessels, and connective tissue. **Primary extracerebral tumors** originate outside the substance of the brain and include meningiomas, acoustic nerve tumors, and tumors of the pituitary and pineal glands. **Metastatic tumors** can be found inside and/or outside the brain substance.

Cranial tumors cause local and generalized clinical manifestations. The local effects are due to the destructive action of a particular site in the brain and to compression that reduces cerebral blood flow. The effects are varied and include seizures, visual disturbances, unstable gait, and cranial nerve dysfunction. The generalized effects result from increased ICP. Intracranial brain tumors do

Classification of Common Primary Brain Tumors

Type	Frequency	Age Group
Astrocytoma	30%	Adults
Meningioma	15%	All ages
Oligodendroglioma	7%	Adults
Ependymoma	5%	All ages

not metastasize as readily as tumors in other organs because there are no lymphatic channels within the brain substance. If metastasis does occur, it is usually through seeding of cerebral blood or cerebrospinal fluid, during cranial surgery, or through artificial shunts.

The principal treatment for cerebral neoplasms is surgical or radiosurgical excision or surgical decompression if total excision is not possible. Chemotherapy and radiotherapy also may be used. Supportive treatment is directed at reducing edema.

An estimated 25 percent of persons with cancer develop metastasis to the brain. One-third of metastatic brain tumors arise from the lung, approximately one-sixth from the breast, and a lesser number from the gastrointestinal tract and kidney. Other tumors metastasize less frequently. Carcinomas are disseminated to the brain by the circulation. Metastatic brain tumors carry a poor prognosis. If a solitary tumor is found, surgery and/or radiation therapy is used; but if multiple tumors exist, symptomatic relief only is pursued.

Spinal cord tumors are classified as **intramedullary tumors**, those originating within the neural tissues, or **extramedullary tumors**, those originating from tissues outside the spinal cord. Intramedullary tumors have the same cellular origins as brain tumors. Extramedullary tumors arise from the meninges, epidural tissue, or vertebral structure. The most common primary extramedullary spinal cord tumors are neurofibromas and meningiomas. Metastatic spinal cord tumors are usually carcinomas, lymphomas, or myelomas. Their location is often extradural.

The acute onset of clinical manifestations suggests a vascular insult caused by thrombosis of vessels supplying the spinal cord. Clinical manifestations fall into three major categories: a compressive syndrome, an irritative syndrome, or, rarely, a syringomyelic syndrome. In the **compressive syndrome**, the motor dysfunction is paresis and spasticity depending on the level of involvement. The sensory manifestations of tingling paresthesias have a similar pattern to that of the motor signs. Pain and temperature dysfunctions are more commonly found than touch, vibration, and proprioceptive changes. Bladder and bowel deficits usually appear when paresis develops in the legs.

The **irritative syndrome** combines the clinical manifestations of a cord compression with radicular pain. This pain is in the sensory root distribution and indicates root irritation. Sensory changes include paresthesia and impaired pain and touch perception; motor disturbances include cramps, atrophy, fasciculation, and decreased or absent deep tendon reflexes.

Intradural-extramedullary tumors are surgically removed or decompressed by excision of the posterior vertebral arch or laminectomy. Laminectomy with decompression and excision is used for gliomas and is followed by radiotherapy. Extradural metastatic tumors are often managed by radiotherapy, chemotherapy, hormonal therapy, or pain management protocols.

Practice Examination

1. In blunt head trauma:

   a. brain tissues are exposed.
   b. only focal injury occurs.
   c. the dura is severed.
   d. the dura remains intact.

2. In an automobile accident, an individual's forehead struck the windshield. The coup/contrecoup injury would be in the:

   a. frontal/parietal region.
   b. frontal/occipital region.
   c. parietal/occipital region.
   d. occipital/frontal region.

3. In moderate diffuse axonal injury:

   a. coma lasts more than 24 hours.
   b. coma lasts less than 24 hours.
   c. disruption of axons occurs in cerebral hemispheres and those extending into the diencephalon and brain stem.
   d. tearing of axons in the cerebral hemisphere occurs.
   e. Both a and d are correct.

Match the injury with its definition.

4. ____ concussion
5. ____ contusion
6. ____ extradural hematoma
7. ____ subdural hematoma
8. ____ intracerebral hematoma

a. bleeding into the brain's parenchyma
b. bruising of part of the brain
c. violent displacement of brain tissue due to acceleration or deceleration
d. arterial bleeding
e. venous bleeding

9. The regions where most spinal cord injuries occur are the:

   a. cervical and thoracic regions.
   b. cervical and lumbar regions.
   c. thoracic and lumbar regions.
   d. lumbar and sacral regions.

10. Injury of the cervical cord may be life-threatening because of:

    a. increased intracranial pressure.
    b. disrupted reflexes.
    c. spinal shock.
    d. loss of bladder and rectal control.
    e. diaphragmatic impairment.

11. Autonomic hyperreflexia is characterized by all of the following except:

    a. hypotension.
    b. slower heart rate.
    c. stimulation of sensory receptors below the level of the cord lesion.
    d. precipitation because of a distended bladder or rectum.

12. Intervertebral disk herniation:

    a. usually occurs at the thoracic level.
    b. in the lumbosacral area causes pain over the gluteal region and into the calf or ankle.
    c. is infrequent in the lumbosacral disks.
    d. Both b and c are correct.
    e. a, b, and c are correct.

13. Transient ischemic attacks (TIAs) are:

    a. unilateral neurological deficits that slowly resolve.
    b. generalized neurological deficits that occur a few seconds every hour.
    c. focal neurological deficits that develop suddenly, last for several minutes, and clear in 24 hours.
    d. neurological deficits that slowly evolve or develop.

14. Which is a risk factor for the development of CVA?

    a. polycythemia vera
    b. hypertension
    c. diabetes mellitus
    d. elevated blood cholesterol
    e. All of the above are risk factors.

15. Which most typically characterizes the victims of a cerebral embolic stroke?

    a. individuals older than 65 years of age with a history of hypertension
    b. individuals with a long history of TIA
    c. middle-aged individuals with a history of heart disease
    d. individuals with gradually occurring symptoms which then rapidly disappear

16. Ruptured aneurysms are most likely in ______ cerebrovascular accidents.

    a. TIA
    b. thrombotic
    c. embolic
    d. hemorrhagic

17. Which is not a primary intracerebral neoplasm?

    a. astrocytoma
    b. meningioma
    c. oligodendroglioma
    d. ependymoma

18. In bacterial meningitis, the CSF has:

    a. normal glucose levels.
    b. an elevated number of lymphocytes.
    c. neutrophilic infiltration.
    d. None of the above is correct.
    e. a, b, and c are correct.

19. Chorea-type movements are:

    a. present in Parkinson disease.
    b. present in Huntington disease.
    c. present in multiple sclerosis.
    d. present in ALS.
    e. the consequence of autosomal recessive disorders.

20. Manifestations in Parkinson disease include which of the following? (*More than one answer may be correct.*)

a. resting tremor
b. muscle flaccidity
c. akinesia
d. early-stage dementia

Match the disease with the site of dysfunction.

21. ____ Parkinson disease
22. ____ myasthenia gravis
23. ____ multiple sclerosis
24. ____ Guillain-Barré syndrome
25. ____ amyotrophic lateral sclerosis

a. cerebral cortex
b. basal ganglia
c. peripheral nerve myelin
d. neuromuscular junction
e. ventricular system of brain
f. corticospinal tracts and anterior roots
g. CNS myelin
h. muscles

Case Study

Mrs. B. is an overweight 71-year-old white female. Upon hospital admission, she exhibited slurred speech and some severe right-handed numbness with a weak hand grip on the left. Her smile was asymmetric with right-sided facial weakness that had persisted for 48 hours. Mrs. B. has a history of smoking moderately for 50 years. Her mother had adult-onset diabetes and died of breast cancer at age 62; one sister died of a subarachnoid hemorrhage at age 63; and another sister is hemiparetic because of a CVA. One brother is hypertensive, and three other younger siblings are apparently healthy.

Vital signs showed a normal temperature, elevated heart rate, and normal respirations but a severely elevated blood pressure. A lumbar puncture was negative for blood with normal protein and glucose levels. A normal electrocardiogram was found. EEG showed localized activity in the left hemisphere. A CT showed increased density on the left. Blood chemistry was normal except for elevated glucose.

How do you assess Mrs. B.'s history, her family history, and her symptoms and signs?

CHAPTER

15

Alterations of Neurologic Function in Children

Foundational Objectives

a. Identify the normal infant neurologic reflexes. Refer to Table 15-1.

> **Memory Check!**
>
> - Many reflex patterns are mediated by the brain stem and spinal cord at birth. As the infant matures, the neonatal reflexes disappear in a predictable order as voluntary motor functions replace them. If these reflexes persist, developmental delays or central motor lesions are likely.

b. Identify the major differences between adult and infant neurological functioning. Review pages 425-427; refer to Figure 15-2.

> **Memory Check!**
>
> - Several differences between adults and children are notable. First, the head of a normal infant accounts for approximately one-fourth of the total height, whereas an adult's head is one-eighth of the total body height. Second, the bones of the infant's skull are separated at the suture line to form anterior and posterior fontanelles, or "soft spots." The posterior fontanelle may be open until two to three months of age, whereas the anterior fontanelle normally closes by 18 months. The adult's cranium is a closed cavity with sutures firmly holding the cranial bones together, while the infant's cranium has room for expansion through the fontanelles and increases in circumference during the first five years of life. An adult's head size cannot expand, regardless of trauma or increased production of cerebrospinal fluid. The head is the fastest-growing body part during infancy. In children, abnormal intracranial conditions characterized by increased intracranial pressure also may increase head circumference in excess of that expected with normal growth. Health care providers carefully monitor head growth during the first five years of life by measuring head circumference and comparing the results with a standardized growth chart.

Objectives

After studying this chapter, the learner will be able to:

1. **Describe the major forms of central nervous system malformation.**
Study pages 427-431; refer to Figures 15-3 through 15-5 and Tables 15-2 and 15-3.

Neural tube defects are caused by an arrest in embryologic development and have an incidence of 0.7 to 1.0 per 1000 live births in the United States. A strong association with fetal death obscures the actual incidence somewhat. These can be subdivided into posterior defects or anencephaly, the myelodysplasias or defects of the vertebral column and spinal cord, and the less frequent anterior midline defects.

Anencephaly is the absence of the skull and parts of the brain. It is a relatively common disorder that is fatal.

Encephalocele is herniation of the brain and meninges through a defect in the skull. Most encephaloceles occur in the occipital area. Others are found in the frontal, parietal, or nasopharyngeal regions.

Meningocele is the protrusion of meninges through a vertebral defect. The spinal cord is not involved. The meningocele is present at birth as a protruding sac at the level of the defect. Meningoceles occur with equal frequency in the cervical, thoracic, and lumbar areas.

Myelomeningocele, or spina bifida, is a herniation of the meninges, spinal fluid, spinal cord, and nerves through a vertebral defect; 80 percent are located in the lumbosacral region. The covering membrane may leak cerebrospinal fluid (CSF), increasing the risks of infection and neural damage. Deficits will be distal to the defect and include weakness, paralysis, spasticity, and either bowel or bladder dysfunction. These deficits may worsen with age because of tethering of the cord with development. Hydrocephalus occurs in 95 percent of cases.

Spina bifida occulta is a less serious form of myelomeningocele, with the defect occurring in the lumbar or sacral area of the spine because of incomplete fusion of the vertebral laminae. Spina bifida occulta is more common than myelomeningocele and usually causes no neurologic deficits; it may occur in 10 to 25 percent of infants. Physical findings may include abnormal hair growth along the spine, a midline sacral dimple with or without a sinus tract, angioma over the defect, or an overlying subcutaneous mass.

Craniosynostosis is the premature closure of cranial sutures during the first 20 months of life. Asymmetry of the skull or interference with brain growth may result if multiple sutures are involved. Brain damage from compression may cause neurological dysfunction.

Microcephaly is a defect in brain growth as a whole. Primary microcephaly may be due to chromosomal abnormality, toxin exposure, radiation, or chemical exposure during periods of induction and major cell migration. Secondary microcephaly may be due to various insults during the third trimester.

Congenital hydrocephalus is characterized by an increase in the volume of CSF that may be due to overproduction, a defect in reabsorption, or blockage of the ventricular drainage system. The incidence rate is approximately 2 of every 1000 live births. Before fusion of the sutures, the skull is able to accommodate the increased fluid, which preserves neuronal function.

2. **Compare and contrast the encephalopathic processes of cerebral palsy, phenylketonuria, and Reye syndrome.**
Study pages 431-434; refer to Figure 15-6 and Table 15-4.

Cerebral palsy (CP) is a static encephalopathy, meaning that the resulting damage does not change over time. Clinical manifestations, however, may change as the child continues to develop. CP can be classified according to the neurologic symptoms produced. These include spasticity, ataxia, dyskinesia, or a combination of all three. Many factors contribute to cerebral palsy, including birth asphyxia, low birth weight, vascular abnormalities, pre- or postnatal trauma, and a host of other insults not well understood.

Phenylketonuria (PKU) is an encephalopathy caused by an inherited metabolic disorder and is progressive in nature. The disorder involves an inability to metabolize the amino acid phenylalanine and occurs once in every 10,000 births worldwide. A high level of phenylalanine causes insufficient amounts of other amino acids to enter the brain, which results in malformation, defective myelination, or cystic degeneration of the white and gray matter. Diagnosis is usually made by nonselective newborn screening. Treatment is to restrict phenylalanine in the diet, which generally results in normal growth and development.

Reye syndrome is an acute encephalopathy caused by an interaction of salicylate, viruses, and liver dysfunction. Clinical manifestations begin with vomiting and lethargy (stage 1) and progress to disorientation, delirium, central neurologic hyperventilation, and stupor (stage 2). Obtundation, coma, and decorticate rigidity ensue (stage 3), followed by rapidly developing seizures, flaccidity, and respiratory arrest (stage 4). Avoiding aspirin administration during viral illnesses in children is the widely accepted preventive measure. Treatment depends on the stage of development.

3. Describe the seizure disorders of children, noting their manifestations.
Study page 433; refer to Table 15-5.

Seizures during infancy and childhood may be the result of asphyxia, intracranial bleeding, CNS infection, electrolyte imbalance, or inborn errors of metabolism. Many seizure disorders are idiopathic, having no known cause. Frequently occurring seizure disorders in infancy and childhood include **infantile spasms**, **Lennox-Gastaut syndrome**, **juvenile myoclonic epilepsy**, and **febrile seizures**.

4. Identify the most common pathogens responsible for bacterial meningitis in infancy and childhood; characterize viral meningitis.
Study page 436.

H. influenzae type B, *S. pneumoniae*, and *N. meningitidis* are responsible for bacterial meningitis in infants and children. *H. influenza* type B is most common in children less than five years of age. *S. pneumoniae* is found in children older than four years of age. *E. coli* is most common in neonates.

The hallmark of **viral meningitis** is a mononuclear response in the CSF instead of a neutrophilic response as in bacterial meningitis and normal sugar levels instead of decreased sugar levels as in bacterial meningitis. The symptoms are similar but milder than those in bacterial meningitis. Malaise, fever, headache, stiff neck, nausea, and vomiting are common.

5. Identify the most common site of infection for human immunodeficiency virus (HIV) in children and identify the common effects of this infection.
Study pages 436-437.

The site most commonly affected by **HIV** in infants and children is the CNS. Manifestations include progressive encephalopathy, deterioration of gross and fine motor skills, developmental and language delays, behavioral impairment, and onset of seizures.

6. Describe the types of brain tumors in children and characterize their presentation.
Study pages 437-441; refer to Figures 15-8 through 15-10 and Tables 15-7 and 15-8.

Brain tumors are the most common solid tumor in childhood and the second most common neoplasm in children; leukemia is the most common neoplasm. Genetic, environmental, and immune factors are all implicated in causation. Parental employment also is a possible etiological factor. Childhood brain tumors arise from any central nervous system cell, with two-thirds of tumors found in the posterior fossa or infratentorial area. Brain tumors are unique in their presentation by virtue of their locations. **Supratentorial tumors** of the cerebral hemispheres are uncommon in children. **Infratentorial tumors** frequently present with localized neurological findings such as truncal ataxia, impaired coordination, gait anomalies, and loss of balance. The most common brain tumors in childhood are **medulloblastoma**, **ependymoma**, **astrocytoma**, **brainstem glioma**, and **optic nerve glioma**. These tumors are generally amenable to a wide range of surgical, chemical, and radiation therapies. Prognosis is variable and specific to the individual process.

Practice Examination

True/False

1. ____ An infant of 11 months of age who displays a strong asymmetric tonic neck is probably just "slow" in development and should be assumed to have normal neurological function.

2. ____ Ninety percent of neural tube defects are anencephaly.

3. ____ Anencephaly is the result of premature closure of the sutures of the skull.

4. ____ Environmental influences play an important role in neural tube defects.

5. ____ Encephalocele is the result of herniation of the brain and meninges through a defect of the lower vertebrae.

6. ____ Neurological function at birth is chiefly at the subcortical level.

7. ____ The prognosis for an individual with meningomyelocele depends on the level and extent of the defect.

8. ____ Hydrocephaly may be due to overproduction of CSF, blockage of CSF flow, or inhibition of reabsorption.

9. ____ Hydrocephaly is almost never a neural tube defect, because such defects usually permit leakage of the CSF out of the defect.

10. ____ Seizure disorders in children are usually static and resolve naturally due to the fact that the neurons and the neuronal pathways are constantly maturing.

11. ____ An obvious "sac" on the back of a newborn should be thoroughly probed and examined in order to determine where it is attached to underlying structures.

Fill-in-the-Blank

12. Aspirin administration during a viral illness has been associated with __________ syndrome, which is considered to be a __________ encephalopathy.

13. Early morning vomiting without associated nausea may be indicative of a __________ fossa brain tumor.

14. Focal neurological findings such as ataxia may be associated with an __________ fossa brain tumor.

15. A child becoming significantly more ill with symptoms of headache, lethargy, and stiff neck after several days of treatment for otitis media may be showing findings consistent with __________.

16. __________ is a disease associated with premature closure of the sutures of the skull.

Match the description with the alteration.

17. ____ may restrict brain growth
18. ____ may result from increased CSF
19. ____ protrusion of the meninges through a vertebral defect
20. ____ may require cesarian section for delivery
21. ____ static disease that has changing findings over time
22. ____ defect in metabolism of an amino acid with severe neurological involvement
23. ____ associated with ingestion of aspirin during upper respiratory infection
24. ____ very small head
25. ____ infectious process that may cause profound damage to cranial nerves

a. meningitis
b. microcephaly
c. Reye syndrome
d. PKU
e. cerebral palsy
f. hydrocephaly
g. meningocele
h. congenital hydrocephaly
i. craniosynostosis

Case Study

Allen S. is an 11-year-old white male who presents to the pediatric nurse practitioner's office for a school physical. His past medical history is unremarkable and the family history also is benign. After the examination has started, his mother requests that the practitioner pay particular attention to her son's lower back. He has an area "down there" that is extremely tender and that has been tender as long as she can remember. The problem worsened this year when Allen was hit from behind while playing sandlot football and was paralyzed and "numb" from the hips down for approximately 15 minutes. When asked about the findings when he was taken to the emergency room for the injury, his mother states that she never sought care for him because his symptoms subsided within a few minutes and he "seemed fine!"

As the physical examination continues, it is noted that he has an exquisitely tender area over the lower lumbar spine and palpation causes pain in both legs. This area feels and appears perfectly normal. He is noted to have a very deep, dime-sized sacral dimple and highly fissured skin over the lower sacral spine. Deep tendon reflexes, strength, and sensation are all within normal limits. Bowel and bladder function are normal as well. Spinal x-rays are ordered.

What do you expect the x-rays to reveal and what is/are the next step(s)?

CHAPTER 16

Mechanisms of Hormonal Regulation

Objectives

After review of this chapter, the learner will be able to:

1. **Identify the functions of the endocrine system and describe the regulation of hormone secretion.**
   Review pages 445-448; refer to Figures 16-2 and 16-3.

2. **Classify the types of hormones, their receptors, and proposed mechanisms of action.**
   Review pages 448-453; refer to Figures 16-4 through 16-9 and Tables 16-1 through 16-4.

3. **State the relationship between the hypothalamus and the pituitary; identify the hormones of the anterior pituitary and posterior pituitary, their target organs, and their functions.**
   Review pages 454-457; refer to Figures 16-11 through 16-13 and Tables 16-5 and 16-6.

4. **Identify the thyroid hormones and state their functions.**
   Review pages 457-460; refer to Figure 16-14 and Table 16-7.

5. **Cite the physiological effects of parathyroid hormone and the variables that affect its secretion.**
   Review page 460; refer to Figures 16-14 and 16-15.

6. **Identify the production sites of pancreatic somatostatin, insulin, and glucagon and state their roles in metabolism.**
   Review pages 460-462; refer to Figures 16-16 and 16-17.

7. **Describe the effects of the adrenal cortical glucocorticoids, mineralocorticoids, and gonadotropins; note the adrenal medullary secretions and their roles.**
   Review pages 462-466; refer to Figures 16-18 through 16-21.

Practice Examination

1. Organs that respond to a particular hormone are called the:

   a. target organs.
   b. integrated organs.
   c. responder organs.
   d. hormone attack organs.
   e. None of the above is correct.

2. A major feature of the "plasma membrane receptor" mechanism of hormonal action is:

   a. action of cyclic AMP.
   b. increased lysosomal activity.
   c. a "second messenger" is required.
   d. All of the above are correct.
   e. Both a and c are correct.

3. A major feature of the "activation of genes" mechanism of hormonal action is:

   a. a "second messenger" is used.
   b. a hormone-golgi complex is used.
   c. the hormone enters the cell.
   d. lysosomal activity increases.
   e. All of the above are correct.

4. A hormone having an antidiuretic effect similar to ADH's is:

   a. insulin.
   b. oxytocin.
   c. hGH.
   d. aldosterone.
   e. ACTH.

5. The hypothalamus controls the adenohypophysis by direct involvement of:

   a. nerve impulses.
   b. prostaglandins.
   c. cerebro-cortical controlling factors (CCCF).
   d. regulating hormones.
   e. None of the above is correct.

6. The target organ of prolactin is the:

   a. melanocyte.
   b. mammary gland.
   c. ovum and sperm.
   d. adrenal medulla.
   e. uterine lining.

7. If calcium levels in the blood were too high, thyrocalcitonin (calcitonin) concentrations in the blood should:

   a. increase, thereby inhibiting osteoclasts.
   b. increase, thereby stimulating osteoclasts.
   c. increase, but this would not affect osteoclasts.
   d. decrease, thereby inhibiting osteoclasts.
   e. decrease, thereby stimulating osteoclasts.

8. In the negative feedback mechanism controlling thyroid hormone secretion, which is the nonregulatory hormone?

   a. TRH
   b. TSH
   c. thyroxine
   d. All of the above are regulatory for thyroid hormone secretion.

9. The control of parathyroid hormone is most accurately described as:

   a. negative feedback controlled by the hypothalamus.
   b. positive feedback controlled by the pituitary.
   c. negative feedback involving the pituitary.
   d. negative feedback not involving the pituitary.
   e. Both a and c are correct.

Match the group of adrenocortical hormones with the function.

10. ____ mineralocorticoids

11. ____ glucocorticoids

a. blood cell formation

b. antiinflammatory

c. aldosterone

d. usually no function

e. bone mineralization

12. The renin-angiotensin-aldosterone system begins to operate when renin is secreted by the:

   a. adrenal cortex.
   b. adrenal medulla.
   c. pancreas.
   d. kidneys.
   e. None of the above is correct.

13. The effects of adrenal medullary hormones and the effects of sympathetic stimulation can be described as:

   a. opposites in all respects.
   b. overlapping in some respects.
   c. opposites in some respects.
   d. variable depending on the sex involved.
   e. overlapping in most respects.

14. Which best describes the respective effects of insulin and glucagon on blood sugar?

a. Insulin raises it; glucagon lowers it.
b. Both raise blood sugar.
c. Insulin lowers it; glucagon raises it.
d. Both lower blood sugar.
e. None of the above is correct.

15. The releasing hormones made in the hypothalamus travel to the anterior pituitary via the:

a. stem neurons.
b. infundibular stem.
c. hypophyseal stalk.
d. hypophyseal arteries.

16. Which is a protein hormone?

a. T_4
b. aldosterone
c. FSH
d. insulin

17. Aldosterone maintains electrolyte balance by:

a. retention of potassium.
b. elimination of sodium.
c. retention of both Na and K.
d. Both a and b are correct.
e. None of the above is correct.

Match the hormone with its target organ.

18. ____ ACTH
19. ____ TSH
20. ____ TRF
21. ____ prolactin

a. mammary glands
b. adrenal cortex
c. adrenal medulla
d. thyroid gland
e. adenohypophysis

Match the hormone with its role.

22. ____ epinephrine
23. ____ glucocorticoids
24. ____ mineralocorticoids
25. ____ gonadocorticoids

a. immunity
b. growth inhibition
c. fight or flight
d. controls Na^+, H_2O, and K^+ excretion
e. normal metabolism and resistance to stress
f. minor sex hormones

CHAPTER 17

Alterations of Hormonal Regulation

Foundational Objectives

a. Diagram the negative-feedback system of hormone secretion. Review page 447.

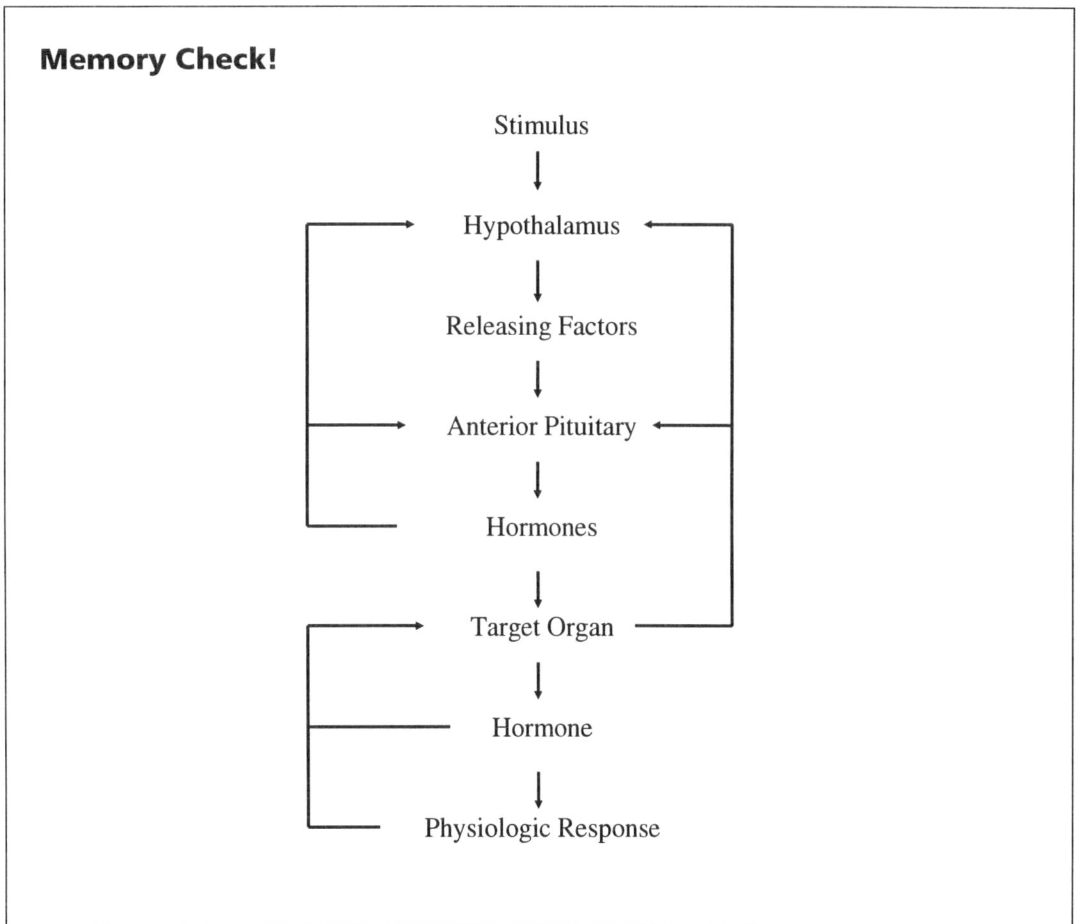

b. Describe hormone receptors as recognizing and signaling mechanisms for hormonal action. Review pages 448-453; refer to Figures 16-4 through 16-9 and Tables 16-3 and 16-4.

Memory Check!

- Hormone receptors are located on the plasma membrane or in the intracellular compartment of a target cell. Water-soluble hormones, which include the protein hormones and epinephrine or norepinephrine, cannot cross the cell membrane and interact or bind with receptors located in or on the cell membrane. Fat-soluble hormones, steroids, vitamin D, and thyroid hormones diffuse freely across the plasma and nuclear membranes to bind primarily with nuclear receptors.
- In the plasma membrane model, the hormones are called "first messengers." The receptors for the water-soluble hormones first recognize the hormone on the plasma membrane and then bind with the hormone. Once recognition and binding have occurred, the hormone-receptor complex initiates the transmission of an intracellular signal by a "second messenger"; the second messenger relays the message inside the cell where a response can occur. The best known second messenger is cyclic AMP (cAMP), although other substances are known as second messengers.
- For cells having cAMP as a second messenger, the purpose of these interactions is to activate the intracellular cyclic nucleotides such as adenylate cyclase. This enzyme converts adenosine triphosphate (ATP) to cAMP. Elevated levels of cAMP alter cell function in specific ways. An example of the function of cAMP as a second messenger can be seen in the action of epinephrine. The epinephrine-receptor complex interaction increases the synthesis of cAMP. Cyclic AMP, in turn, activates an elaborate enzyme cascade in which inactive enzymes are converted in sequence to active enzymes that lead to glycogen breakdown into glucose.
- In the lipid-soluble hormonal model, relatively small hydrophobic molecules cross the plasma membrane by simple diffusion. Once inside the cytosol, some hormones bind to receptor molecules in the cytoplasm and then diffuse into the nucleus. Hormones without cytoplasmic receptors diffuse directly into the nucleus and bind with an acceptor molecule. Once activated by hormones, the first messengers, the receptor likely binds to specific sites on the chromatin of the target cell. This causes RNA transcription and increased synthesis of specific proteins.

c. Identify the origins and functions of hormones. Review the structure and function of endocrine glands in summary of Chapter 16 on pages 468-469; refer to Tables 16-5 through 16-7.

Memory Check!

Site of Origin and Effects of Hormones

Site	Hormone	Effect
Hypothalamus	Releasing hormones	Act on anterior pituitary to release specific hormones
Posterior pituitary	Antidiuretic hormone (ADH)	Causes conservation of body water by promoting water resorption by renal tubules
	Oxytocin	Stimulates uterine contraction and lactation

(Continued)

Memory Check! (cont'd)

Site	Hormone	Effect
Anterior pituitary	Adrenocorticotropic hormone (ACTH)	Stimulates production of glucocorticoids by adrenal cortex
	Melanocyte-stimulating hormone (MSH)	Stimulates pigment production in skin
	Growth hormone (GH)	Promotes growth of body tissues
	Thyroid-stimulating hormone (TSH)	Stimulates production and release of thyroid hormones
	Follicle-stimulating hormone (FSH)	Initiates maturation of ovarian follicles Stimulates spermatogenesis
	Prolactin	Stimulates secretion of breast milk
	Luteinizing hormone (LH)	Causes ovulation and stimulates ovary to produce estrogen and progesterone Stimulates androgen production by interstitial cells of testes
Thyroid	Thyroxine (T_3, T_4)	Increases rate of cellular metabolism
	Calcitonin	Osteoblastic, lowers serum calcium
Parathyroid	Parathyroid hormone (PTH)	Osteoclastic, raises serum calcium
Pancreatic islets of Langerhans	Insulin	Promotes utilization of glucose, lowers serum glucose
	Glucagon	Promotes utilization of glycogen, raises serum glucose
Adrenal cortex	Glucocorticoids, mostly cortisol	Antagonizes effects of insulin, inhibits inflammatory response and fibroblastic activity
	Mineralocorticoid, mostly aldosterone	Promotes retention of sodium by renal tubules
	Androgens and estrogens	Secondary sex characteristics
Adrenal medulla	Catecholamines (epinephrine and norepinephrine)	Regulation of blood pressure by effects on vascular smooth muscle and heart

Objectives

After studying this chapter, the learner will be able to:

1. Identify the mechanisms causing hormonal alterations.
Study pages 472-473; refer to Figure 17-1.

Any significantly elevated or depressed hormone levels have a variety of causes. Feedback systems may fail to function properly or may respond to inappropriate signals. Inadequate amounts of biologically free or active hormone occur when the secretory cells are unable to produce. A gland also may synthesize or release excessive amounts of hormone. Once in the circulation, hormones may be degraded too fast or too slow, or they may be inactivated by antibodies before reaching their target cell. Hormones produced by nonendocrine tissues may also result in abnormally elevated hormone levels.

The target cell may fail to respond to its hormone. The general types of abnormal target cell responses are receptor-associated disorders and intracellular disorders. **Receptor-associated disorders** may exhibit any of the following: decreased numbers of receptors, defective hormone-receptor binding, impaired receptor function with insensitivity to the hormone, presence of antibodies against specific receptors that either reduce available binding sites or mimic hormone action, or unusual expression by some tumor cells having abnormal receptor activity.

Intracellular disorders may involve inadequate synthesis of the second messenger, such as cAMP, needed to signal intracellular events. The target cell for water-soluble hormones such as insulin may not respond to hormone-receptor binding and thus fail to generate the required second messenger. The cell also may fail to respond to the second messenger if levels of intracellular enzymes or proteins are altered.

The target cell response for lipid-soluble hormones such as thyroid hormone are thought to occur less frequently than those affecting the water-soluble hormones. For lipid-soluble hormones, the number of intracellular receptors may be decreased or their receptors may have an altered affinity for hormones. Alterations of new messenger RNA or absence of substrates for new protein synthesis also may alter target cell response.

2. Distinguish between SIADH and diabetes insipidus.
Study pages 473-474.

Diseases of the posterior pituitary are rare, but when occurring, they are usually related to abnormal antidiuretic hormone (ADH/vasopressin) secretion. **Syndrome of inappropriate ADH secretion** (SIADH) is characterized by high levels of ADH without normal physiologic stimuli for its release.

SIADH is associated with several forms of cancer because of the ectopic secretion of ADH by tumor cells. Tumors associated with SIADH include oat cell adenocarcinoma of the lung, carcinoma of the duodenum and pancreas, leukemia, lymphoma, and Hodgkin disease. Transient SIADH may follow pituitary surgery as stored ADH is released in an unregulated fashion. SIADH may be seen in infectious pulmonary diseases because of the ectopic production of ADH by infected lung tissue or by increased posterior pituitary secretion of ADH in response to hypoxia. SIADH also may be associated with psychiatric disease and may occur after treatment with a variety of drugs that stimulate ADH release.

The main features of SIADH are water retention and solute loss, particularly sodium. This leads to hyponatremia and hypoosmolality. As ADH is released continually, water retention results from the normal action of ADH on the renal tubules and collecting ducts. This action increases their permeability to water, thus increasing water reabsorption. Hyponatremia suppresses renin and aldosterone secretion, thus decreasing proximal tubule reabsorption of sodium.

Thirst, impaired taste, anorexia, dyspnea on exertion, fatigue, and dulled consciousness occur when the serum sodium falls from 140 to 130 mEq/L. Vomiting and abdominal cramps occur with a drop in sodium levels from 130 to 120 mEq/L. With a serum sodium level below 113 mEq/L, confusion, lethargy, muscle twitching, and convulsions may occur. Symptoms usually resolve with correction of hyponatremia. The treatment of SIADH involves the correction of any underlying casual problems, correction of severe hyponatremia by administration of hypertonic saline, and fluid restriction to 600 to 800 ml/day.

Diabetes insipidus is related to an insufficiency of ADH leading to polyuria and polydipsia. There are three forms of diabetes insipidus: a neurogenic or central form, a nephrogenic form, and a psychogenic form. The **neurogenic form of diabetes insipidus** occurs when any organic lesion of the hypothalamus, infundibular stem, or posterior pituitary interferes with ADH synthesis, transport, or release. This results in too little ADH. **Nephrogenic diabetes insipidus** is an insensitivity of the renal tubule to ADH, particularly the collecting tubules. This diabetes is generally related to disorders and drugs that damage the renal tubules or inhibit the generation of cAMP in the tubules. The **psychogenic form** is caused by extremely large volume fluid intake.

The clinical manifestations of diabetes insipidus are due to the absence of ADH. These signs and symptoms include polyuria, nocturia, continuous thirst, polydipsia, low urine osmolality, and high-normal plasma osmolality. Individuals with long-standing diabetes insipidus develop a large bladder capacity and distention of the kidney pelvis and calices with urine.

Individuals who have excessive urine output and a low urine osmolality after a dehydration or water restriction test generally require ADH replacement with a synthetic vasopressin analogue. Drugs that potentiate the action of otherwise insufficient amounts of endogenous ADH may be used to stimulate ADH release from the hypothalamus in less severely affected individuals.

3. **Describe the disorders of the anterior pituitary as either hypofunctions or hyperfunctions of the gland.**
   Study pages 475-478; refer to Figures 17-3 through 17-5.

Anterior pituitary hypofunction may develop from infarction of the gland, removal or destruction of the gland, or vasospasm of artery supplying the gland. **Hyperfunction of the anterior pituitary** generally involves an adenoma composed of secretory pituitary cells. An adenoma may lead to hypersecretion of the hormone produced by the adenoma and hyposecretion of another hormone due to the compressive effects of the tumor.

The pituitary gland is extremely vascular and is therefore extremely vulnerable to infarction and subsequent hypopituitarism. The pituitary gland may be susceptible to necrosis because its blood supply through the portal system is already partially deoxygenated. The likelihood of infarction is increased during pregnancy. The primary pathologic mechanism in postpartum pituitary infarction, or **Sheehan syndrome**, is vasospasm of the artery supplying the anterior pituitary. Following tissue necrosis, edema occurs which expands the pituitary within the fixed confines of the sella turcica. This further impedes blood supply to the pituitary and promotes hypofunction.

The signs and symptoms of hypofunction of the anterior pituitary are highly variable and depend on which hormones are affected. If all hormones are absent, a condition termed **panhypopituitarism** develops. The individual suffers from cortisol deficiency from lack of ACTH, thyroid deficiency from lack of TSH, diabetes insipidus from lack of ADH, and gonadal failure and loss of secondary sex characteristics from absence of FSH and LH. Growth hormone and somatomedin levels are low and may affect children. These deficiencies do not generally develop in adults. When there is a growth hormone deficiency in children, hypopituitary **dwarfism** infrequently occurs. A dwarf has a normal face with normal proportions of head, trunk, and limbs; the dwarf also has normal intelligence.

In cases of hypopituitarism, the underlying disorder should be corrected as quickly as possible. Thyroid and cortisol replacement therapy may need to be initiated and maintained. Sex steroid replacement may be required depending on the needs and desires of the individual.

Pituitary adenomas that cause **hyperpituitarism** are usually benign, slow-growing tumors. Effects from an increase in tumor size include nonspecific complaints of headache, fatigue, neck pain or stiffness, and seizures. Visual changes produced by pressure on the optic chiasma include visual field impairments. If the tumor infiltrates other cranial nerves, various neuromuscular functions are affected. Hypersecretion of hormones secreted by the adenoma leads to symptoms associated with the particular hormone that is affected.

Acromegaly occurs in adults who are exposed to continuously excessive levels of growth hormone (GH). Acromegaly is uncommon. The most common cause of acromegaly is a primary autonomous GH-secreting pituitary adenoma. Acromegaly occurs more frequently in women than men and is a slowly progressive disease. If untreated, it is associated with a decreased life expectancy due to an increased occurrence of hypertension, congestive heart failure, and diabetes mellitus.

In the adult, after epiphyseal closure has occurred, increased amounts of GH and somatomedins cause connective tissue and cytoplasm increases.

Bony proliferation involves periosteal vertebral growth and enlargement of the facial bones and the bones of the hands and feet. The associated growth results in protrusion of the lower jaw and forehead. Because somatomedins stimulate cartilaginous growth, there is elongation of ribs at the bone-cartilage junction, causing a barrel-chested appearance and increased proliferation of cartilage in joints. Because of bony and soft tissue overgrowth, nerves may be entrapped and damaged. This may be manifested by weakness, muscular atrophy, foot drop, and sensory changes in the hands. Because of a space-occupying lesion, central nervous system symptoms of headache, seizure activity, and visual disturbances may develop. The metabolic effects of GH hypersecretion include impaired carbohydrate tolerance and increased metabolic rate. Diabetes mellitus occurs when the pancreas is unable to secrete enough insulin to offset the effects of GH.

In children and adolescents whose epiphyseal plates have not yet closed, the effect of increased GH levels is **giantism**. It occurs when high levels of somatomedins stimulate excessive skeletal growth.

The goal of treatment is to protect the individual from the effects of tumor growth and to control hormone hypersecretion while minimizing damage to appropriately secreting portions of the pituitary. Surgery and radiation therapy are used, depending on the extent of tumor growth.

4. Characterize the manifestations of hypothyroidism and hyperthyroidism.
Refer to Tables 17-1 and 17-2.

Manifestations of Hypothyroid and Hyperthyroid States

Characteristic	Hypothyroidism	Hyperthyroidism
Basal metabolic rate	Decreased	Increased
Sympathetic response	Decreased	Increased
Weight	Gain	Loss
Temperature tolerance	Cold intolerance Decreased sweating	Heat intolerance Increased sweating
Gastrointestinal function	Constipation Decreased appetite	Diarrhea Increased appetite
Cardiovascular function	Decreased cardiac output Bradycardia	Increased cardiac output Tachycardia and palpitations
Respiratory function	Hypoventilation	Dyspnea
Muscle tone and reflexes	Decreased	Increased
General appearance	Myxedematous Deep voice Impaired growth (child)	Exophthalmos Lid lag Decreased blinking Enlarged thyroid gland
General behavior	Mental retardation (infant) Mental and physical sluggishness Somnolence	Restlessness, irritability, anxiety Hyperkinesis Wakefulness

Note: Hypothyroidism is more common than hyperthyroidism.

5. Describe the disorders of hyperthyroidism; note the progressive states of severity.
Study pages 478-480; refer to Figure 17-6.

Whenever thyroid hormones (TH) from any source exert greater-than-normal responses, **thyrotoxicosis** exists. **Hyperthyroidism** is a form of thyrotoxicosis in which excess thyroid hormones are secreted by the thyroid gland. Specific diseases that can cause hyperthyroidism include Graves disease and toxic multinodular goiter. Thyrotoxicosis other than hyperthyroidism is seen in subacute thyroiditis, increased TSH secretion, ectopic thyroid tissue, and ingestion of excessive TH. All forms of thyrotoxicosis share some common characteristics because of increased circulating levels of thyroid hormones. The major types of therapy used to control the elevated levels of TH include drug therapy, radioactive iodine therapy, and surgery.

Graves disease is the most common form of hyperthyroidism and is likely associated with autoimmune abnormalities. Thyroid receptor antibody of the IgG class binds to the plasma membrane and initiates thyroid growth, vascularity, and hypersecretion of hormone. Ophthalmopathy is characterized by edema of the orbital contents, exophthalmos, and extraocular muscle weakness that sometimes leads to diplopia and pain, lacrimation, photophobia, and blurred vision.

Diffuse toxic goiter occurs when the thyroid gland enlarges in response to increased demand for TH. The demand for TH increases in puberty, pregnancy, iodine deficiency, and immunologic, viral, or genetic disorders. The thyroid gland returns to its original size when the stimulus for increased TH no longer exists. During the demand status, some follicular cells may produce less TH than the body requires. The remainder of the gland then functions to supply the body's need. If hyperthyroidism develops, the manifestations are similar to those of Graves disease.

Thyrotoxic crisis is rare but a dangerous worsening of the thyrotoxic state; death can occur within 48 hours without appropriate treatment. This condition occurs most frequently in individuals who have undiagnosed or partially treated severe hyperthyroidism and who are subjected to excessive stress from other causes. The systemic symptoms of thyrotoxic crisis include hyperthermia, tachycardia, high-output heart failure, agitation or delirium, and nausea, vomiting, or diarrhea contributing to fluid depletion. The symptoms may be attributed to increased beta-adrenergic receptors and catecholamines. The treatment is to reduce circulating TH levels by blocking thyroid hormone synthesis.

6. Describe the disorders of hypothyroidism.
Study pages 480-483; refer to Figures 17-7 and 17-8.

Deficient production of TH by the thyroid gland results in **hypothyroidism**, which may be either primary or secondary. Primary causes include congenital defects or loss of thyroid tissue following treatment for hyperthyroidism and defective hormone synthesis resulting from antithyroid antibodies or endemic iodine deficiency. Causes of the less common secondary hypothyroidism are insufficient pituitary stimulation of the normal gland and peripheral resistance to TH.

Hypothyroidism can result from three distinct rare disorders. **Acute thyroiditis** is caused by bacterial infection of the thyroid gland. **Subacute thyroiditis** is a nonbacterial inflammation of the thyroid often preceded by a viral infection. Both conditions are accompanied by fever, tenderness, and enlargement of the thyroid. **Autoimmune thyroiditis**, or **Hashimoto disease**, results in destruction of thyroid tissue by circulating thyroid antibodies and infiltration of lymphocytes. Autoimmune thyroiditis may also be caused by an inherited immune defect.

Myxedema coma is a medical emergency associated with severe hypothyroidism. Symptoms include hypothermia without shivering, hypoventilation, hypotension, hypoglycemia, and lactic acidosis. Older patients with severe vascular disease and with moderate or untreated hypothyroidism are particularly at risk for developing myxedema coma. It may also occur after overuse of narcotics or sedatives or after an acute illness in hypothyroid individuals.

Hypothyroidism in infants (congenital hypothyroidism) occurs because of absent thyroid tissue and hereditary defects in thyroid hormone synthesis. Signs may not be evident for at least four months after birth but include abdominal protrusion, umbilical hernia, subnormal temperature, lethargy, excessive sleeping, and slow pulse. Skeletal growth is stunted and the child will be dwarfed with short limbs if not treated. These signs constitute **cretinism**. Mental retardation in cretins is a function of the severity of hypothyroidism and the delay before initiation of thyroxine treatment.

Hypothyroidism is difficult to identify at birth, but high birth weight, hypothermia, delay in passing meconium, and neonatal jaundice are suggestive signs. There is a high probability of normal growth and intellectual function if treatment is started immediately after birth.

Thyroid carcinoma is the most common endocrine malignancy but is still relatively rare. In approximately 10 percent of cases, any hyperplasia of the thyroid gland leads to thyroid carcinoma. The most consistent causal risk factor for the development of thyroid cancer is exposure to ionizing radiation. Changes in voice and swallowing and difficulty in breathing are related to tumor growth impinging on the esophagus or trachea. Treatment for this rare entity may include partial or total thyroidectomy, TSH suppressive therapy, radioactive iodine therapy, postoperative radiation therapy, and chemotherapy.

7. Distinguish between primary, secondary, and tertiary hyperparathyroidism and hypoparathyroidism.
Study pages 483-485.

Approximately 80 percent of **primary hyperparathyroidism** disorders result from a chief cell adenoma with an increased secretion of parathyroid hormone (PTH). This causes hypercalcemia and decreased serum phosphate levels.

Secondary hyperparathyroidism may be a compensatory response of the parathyroid glands to chronic hypocalcemia. Loss of calcium by failing kidneys leads to increased secretion of PTH.

Tertiary hyperparathyroidism develops with hyperplasia of the parathyroid glands and a loss of sensitivity to normal circulating calcium levels. This hyperthyroidism frequently occurs in individuals with chronic renal failure.

Hypersecretion of PTH causes excessive osteoclastic and osteolytic activity resulting in bone resorption. Pathologic fractures, kyphosis of the dorsal spine, and compression fractures of the vertebral bodies may occur. Chronic hypercalcemia may be associated with kidney stones, gastrointestinal disturbances, and muscle weakness and lethargy.

Long-term management of hypercalcemia uses drugs that decrease resorption of calcium from bone. Definitive treatment requires the surgical removal of the hyperplastic parathyroid glands.

Hypoparathyroidism is most commonly caused by damage to the parathyroid glands during thyroid surgery. In the absence of PTH, the ability to resorb calcium from bone and to regulate calcium reabsorption from the renal tubules is impaired. Hypocalcemia lowers the threshold for nerve and muscle excitation. Muscle spasms, hyperreflexia, clonic-tonic convulsions, laryngeal spasms, and, in severe cases, death from asphyxiation are seen with hypocalcemia.

The treatment of hypoparathyroidism involves administration of calcium and vitamin D. Hypoplastic dentition, cataracts, bone deformities, and basal ganglia calcifications do not respond to the correction of hypocalcemia, but the other symptoms of hypocalcemia are reversible.

8. Describe the similarities and differences between insulin-dependent and non-insulin-dependent diabetes mellitus; note other types of diabetes mellitus.
Study pages 485-490; refer to Tables 17-3 through 17-6.

Diabetes mellitus encompasses many etiologically unrelated diseases and includes many different causes of disturbed glucose tolerance. Diabetes mellitus is a syndrome characterized by chronic hyperglycemia and other disturbances of carbohydrate, fat, and protein metabolism. The four major classes of diabetes mellitus are insulin-dependent diabetes mellitus (IDDM or type I diabetes mellitus), non-insulin-dependent diabetes mellitus (NIDDM or type II diabetes mellitus), malnutrition-related diabetes mellitus (MRDM), and other types of diabetes mellitus. Types I and II are the most common.

The diagnosis of diabetes is based on three observations: first, more than one fasting plasma glucose level greater than 140 mg/dl; second, elevated plasma glucose levels in response to an oral glucose tolerance test; and third, random plasma glucose levels above 200 mg/dl combined with classical symptoms or polydipsia, polyphagia, and polyuria. In individuals with poorly controlled diabetes, increases in the quantities of glycosylated hemoglobins are seen. Once a hemoglobin molecule is glycosylated, it remains that way.

Type I diabetes mellitus is characterized by a lack of insulin and a relative excess of glucagon and is most commonly diagnosed in individuals under 18 years of age. In type I diabetes mellitus, beta cells are destroyed and islet cell antibodies appear. These antibodies tend to disappear with time. This disease seems to be caused by gradual process of autoimmune destruction in genetically susceptible individuals. Because of decreased use of glucose, glucose accumulates in the blood and is subsequently released in the urine. This in turn causes polyuria and polydipsia resulting from osmotic diuresis. Ketoacidosis, caused by increased levels of circulating ketones without the inhibiting effects of insulin; increased levels of circulating fatty acids; and weight loss are all manifestations of type I diabetes mellitus.

Type II diabetes mellitus, which is more common than type I, is probably caused by genetic susceptibility that is triggered by environmental factors. It primarily affects individuals after the age of 40. The greatest risk factor for this diabetes is obesity. In the obese, insulin has a diminished ability to influence glucose uptake and metabolism. In type II diabetes, amyloid deposits in the islets, fatty atrophy of the pancreas and liver, and vascular sclerosis are generally present. Some insulin production continues in type II diabetes mellitus, but the mass and number of beta cells is decreased.

The treatment of the individual with type II diabetes requires appropriate meal planning as in type I diabetes; however, oral medication may be needed for optimal management. Insulin may also be required in the treatment of some individuals with type II diabetes. Exercise is an important aspect of treatment for the individual with type II diabetes. Exercise reduces after-meal blood glucose levels and diminishes insulin requirement. Also, exercise adds to weight loss in the overweight individual.

Classifications of Diabetes and Glucose Intolerance States

Classification	Former Terminology	Characteristics
Diabetes mellitus (DM)		
Type I Insulin-dependent diabetes mellitus (IDDM)	Juvenile-onset diabetes	Few islet cells, acute onset at puberty, long preclinical record, insulin-dependent, ketosis prone, autoimmune and genetic-environment etiology
Type II Non-insulin-dependent diabetes mellitus (NIDDM)	Adult-onset, maturity-onset diabetes (over age 40)	Usually not insulin-dependent but they may use insulin, decreased islet cells because of age, not ketosis prone, frequently obese, likely an autosomal recessive disorder
Malnutrition-related diabetes mellitus (MRDM)	Pancreatic diabetes, tropical diabetes	Severe protein malnutrition in tropical and developing countries, severe hyperglycemia, glycemia without ketosis, etiology unknown
Other types		
Pancreatic disease Hormonal Drug- or chemical-induced insulin receptor abnormalities	Secondary diabetes	Presence of diabetes and associated conditions
Impaired glucose tolerance (IGT)	Asymptomatic, chemical, subclinical, borderline, latent diabetes	Abnormal fasting glucose levels and glucose tolerance tests, 10-15% will convert to type II diabetes within 10 years
Gestational diabetes mellitus (GDM)	Same as above	Glucose intolerance develops during pregnancy (third trimester), increased risk of perinatal complications, increased risk of developing diabetes within 10-15 years after parturition

9. Identify the acute complications of diabetes mellitus; describe the features of each.
Study page 490; refer to Figure 17-9 and Table 17-7.

Acute complications of diabetes mellitus include hypoglycemia or insulin shock, diabetic ketoacidosis (DKA), and hyperosmolar hyperglycemic nonketotic coma (HHNK).

Acute Complications of Diabetes Mellitus

Variable	**Insulin Shock Hypoglycemia**	**DKA**	**HHNK**
Onset	Rapid	Slow	Slowest
Symptoms	Weak, anxious, confused	Nausea, vomiting, polyuria, polyphagia, polydipsia, headache, irritable, comatose	Similar to DKA; stuporous, focal motor seizures
Skin	Cold, moist, pale	Hot, flushed, dry	Very dry
Mucous membranes	Normal	Dry	Extremely dry
Respiration	Normal	Hyperventilation, "fruity" or acetone odor to breath	Normal
Those at risk	Type I and II DM, fluctuating blood glucose levels, insufficient food intake, excessive exercise, oral medication, excessive insulin	Type I DM, stressful situations, omission of insulin	High carbohydrate diets, diuresis, hyperosmolar dialysis
Blood sugar/dl	30 mg or less in newborns, 60 mg or less in adults	300-750 mg	600-2000 mg
Treatment	Fast-acting carbohydrate, intravenous glucose, subcutaneous glucagon	Low-dose insulin, electrolyte and fluid replacement	Fluid replacement with crystalloids and colloids

10. Describe the chronic complications of diabetes mellitus.
Study pages 490-494; refer to Figure 17-10.

Before the discovery of long-term insulin, the survival time of diabetics was short, especially for individuals with type I diabetes. Today, long-term survival is common. As a result, the problems of neuropathy, vascular disease, and infection have become important in clinical management of diabetic individuals.

Chronic Complications of Diabetes Mellitus

Insulin Deficiency

* Lipid mobilization

* Decreased glucose utilization

* Increased glucose production

Diabetic Neuropathies	**Microvascular Disease**	**Macrovascular Disease**	**Infection**
axonal and Schwann cell degenerations, altered motor nerve conduction, sensory alterations	* retinopathy * nephropathy capillary basement membrane thickening, decreased tissue perfusion or ischemia, hypertension	*coronary heart disease *CVA *peripheral vascular disease proliferation of fibrous plaques, atherosclerosis because of high serum lipids, ischemia	sensory impairment, atherosclerosis, ischemia, hypoxia, leukocytic impairment

* *major consequences*

11. Describe the etiology, pathogenesis, and manifestations of hyperfunction and hypofunction of the adrenal cortex.
Study pages 495-500; refer to Figures 17-11 through 17-14 and Tables 17-8 and 17-9.

Cushing syndrome refers to excessive levels of circulating cortisol caused by hyperfunction of the adrenal cortex with or without pituitary involvement. **Cushing disease** refers specifically to pituitary-dependent hypercortisolism. Cushing-like syndrome may also develop as a result of the exogenous administration of cortisone. Elevated levels of pituitary ACTH and adrenal neoplasms account for many cases of hypercorticoadrenalism.

Two observations consistently apply to individuals with Cushing syndrome: they lack diurnal or circadian secretion patterns of ACTH and cortisol, and they do not increase ACTH and cortisol secretion in response to a stressor.

Most of the clinical signs and symptoms of Cushing syndrome are caused by hypercortisolism. The most common feature is the accumulation of adipose tissue in the trunk, facial, and cervical areas. These have been described as "truncal obesity," "moon face," and "buffalo hump." Protein wasting is commonly observed in hypercortisolism and is caused by the catabolic effects of cortisol on peripheral tissues. Muscle wasting is especially obvious in the muscles of the extremities. Loss of the protein matrix in bone leads to osteoporosis and accompanying pathologic fractures, vertebral compression fractures, bone and back pain, kyphosis, and reduced height. Loss of collagen also leads to thin, weakened integumentary tissues through which capillaries are more visible. This accounts for the characteristic purple striae observed in the trunk area. Loss of collagenous support around small vessels makes them susceptible to rupture and easy bruising.

With elevated cortisol levels, vascular sensitivity to catecholamines is significantly increased, which leads to vasoconstriction and hypertension. Chronically elevated cortisol levels also cause suppression of the immune system and increased susceptibility to infections.

Approximately 50 percent of individuals with Cushing syndrome experience irritability and depression. Without treatment, approximately 50 percent of individuals with Cushing syndrome die within five years of onset because of infection, suicide, complications from generalized arteriosclerosis, and hypertensive disease. Treatment is specific for the cause of hypercorticoadrenalism and includes medication, radiation, and surgery.

Hyperaldosteronism is characterized by excessive aldosterone secretion by the adrenal glands. An aldosterone-secreting adenoma or excessive stimulation of the normal adrenal cortex by substances such as angiotensin, ACTH, or elevated potassium may cause hypersecretion.

Conn disease, or **primary aldosteronism**, presents a clinical picture of hypertension, hypokalemia, renal potassium wasting, and neuromuscular manifestations. The most common cause of primary aldosteronism is the benign, single adrenal adenoma followed by multiple tumors or idiopathic hyperplasia of the adrenals.

Because aldosterone secretion is normally stimulated by the renin-angiotensin system, **secondary hyperaldosteronism** can result from sustained elevated renin release and activation of angiotensin. Increased renin-angiotensin secretion occurs with decreased circulating blood volume and decreased delivery of blood to the kidneys.

Hypertension and hypokalemia are the essential manifestations of hyperaldosteronism. Hypertension usually results from increased intravascular volume and from altered serum sodium concentrations. If hypertension is sustained, left ventricular hypertrophy and progressive arteriosclerosis develop. Aldosterone-stimulated potassium loss can result in the typical manifestations of hypokalemia: hypokalemic alkalosis as potassium moves from intracellular to extracellular space in exchange for hydrogen ions as well as renal loss of hydrogen ions to facilitate sodium reabsorption. Individuals with hypokalemic alkalosis may experience (1) tetany and paresthesia, (2) skeletal muscle weakness, (3) cardiovascular alterations, and (4) loss of urine-concentrating mechanisms leading to poly-uria or nocturia.

Treatment manages hypertension and hypokalemia with correction of any underlying causal abnormalities. If an aldosterone-secreting adenoma is present, it must be surgically removed.

Hypersecretion of adrenal androgens and estrogens may be caused by adrenal tumors, Cushing syndrome, or defects in steroid synthesis. The clinical manifestations depend on the hormone secreted, the sex of the individual, and the age at which the hypersecretion occurs. Hypersecretion of estrogens causes **feminization**, or the development of female sex characteristics. Hypersecretion of androgens causes **virilization**, or the development of male sex characteristics.

The effects of an estrogen-secreting tumor are most evident in males and cause gynecomastia, testicular atrophy, and decreased libido. In female children, such tumors may lead to early development of secondary sex characteristics. Androgen-secreting tumor changes are more easily observed in females and include excessive face and body hair growth or hirsutism, clitoral enlargement, deepening of the voice, amenorrhea, acne, and breast atrophy. In children, virilizing tumors promote precocious sexual development and bone aging. Treatment of androgen-secreting tumors usually involves surgical excision.

Hypocortisolism develops either because of inadequate stimulation of the adrenal glands by ACTH or because of an inability of the adrenals to produce and secrete the adrenal cortical hormones. Hypofunction of the adrenal cortex may affect glucocorticoid or mineralocorticoid secretion or a combination of both. Primary adrenal insufficiency is termed **Addison disease**, a relatively rare adult disease.

Addison disease is characterized by elevated serum ACTH levels with inadequate corticosteroid synthesis and output. The most common cause is idiopathic organ-specific autoimmune disease. A combination of cell membrane and cytoplasmic antibodies and cell-mediated immune mechanism contribute to the pathology of the disease. Apparently, a genetic defect in immune surveillance mechanisms causes a deficiency of immune suppressor cells. The symptoms of Addison disease are primarily a result of hypocortisolism and hypoaldosteronism. These manifestations include weakness, gastrointestinal disturbances, hypoglycemia, hyperpigmentation from increased ACTH secretion, and hypotension.

The treatment of Addison disease involves glucocorticoid and possibly mineralocorticoid replacement therapy and dietary modifications to include adequate sodium. Hypocortisolism requires daily chronic glucocorticoid replacement therapy, and additional cortisol must be administered during acute stress.

12. Characterize adrenal medulla hyperfunction.
Study page 501.

The most prominent cause of adrenal medulla hypersecretion is **pheochromocytoma**. Fewer than 10 percent of these tumors metastasize; if they do, they are usually found in the lungs, liver, bones, or paraaortic lymph glands. Most pheochromocytomas produce norepinephrine, although large tumors secrete both epinephrine and norepinephrine. Pheochromocytomas cause excessive production of epinephrine and norepinephrine due to autonomous functioning of the tumor. The clinical manifestations of a pheochromocytoma include persistent hypertension associated with flushing, diaphoresis, tachycardia, palpitations, and constipation. Hypermetabolism may develop because of stimulation of the thyroid gland by the catechol-amines. Glucose intolerance may occur because of catecholamine-induced inhibition of insulin release by the pancreas.

The usual treatment of pheochromocytoma is surgical excision of the tumor. Medical therapy with adrenergic blocking agents is used to stabilize blood pressure prior to surgery.

Practice Examination

1. Which laboratory values would be expected in an individual with SIADH?

   a. serum sodium = 150 mEq/L and urine hypoosmolality
   b. serum potassium = 5 mEq/L and serum hypoosmolality
   c. serum sodium = 120 mEq/L and urine hypoosmolality
   d. serum potassium = 3 mEq/L and serum hyperosmolality

2. Hypopituitarism in an adult male likely includes all of the following except:

   a. dwarfism.
   b. impotence.
   c. muscular mass decrease.
   d. skin pallor.

3. Excessive secretion of GH in an adult may cause:

   a. acromegaly.
   b. giantism.
   c. hypoglycemia.
   d. decreased metabolic rate.

4. A characteristic shared by both diabetes mellitus and diabetes insipidus is:

   a. elevated blood and urine glucose levels.
   b. inability to produce ADH.
   c. inability to produce insulin.
   d. polyuria.
   e. elevated blood urine and ketone body levels.

5. The manifestations of hyperthyroidism include all of the following except:

   a. diarrhea.
   b. constipation.
   c. heat intolerance.
   d. weight loss.
   e. wakefulness.

6. Hypothyroidism crisis is:

   a. myxedema coma.
   b. Addison disease.
   c. Cushing disease.
   d. Graves disease.
   e. cretinism.

7. Graves disease is:

   a. hyperthyroidism.
   b. associated with autoimmunity.
   c. manifested by ophthalmopathy.
   d. All of the above are correct.

8. Inadequate levels of thyroid hormones at birth may cause:

   a. CNS abnormalities.
   b. immediate death.
   c. thyroid crisis.
   d. myxedema.
   e. dwarfism.

9. Hyperparathyroidism causes:

   a. increased osteoclastic activity.
   b. decreased plasma calcium.
   c. increased phosphorus absorption from GI tract.
   d. hypocalcemia.

10. A manifestation of hypocalcemia is:

    a. myopathy.
    b. lethargy.
    c. hypertension.
    d. tetany.
    e. bone cysts.

11. What is the most common cause of acromegaly?

    a. anterior pituitary adenoma
    b. overproduction of ACTH
    c. overproduction of TSH
    d. pituitary atrophy

12. If a 19-year-old woman were suffering from shortness of breath, weight loss, excessive sweating, exophthalmos, and irritability, which hormone would you expect to find elevated in her serum?

    a. cortisol
    b. thyroxine
    c. ACTH
    d. 17-ketosteroid

13. A 24-year-old female with a history of "juvenile-onset" diabetes is found in a stuporous state. She is hypotensive and has cold, clammy skin. What is the likely etiology of her condition?

    a. hyperglycemia
    b. insulin reaction
    c. renal failure
    d. peripheral neuropathy

14. A 10-year-old male came into the emergency room comatose, suffering from metabolic acidosis and blood glucose of 800 mg/dl. The most probable disease is:

    a. cretinism.
    b. IDDM.
    c. NIDDM.
    d. IGT.
    e. GDM.

15. Your neighbor has not previously been diabetic but has gained 80 pounds in the past year and is able to produce some insulin. Her fasting blood sugar is always elevated. She is being treated with oral insulin-stimulating drugs. This likely is:

    a. diabetes insipidus.
    b. IDDM.
    c. NIDDM.
    d. IGT.
    e. GDM.

16. Common symptoms and signs of diabetes mellitus include all of the following except:

    a. hyperglycemia.
    b. blurred vision.
    c. increased muscle anabolism.
    d. persistent infection.
    e. polyuria.

17. Which laboratory finding is inconsistent with a diagnosis of insulin-dependent diabetes mellitus (IDDM)?

    a. FBS (fasting blood sugar) of 90 mg/dl
    b. ketonuria
    c. blood glucose of 210 mg/dl after one hour following ingestion of 100 gm glucose
    d. decreased serum insulin level
    e. All of the above are consistent with IDDM.

18. Common complications to diabetes mellitus include all of the following except:

    a. retinopathy.
    b. peripheral neuropathy.
    c. nephropathy (kidney disease).
    d. None of the above is common.
    e. All of the above are common.

19. An individual with type I diabetes mellitus experiences hunger, lightheadedness, headache, confusion, and tachycardia while cross-country running. The likely cause of these manifestations is:

    a. hyperglycemia.
    b. eating a snack before running.
    c. hypoglycemia because of running.
    d. Both a and b are correct.
    e. None of the above is correct.

20. Which is expected during hyperinsulinism?

    a. excess insulin
    b. high serum glucose
    c. epinephrine release
    d. All of the above are correct.
    e. Both a and c are correct.

21. Long-term corticosteroid therapy may cause which of the following? (*More than one answer may be correct.*)

    a. delayed wound healing
    b. osteoporosis
    c. peptic ulcers
    d. hyperkalemia

22. Which electrolyte changes occur in Addison disease?

    a. hypokalemia
    b. hypernatremia
    c. hyponatremia
    d. hypocalcemia

23. A benign tumor of adrenal glands which causes hypersecretion of aldosterone is:

    a. Addison disease.
    b. a pheochromocytoma.
    c. Cushing disease.
    d. Cushing syndrome.
    e. Conn disease.

Match the hypersecretion with the circumstance.

24. ____ hypersecretion of aldosterone

25. ____ hypersecretion of glucocorticoids

a. decreased cardiac output

b. hyperglycemia and/or osteoporosis

c. BMR (basal metabolic rate) increases

d. hypernatremia

e. hyponatremia

Case Study

Scott, a 17-year-old high school football player, was brought to the hospital emergency room in a coma. According to his mother, he had lost weight during the last month in spite of eating large amounts of food. Besides losing weight, he was excessively thirsty and had frequently awakened his younger brother as he noisily voided several times during the night. The family history revealed others with diabetes mellitus. Physical examination was not significant except for tachycardia and hyperpnea.

Laboratory serum studies revealed:

Glucose on admission = 1000 mg/dl (high)
pH = 7.25 (low)
pCO_2 = 30 mm Hg (low)
HCO_3^- = 12 mEq/L (low)
Glycosylated hemoglobin = 9% (high)

What do you think Scott's symptoms, signs, and diagnostic studies suggest?

CHAPTER 18

Structure and Function of the Hematologic System

Objectives

After review of this chapter, the learner will be able to:

1. **Identify the constituents of blood plasma.**
   Review page 509; refer to Table 18-1.

2. **Identify the structural characteristics, normal values, and functions of the cellular elements of blood.**
   Review pages 509-512; refer to Figures 18-1 through 18-4 and Table 18-2.

3. **Describe lymphoid organs and the mononuclear phagocyte system; note the effects of colony-stimulating factors (CSFs).**
   Review pages 513-516; refer to Figure 18-5 and Table 18-3.

4. **Describe hematopoiesis and erythropoiesis and identify the CSFs and the nutritional requirements necessary for these processes.**
   Review pages 516-523; refer to Figures 18-6 through 18-11 and Tables 18-4 through 18-6.

5. **Describe the mechanisms and the sequence of events in hemostasis.**
   Review pages 523-526; refer to Figures 18-12 through 18-15.

6. **Diagram the fibrinolytic system.**
   Review pages 526-527; refer to Figure 18-16.

7. **Identify various hematologic values at different ages.**
   Refer to Table 18-7.

Practice Examination

1. Which does not constitute a plasma component?

   a. colloids
   b. electrolytes
   c. gases
   d. glucose
   e. platelets

2. Which is the most abundant protein in blood plasma?

   a. fibrinogen
   b. albumins
   c. globulins
   d. immunoglobulins
   e. hormones

3. A fragment of megakaryocyte cytoplasm is the:

   a. reticulocyte.
   b. normoblast.
   c. promyelocyte.
   d. proerythroblast.
   e. platelet.

4. The progenitor of granulocytes is a:

   a. pronormoblast.
   b. promegakaryocyte.
   c. prolymphoblast.
   d. myeloblast.

5. Identify the correct sequence in the development of erythrocytes.

   a. polychromatophilic erythroblast, normoblast, reticulocyte
   b. normoblast, reticulocyte, basophilic erythroblast
   c. normoblast, committed proerythroblast, reticulocyte
   d. normoblast, basophilic erythroblast, reticulocyte

6. A differential count of WBCs includes all of the following except:

   a. granulocytes.
   b. agranulocytes.
   c. reticulocytes.
   d. monocytes.
   e. lymphocytes.

7. The purpose of erythropoietin is to:

   a. decrease maturation of erythroblasts.
   b. detect hypoxia.
   c. control erythrocyte production.
   d. control the size of platelets.

8. The normal platelet count/mm^3 of blood is about:

   a. 4-10 $\times$ 10^3.
   b. 50-100 $\times$ 10^3.
   c. 150-300 $\times$ 10^3.
   d. 5 $\times$ 10^6.
   e. 150-300 $\times$ 10^6.

9. About how many times more RBCs than WBCs are there in a mm^3 of blood?

   a. 15
   b. 90
   c. 100
   d. 1000
   e. None of the above is correct.

10. If the total leukocytic count of an individual was 7000/mm^3, about how many neutrophils would normally be present in a mm^3 of blood?

   a. 400
   b. 700
   c. 2100
   d. 3000
   e. 4200

11. Which granulocyte functions in antibody-mediated defense against parasites?

   a. lymphocytes
   b. monocytes
   c. neutrophils
   d. eosinophils
   e. basophils

12. Erythropoietin:

   a. is secreted by the kidney.
   b. is a glycoprotein.
   c. causes recycling of iron for production of RBCs.
   d. is released by the kidney to stimulate erythrocyte and platelet formation.
   e. Both a and b are correct.

13. Which is not an agranulocyte?

   a. basophil
   b. lymphocyte
   c. monocyte
   d. reticulocyte
   e. Both a and d are correct.

14. Which are the most effective phagocytes?

   a. neutrophils and basophils
   b. lymphocytes and eosinophils
   c. basophils and monocytes
   d. neutrophils and monocytes
   e. None of the above is correct.

15. Which vitamins are needed for erythropoiesis?

a. C and E
b. B_2 and B_{12}
c. A and D
d. Both a and b are correct.
e. a, b, and c are correct.

Match the colony-stimulating factor with the cell that is stimulated.

16. ____ IL-3
17. ____ G-CSF

a. erythrocytes
b. macrophage, neutrophil
c. neutrophil, eosinophil, and basophil
d. normoblast
e. erythroblast

18. Which is not used to measure RBC indices?

a. differential count
b. reticulocyte count
c. erythrocyte count
d. hemoglobin determination

19. Which test reflects bone marrow activity?

a. reticulocyte count
b. hemoglobin mean
c. hematocrit mean
d. g/dl

20. As an individual ages:

a. the erythrocyte life span is shortened.
b. lymphocytic function decreases.
c. platelet numbers decrease.
d. All of the above are correct.

21. Hemostasis involves all of the following except:

a. vasoconstriction.
b. platelet plug formation.
c. intrinsic pathway activities.
d. clot formation.
e. erythropoiesis.

22. When a blood vessel is damaged:

a. subendothelial collagen is exposed.
b. platelets are attracted to collagen.
c. platelets degranulate.
d. Both a and b are correct.
e. a, b, and c are correct.

23. The biochemical mediators released by adhering platelets cause:

    a. vasodilation of the injured vessel.
    b. vasoconstriction of the injured vessel.
    c. the inflammatory process to proceed.
    d. All of the above are correct.

24. Which is a correct sequence in coagulation?

    a. X, tissue thromboplastin, XA
    b. prothrombin activator complex, X, XA
    c. fibrinogen, thrombin, stabilizer fibrin
    d. damaged tissue, tissue thromboplastin, X

25. Which is a correct sequence in fibrinolysis?

    a. fibrin, plasminogen
    b. FDP, fibrinogen
    c. plasminogen, XIIa
    d. plasmin, fibrin

CHAPTER

19

Alterations of Hematologic Function

Foundational Objectives

a. Identify the differentiation sequence, function, and normal values for erythrocytes. Review pages 509-518; refer to Figures 18-6, 18-7, and 18-10 and Table 18-2.

Memory Check!

Differentiation of Erythrocytes

Uncommitted Pluripotential Stem Cell

↓ ← Erythropoietin

Proerythroblast (Very large nucleus)

↓

Basophilic Erythroblast (Hemoglobin synthesis begins)

↓

Intermediate Polychromatic Erythroblast
(Last stage of DNA synthesis and cell division, hemoglobin synthesis continues)

↓

Orthochromatic Normoblast
(The nucleus shrinks and undergoes autolysis and resorption, additional hemoglobin is synthesized)

↓

Reticulocyte
(Larger than mature RBC, no nucleus, enters vascular circulation of the bone marrow by diapedesis)

↓

Erythrocyte
(Reticulum of the nucleus resorbed, disk shape achieved)

- The function of erythrocytes is to transport gas to and from the tissue cells and lungs. The normal adult range of values for erythrocytes is:

Number = 4.2-6.2 million/mm^3

Hematocrit = 42-48%

Hemoglobin = 12-16.5 g/dl

Note: Reticulocytes normally comprise less than 1 percent of the RBCs found in blood.

(Continued)

Memory Check! (cont'd)

- The rate of erythropoiesis or formation of RBCs is measured by the reticulocyte count. A low count may indicate the inability of bone marrow to respond. A high count may indicate a good marrow response to low numbers of RBCs. Erythropoietin is secreted by the kidney in response to tissue hypoxia from anemia, high altitude, or pulmonary disease. Erythropoietin stimulates proliferation of stem cells in the marrow and accelerates maturation of erythroblasts.

b. Identify the differentiation sequence for granulocytes, agranulocytes, and platelets. Refer to Figure 18-6 and Tables 18-2 and 18-7.

Memory Check!

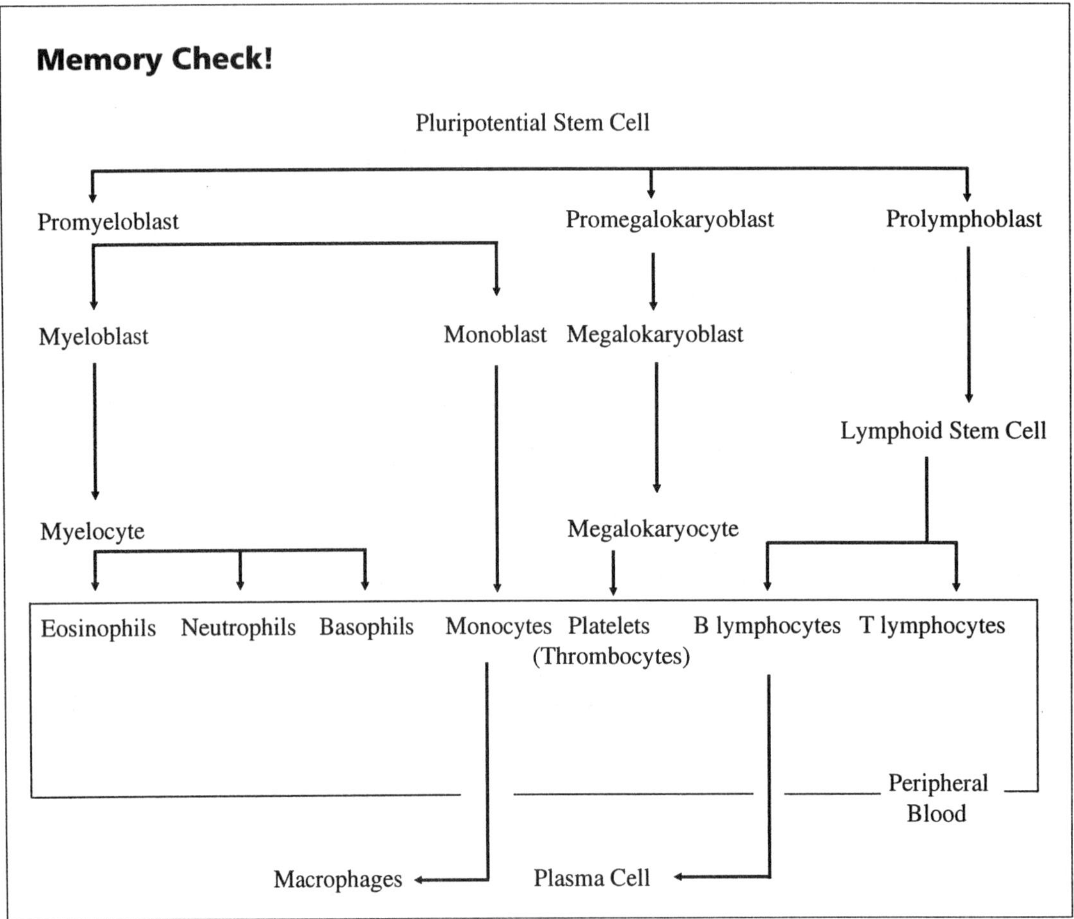

c. Identify the normal numbers in circulating blood, the function, and the life span of leukocytes and platelets. Refer to Table 18-2.

Memory Check!

Cellular Components of the Blood

Cell	Normal Amounts in	Function	Life Span
Leukocyte	5,000-10,000/mm^3	Bodily defense mechanisms	
Lymphocyte	25% to 33% of leukocytes	Immunity	Days or years
Monocyte and macrophage	3% to 7% of leukocytes	Phagocytosis, mononuclear phagocyte system	Months or years
Eosinophil	1% to 4% of leukocytes	Phagocytosis, antibody-mediated defense against parasites, allergic reactions, recovery phase of infection	Unknown
Neutrophil	57% to 67% of leukocytes	Phagocytosis, particularly during early phase of inflammation/infection	4 days
Basophil	0% to 0.75% of leukocytes	Unknown, but associated with allergic reactions and mechanical irritation	Unknown
Platelet	140,000-340,000/mm^3	Hemostasis following vascular injury, normal coagulation and clot formation/reactions	8 to 11 days

d. Briefly summarize the coagulation cascade and the fibrinolytic system. Refer to Figures 18-15 and 18-16.

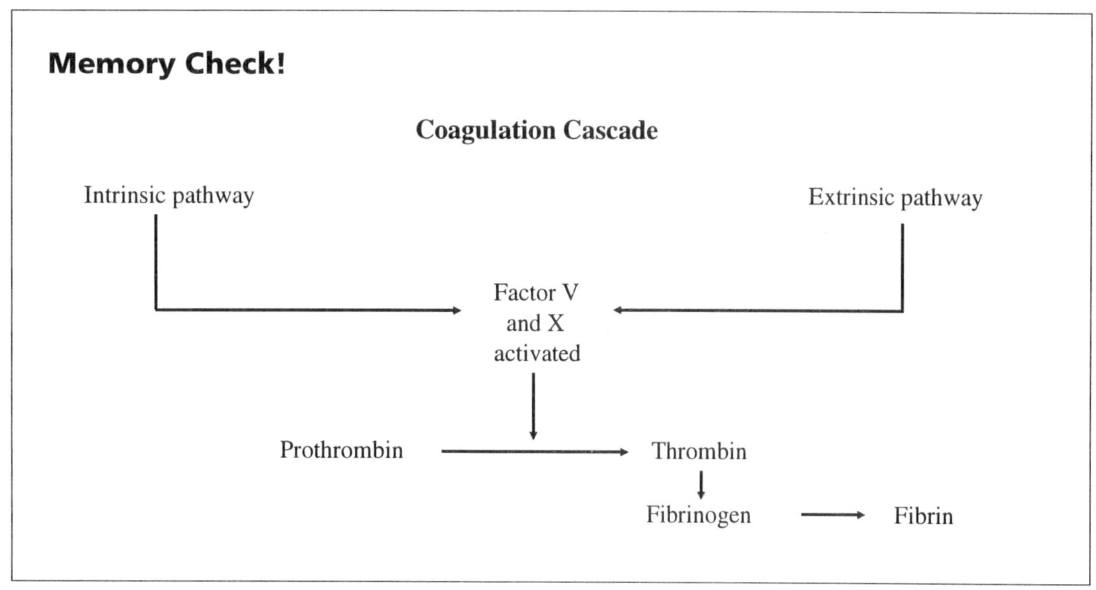

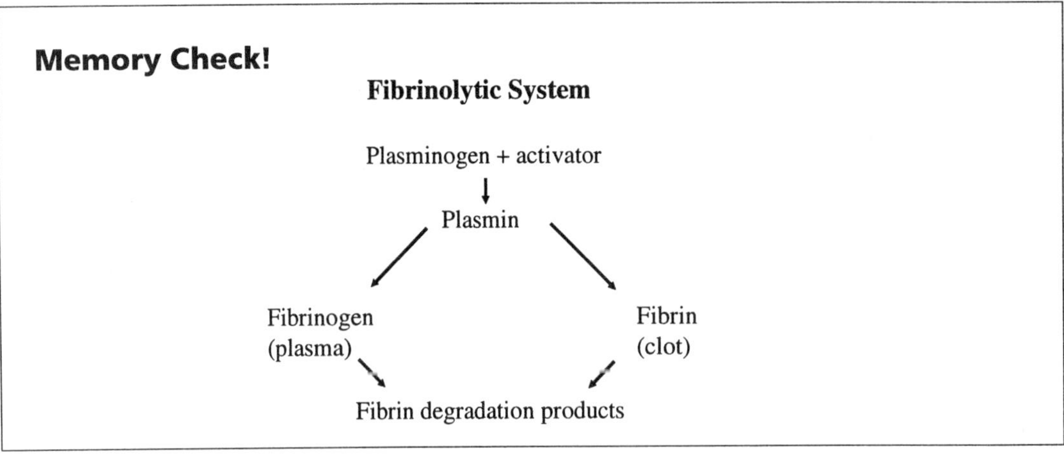

Objectives

After studying this chapter, the learner will be able to:

1. **Define and classify anemia.**
   Study page 533; refer to Figure 19-1 and Tables 19-1 through 19-3.

Anemia is a reduction in the total number of circulating erythrocytes or a decrease in the quality or quantity of hemoglobin. Anemic conditions are usually a result of impaired erythrocyte production, blood loss, increased erythrocyte destruction, or a combination of the three.

Whether there is decreased/defective production or destruction of erythrocytes, anemias are classified according to their **etiologic basis** or **morphologic appearance**. Descriptions of anemias based on erythrocyte cellular structure refer to the cell's size and hemoglobin content. The morphologic classification is widely used. Terms that refer to cellular size end with "cytic." Terms that describe hemoglobin content end with "chromic." An erythrocyte can be **macrocytic**, meaning abnormally large, or **microcytic**, meaning abnormally small, and **hyperchromic**, containing an unusually high concentration of hemoglobin within its cytoplasm, or **hypochromic**, containing an abnormally low concentration of hemoglobin. For comparison, cells of normal size are termed **normocytic** and cells with normal amounts of hemoglobin are termed **normochromic**. In some anemias, the erythrocytes take on various sizes or they have various shapes; this is **anisocytosis** and **poikilocytosis**, respectively.

2. **Describe the pathophysiology of the clinical manifestations of anemias.**
   Study page 533.

Compensation for reduced oxygen-carrying capacity of the blood requires the cardiovascular, respiratory, and hematologic systems to respond. A reduction in the number of circulating erythrocytes after hemorrhage affects the consistency and volume of the blood. To compensate for reduced blood volume, fluids from the interstitium move into the blood vessels and plasma volume expands. The thinner, less viscous blood flows faster and more turbulently than normal blood. Increased blood flow within the heart can cause ventricular dysfunction, cardiac dilation, and heart valve insufficiency.

Hypoxia of anemia causes arterioles, capillaries, and venules to dilate, which speeds blood flow even more. As venous return to the heart increases, the heart must pump harder and faster to meet normal oxygen demand and to prevent cardiopulmonary congestion. Congestive heart failure can develop.

Tissue hypoxia also causes the rate and depth of breathing to increase in an attempt to make more oxygen available to the remaining erythrocytes. When anemia is severe or sudden in onset, peripheral blood vessels constrict to direct available blood flow to the vital organs. A number of systemic symptoms occur subsequent to this shunting of blood.

Decreased blood flow is sensed by the kidneys, and in an effort to improve kidney perfusion, the renal renin-angiotensin response is activated. This results in salt and water retention, causing increased workload for the heart. The individual will experience shortness of breath or dyspnea, a rapid pounding heartbeat, dizziness, and fatigue even when at rest.

The skin, mucous membranes, lips, nailbeds, and conjunctivae become pale due to reduced hemoglobin concentration or yellowish due to accumulation in the skin of products of red blood cell breakdown or hemolysis. Decreased oxygen delivery to the skin results in impaired healing and loss of elasticity. Thinning and early graying of the hair can occur.

If the anemia is due to vitamin B_{12} deficiency, the nervous system is affected. Myelin degeneration may occur with loss of nerve fibers in the spinal cord. Paresthesias, gait disturbances, extreme weakness, spasticity, and reflex abnormalities may then result.

Decreased oxygen supply to the gastrointestinal tract often produces abdominal pain, nausea, vomiting, and anorexia. Low-grade fever, less than 101° F, occurs in some anemic individuals and may be the result of leukocytic pyrogens being released from ischemic tissues. Therapeutic intervention for any anemic condition requires treatment of the underlying disorder and palliation of symptoms. Therapies for anemia include transfusions, dietary corrections, and administration of supplemental vitamins or iron.

3. Develop a comparative chart of the macrocytic-normochromic, microcytic-hypochromic, and normocytic-normochromic anemias.

Study pages 533-540; refer to Tables 19-1 through 19-3.

Anemias

Anemia	Etiology	High-Risk Groups	Symptoms
	Macrocytic-normochromic		
Pernicious	Insufficient influence of vitamin B_{12} on developing cells because of deficient IF, antibodies develop against parietal cells, gastrectomy or ilectomy therapies, chronic gastritis	Anglo-Saxon and Scandinavian populations	*Typical, digestive symptoms from lack of HC1 and enzymes, glossitis, peripheral neuropathy: tingling numbness, loss of vibratory sense
Folate (folic acid)	Dietary deficiency inhibits DNA synthesis	Alcoholics, chronically malnourished	*Typical, similar to pernicious except no neurologic disorders
	Microcytic-hypochromic		
Iron deficiency	Excessive bleeding which depletes iron, poor diet, no meat	Profuse menstruation, adolescents, children, minor blood loss, elderly	*Typical
Sideroblastic	Dysfunctional iron uptake by erythroblasts, decreased heme synthesis, enzymes, etc., genetic	Acquired from drugs: ethanol, lead, chloramphenicol,	*Typical, mild hepatomegaly and splenomegaly
Thalassemia	Genetics, persistence of fetal hemoglobin (HbF) after birth, phagocytosis of cell	Italians, Greeks	*Typical

(Continued)

Anemias (cont'd)

Anemia	Etiology	High-Risk Groups	Symptoms
	Normocytic-normochromic		
Aplastic	Radiation, drugs, lesions within red bone marrow, immune response that halts erythropoiesis	Anyone	*Typical, infection, bleeding
Post-hemorrhagic	Sudden blood loss	Surgery, trauma	Shock, acidosis
Hemolytic	Premature dysfunction of mature erythrocytes in circulation, genetics result in fragile cells, acquired from infections, drugs, IgG of warm or cold, IgM, antibodies	Anyone	Splenomegaly, jaundice
Chronic inflammation	Bacterial toxins, cytokines from activated macrophages and lymphocytes, reduced iron in blood	AIDS, autoimmunity, neoplasms	Mild because of disability caused by chronic condition
Sickle cell	Genetic trait causes abnormal hemoglobin and increased lysis of sickled cells	8% of African Americans	*Typical, develop during heavy exercise

* *typical symptoms and signs: fatigue, weakness, dyspnea, pallor*

4. Describe the types, causes, manifestations, and treatment of polycythemia vera.
Study pages 540-541; refer to Table 19-4.

Polycythemia vera is an unusual disease that causes excessively large numbers of erythrocytes in the blood. It is typically accompanied by increased circulating platelets and granulocytes. There are essentially two types of polycythemia vera: primary or absolute and secondary or relative. The primary form of polycythemia vera is relatively rare and tends to occur in men between the ages of 40 and 60 of Jewish or European ancestry. Rarely is polycythemia vera found in children or multiple members of a single family. The cause of secondary polycythemia, the more common form, is essentially a physiologic response to hypoxia. It is not uncommon to find an increased red cell count in individuals living at high altitudes, in smokers, and in individuals with congestive heart failure or chronic obstructive pulmonary disease.

The clinical signs of polycythemia vera include ruddy, red color of the face, hands, feet, ears, and mucous membranes; engorgement of retinal and sublingual veins; elevated blood pressure; splenomegaly; and hepatomegaly. Symptoms include headache, a feeling of fullness in the head, dizziness, weakness, itching, sweating, epigastric distress, fatigue on exertion, backache, and visual disturbances. The clinical manifestations of vascular disease likely predominate. Angina pectoris, calf pain associated with vasospasms during walking, thrombosis, and cerebral insufficiency can occur.

Treatment for polycythemia vera consists of reducing erythrocytosis and blood volume, controlling symptoms, and preventing thrombosis. Erythrocytosis and blood volume are reduced by phlebotomy, wherein a vein is opened and blood is removed according to need. Smokers should be urged to quit, and patients with congestive heart failure and chronic obstructive pulmonary disease require appropriate pharmaceutical intervention.

5. Describe terms associated with high or low leukocyte counts and the causes of the alterations.
Study pages 541-544; refer to Tables 19-5 and 19-6.

Leukocytosis exists when the leukocyte count is higher than normal; leukopenia is a condition in which the leukocyte count is lower than normal. Leukocytosis is a normal, protective response to invading microorganisms, strenuous exercise, emotional changes, temperature changes, anesthesia, surgery, pregnancy, some drugs, hormones, and toxins. Malignancies and hematologic disorders also cause leukocytosis. Increased levels of circulating neutrophils, eosinophils, basophils, and monocytes are chiefly a physiologic response to infection. Elevations can also occur as a result of polycythemia vera and chronic myelocytic leukemia that increase stem cell proliferation in the bone marrow.

Leukopenia is never beneficial. As the leukocyte count falls below 1000 per cubic millimeter, the individual is at risk for infection. The risk for very serious life-threatening infections develops with counts below 500/mm3. Leukopenia can be caused by radiation, anaphylactic shock, systemic lupus erythematosus, and certain chemotherapeutic agents. Decreased leukocytic counts occur when infectious processes delete the circulating granulocytes and monocytes. Infectious agents draw them out of the circulation and into infected tissues faster than they can be replaced. Decreases can also be caused by disorders that suppress marrow function.

Granulocytosis or **neutrophilia** is prevalent in the early stages of infection or inflammation when stored neutrophils from the venous sinuses are released into the circulating blood. Emptying of the venous sinuses stimulates granulopoiesis to replenish normal stores of granulocytes in the marrow. **Neutropenia**, or low neutrophilic count, may be caused by decreased or ineffective neutrophil production because the marrow is producing other formed elements. Also, autoimmunity, reduced neutrophil survival, and abnormal neutrophil distribution and sequestration in tissues lead to neutropenia. When the demand for neutrophils exceeds the circulatory supply, the marrow releases immature neutrophils and other leukocytes into the blood; this is called a **shift to the left**. The shift to the left is sometimes called a leukemoid reaction because the morphologic findings in blood smears are similar to those of individuals with leukemia. As infection or inflammation diminishes and granulopoiesis replenishes the circulating granulocytes, a **shift to the right** or back to normal occurs. Neutropenia exists when the neutrophil count is less than $2000/mm^3$. If neutrophils are reduced to below $500/mm^3$ and the entire granulocyte count is extremely low, a very serious condition called **agranulocytosis** results. The usual cause of agranulocytosis is interference with hematopoiesis in the bone marrow or increased cell destruction in the circulation. Chemotherapeutic agents used in the treatment of hematologic and other malignancies and some drugs cause bone marrow suppression. Clinical manifestations of agranulocytosis include respiratory infection, general malaise, septicemia, fever, tachycardia, and ulcers in the mouth and colon. If untreated, sepsis caused by agranulocytosis can result in death within three to six days.

Eosinophilia is an absolute increase in the total numbers of circulating eosinophils. Allergic disorders associated with asthma, hay fever, parasitic invasion, and drug reactions are frequently the cause of eosinophilia. Chemotactic factor of anaphylaxis (CTF-A) and histamine released from mast cells attract eosinophils to the area. **Eosinopenia** is a decrease in circulating eosinophils generally due to migration of eosinophils into inflammatory sites. It may also be seen in Cushing syndrome as a result of stress due to surgery, shock, trauma, burns, or mental distress.

Basophilia is quite rare and is generally seen as a response to inflammation and hypersensitivity reactions of the immediate type. An increase in basophils is also seen in chronic myeloid leukemia and myeloid metaplasia. **Basopenia** is seen in hyperthyroidism, acute infection, and long-term therapy with steroids, as well as during ovulation and pregnancy.

Monocytosis, an increase in monocytes, is often transient and correlates poorly with disease states. When present, it is most commonly associated with bacterial infections during the late stages of recovery when needed to phagocytize any surviving microorganisms and debris. Monocytosis is seen in chronic infections such as tuberculosis and subacute bacterial endocarditis. **Monocytopenia**, a decrease in monocytes, is rare but has been identified with hairy cell leukemia and prednisone therapy.

A **lymphocytosis** is rare in acute bacterial infections and occurs most often in acute viral infections, especially those caused by the Epstein-Barr virus (EBV). **Lymphocytopenia** may be associated with neoplasias, immune deficiencies, and destruction by drugs. It may be that the lymphocytopenia associated with heart failure and other acute illnesses is caused by elevated levels of cortisol. Lymphocytopenia is a major problem in AIDS. The lymphocytopenia seen with this condition is caused by the HIV virus, which is cytopathic for T-helper lymphocytes.

6. Describe the pathogenesis of infectious mononucleosis.
Study page 544.

Infectious mononucleosis is an acute infection of B lymphocytes. The most common etiologic virus is the Epstein-Barr virus (EBV); however, cytomegalovirus (CMV) and other viruses as well as *Toxoplasma gondii* have been identified as causative agents for this disease.

Infectious mononucleosis usually affects young adults between the ages of 15 and 30. The proliferation of clones of B and T cells and removal of dead and damaged leukocytes are largely responsible for the swelling of cervical lymphoid tissues. The incubation period for infectious mononucleosis is approximately 30 to 50 days. The accompanying sore throat is caused by inflammation at the site of viral entry. Splenomegaly occurs in about one-half of affected individuals.

Laboratory findings include an increase in relative and absolute lymphocyte and monocyte counts with 10 to 20 percent being atypical in form. The atypical lymphocytes are large with oval, horseshoe-shaped or indented nuclei and vacuolated, spongy cytoplasm. During the first week of infection, the leukocyte count may be normal or slightly low. After the first week, the leukocyte count, which is predominantly lymphocytes and monocytes, rises to 10,000 to 20,000 per cubic millimeter and persists at this level from four to eight weeks. Platelet counts are low.

Infectious mononucleosis is usually self-limiting with recovery occurring in few weeks. Treatment consists of rest and alleviation of symptoms with analgesics.

7. Classify, contrast, and describe the manfestations of leukemia.
Study pages 545-547; refer to Figures 19-2 and 19-4.

Leukemia is a malignant disorder of the blood and blood-forming organs, exhibiting an uncontrolled proliferation of dysfunctional leukocytes. The excessive proliferation of leukemic cells crowds the bone marrow and causes decreased production and function of normal hematopoietic cells.

The two major forms of leukemia are acute and chronic. They are classified by predominant cell type; the type is named according to the point of arrested cell maturation. Acute leukemia is characterized by undifferentiated immature or blastic cells. The onset of disease is abrupt and rapid, and the affected individual has a short survival time. In chronic leukemia, the predominant cell appears mature but does not function normally. The onset of disease is gradual and the prolonged clinical course results in a relatively longer survival time. Leukemia occurs with varying frequencies at different ages and is about ten times more frequent in adults than in children in the United States.

Causal risk factors acting together with a genetic predisposition can alter nuclear DNA of a single cell, and then the leukemic cell proliferates. The leukemic cell is unable to mature and respond to normal regulatory mechanisms. Abnormal chromosomes are reported in 40 to 50 percent of patients with acute leukemia. Studies indicate a significant tendency for leukemia to recur in families. Hereditary abnormalities are also associated with an increased incidence of leukemia.

Acquired disorders that progress to acute leukemia include chronic myelocytic leukemia (CML), polycythemia vera, Hodgkin disease, multiple myeloma, ovarian cancer, chronic lymphocytic leukemia (CLL), and sideroblastic anemia. Large doses of ionizing radiation also are associated with an increased incidence in myelogenous leukemia. Drugs such as chloramphenicol and certain alkylating agents cause bone marrow depression and also can predispose an individual to leukemia. Acute myelogenous leukemia (AML) is the most frequently reported secondary cancer following high doses of chemotherapy used for some other cancers.

Leukemias

Variable	Myelogenous AML or ANLL	CML	Lymphocytic ALL	CLL
Age	Adults or children	Adults, < 50 years of age	Children	Adults, > 50 years of age
Onset	Acute	Gradual	Acute	Gradual
Sign/symptoms	Pallor, petechial hemorrhage, lymphadenopathy	Splenomegaly, hepatomegaly, Philadelphia chromosome	Same as AML or ANLL	Splenomegaly, hepatomegaly, lymphadenopathy
Presence of blasts	High	Low	High	Rare
Treatment	Chemotherapy, marrow transplants	No cure: chemotherapy, marrow transplants	Chemotherapy, marrow transplants	No cure: chemotherapy, marrow transplants
Survival	Days to months	Months to years	Months (untreated) Years (treated)	Years

8. Differentiate multiple myeloma from the leukemias.
Study pages 547-549; refer to Figure 19-3.

Multiple myeloma is a B cell cancer arising from a hematopoietic stem cell that is associated with mature plasma cell structure and function. This disorder likely originates in the bone marrow and moves through the circulation to lymph nodes. The nodes are required for their cellular development. Subsequently, the neoplastic cells return to the bone marrow or soft tissue sites. Development of myeloma is governed by cytokines; IL-6 is likely the major myeloma growth factor.

Multiple Myeloma/Common Leukemias

Characteristic	Multiple Myeloma	Common Leukemias
Malignant proliferation of WBC in the bone marrow	Yes	Yes
Anemia	Yes	Yes
Bleeding	Yes	Yes
Recurrent infections	Yes	Yes
Plasma cells	Yes	No
Ineffective immunoglobulins	Yes	No
Bence-Jones protein in urine	Yes	No
Pathologic bone fractures	Yes	No
WBC blood elevation	No	Yes
Osteocytic lesions	Yes	Possible
Elevated calcium serum	Yes	Possible
Bone pain	Yes	Possible
Renal disease	Yes	Possible

Chemotherapy, radiation therapy, plasmapheresis, and marrow transplant have been used for treatment. With chemotherapy and aggressive management of complications, a median survival of 24 to 30 months and a ten-year survival rate of 3 percent can be achieved.

9. Compare Hodgkin disease and non-Hodgkin lymphomas.
Study pages 549-553; refer to Figures 19-5 through 19-8 and Table 19-7.

Lymphomas are tumors of (1) primary lymphoid tissue or the thymus and bone marrow and (2) secondary lymphoid tissue or lymph nodes, spleen, tonsils, and intestinal lymphoid tissue. Most lymphomas are neoplasms of secondary lymphoid tissue involving mostly lymph nodes and/or spleen. The major types of malignant lymphomas are **Hodgkin disease** and **non-Hodgkin lymphoma.** Bone marrow involvement occurs more often in non-Hodgkin lymphoma than in Hodgkin disease. Hodgkin disease uses one of four histologic types for classification. Non-Hodgkin lymphoma has several classifications that eventually may become standardized into three types having histologic subdivisions within each type.

Malignant Lymphomas

Variable	Hodgkin	Non-Hodgkin
Cause	Unknown: herpes virus, Epstein-Barr virus	Unknown: immunosuppression
Cellular deviation	*Monocyte-macrophage (Reed-Sternberg cells), T cells	B cells
Age of onset	2 peaks 20s and 30s 60s and 70s	> 50
Nodes involved	Cervical, inguinal, axillary, retroperitoneal	Cervical, axillary, inguinal, femoral
Extranodal involvement	Uncommon	More common
Symptoms	Painless mass, fever, night sweats, weakness, weight loss	Similar to Hodgkin plus pleural effusion, abdominal pain, splenomegaly
Curability	> 75%	< 25%
Treatment	Radiotherapy or surgery for localized, chemotherapy for generalized for both lymphomas	

** Reed-Sternberg cell is a malignant tissue macrophage that is scattered among normal cells.*

10. Describe thrombocytopenia and thrombocytosis.
Study pages 554-555.

Thrombocytopenia exists when the platelet count is below 100,000 platelets per cubic millimeter of blood. Hemorrhage from minor trauma can occur with counts of 50,000 or less. Spontaneous bleeding can occur with counts between 20,000 and 10,000. Severe bleeding results if the count is below 10,000. Such bleeding can be fatal if it occurs in the gastrointestinal tract, respiratory system, or central nervous system.

Primary idiopathic thrombocytopenic purpura (ITP) may be either acute or chronic. It is thought to be an autoimmune disorder in which an IgG autoantibody is formed that binds to and destroys the platelets. The acute form is most common in children and young adults and is usually preceded by a viral infection. Chronic ITP is more common in females between the ages of 10 and 50. The individual most commonly presents with mucosal or skin bleeding, which often is manifested as menorrhagia, purpura, and petechiae.

Secondary thrombocytopenia is caused by conditions associated with drug hypersensitivities that produce antibodies, viral and bacterial infections, and some autoimmune conditions. Viruses inhibit platelet production, destroy circulating platelets, or form viral antigen-antibody complexes.

Thrombocytosis has a platelet count greater than 400,000 per cubic millimeter of blood. Transient thrombocytosis is a normal, physiologic response to stress, infection, trauma, exercise, and ovulation. It is usually asymptomatic until the count exceeds 1 million/mm^3. Then, intravascular clot formation or thrombosis, hemorrhage, or other abnormalities can occur.

Primary thrombocytosis is a myeloproliferative disorder in which megakaryocytes in the marrow are produced in excess. Clinical manifestations of primary thrombocytosis include thrombosis of peripheral blood vessels or, in severe cases, thrombosis of hepatic, mesenteric, or pulmonary vessels. Splenomegaly and easy bruising also occur. In individuals with thrombotic and hemorrhagic complications, the platelet count is lowered by use of chemotherapy agents or phlebotomy.

Secondary thrombocytosis occurs following splenectomy because platelets that normally would be stored in the spleen remain in circulating blood. Secondary thrombocytosis may be seen in conjunction with hemolytic anemias and some polycythemias or as a compensation following thrombocytopenia.

11. Identify the causes of coagulation disorders; characterize disseminated intravascular coagulation.
Study pages 555-557; refer to Figure 19-9.

Disorders of coagulation are usually caused by defects or deficiencies of one or more of the clotting factors. Two common inherited disorders are the **hemophilias** and von Willebrand disease. These are caused by deficiencies of clotting factors. The hemophilias lack the clotting factors VIII and IX, while **von Willebrand** has low levels of factor VIII and impaired platelet function. The partial thromboplastin time (PTT), which measures the intrinsic pathway, likely would be prolonged.

Other coagulation defects are acquired and usually result from deficient synthesis of clotting factors by an impaired liver. A deficiency of vitamin K, which is necessary for normal synthesis of the clotting factors by the liver, is an acquired coagulation defect. Deficiencies of vitamin K occur because of insufficient dietary intake, the absence of bile salts necessary for vitamin K absorption, intestinal malabsorption syndromes, and oral antibiotics that kill resident intestinal bacteria that normally provide a source of vitamin K.

Any cardiovascular abnormality that speeds, slows, or obstructs blood flow can create conditions for coagulation within the vessels. Coagulation is also stimulated by tissue thromboplastin that is released by damaged or dead tissue; any condition of tissue decay or damage releases tissue thromboplastin and can cause coagulation. Damage to inflamed vessels causes platelet activation, which in turn activates the coagulation cascade. In these acquired conditions, normal hemostatic function proves detrimental to the body by excessively consuming coagulation factors or by overwhelming normal control of clot formation and breakdown.

Disseminated intravascular coagulation (DIC) is an acquired coagulation disorder having a variety of predisposing conditions. DIC is a paradoxical condition in which clotting and hemorrhage occur within the vascular system simultaneously. The development of DIC is generally associated with three pathologic processes, including endothelial damage, release of tissue thromboplastin (TTP), and direct activation of factor X. Gram-negative sepsis, septic shock, hypoxia, and low flow states associated with cardiopulmonary arrest can damage the endothelium and precipitate DIC by activating the intrinsic clotting pathway. Endotoxins of gram-negatives activate both intrinsic and extrinsic clotting pathways.

Release of tissue thromboplastin is associated with burns, brain injury, myocardial infarctions, surgeries, obstetric accidents, and malignancies. Excessive amounts of TTP in the circulation activate the extrinsic clotting pathway.

Activation of factor X is stimulated by various substances that enter the bloodstream. Pancreatic and hepatic enzymes and venom from snakebites act in this manner.

DIC also can be precipitated by blood transfusion. Transfused blood dilutes the clotting factors and circulating, naturally occurring antithrombins. Antigen-antibody reactions are responsible for the development of DIC following anaphylaxis as procoagulant material is released from disrupted platelets.

In DIC, the extrinsic system is most often involved. When either system is activated, widespread, unrestricted coagulation occurs throughout the body, leading to thrombic events within the vasculature. The clotting factors are consumed as widespread clotting develops. Thrombosis in the presence of hemorrhage comprises this paradoxical alteration.

The amount of thrombin that enters the systemic circulation during DIC greatly exceeds the ability of the body's naturally occurring antithrombins. The obstruction that results from circulatory deposition of thrombin interferes with blood flow and causes widespread organ hypoperfusion that can lead to ischemia, infarction, and necrosis with manifestations of multisystem organ dysfunction.

Plasmin, which is present because of overstimulation of the clotting cascade, begins to degrade fibrin before a stable clot can develop. As fibrin is broken down by plasmin, fibrin degradation products (FDPs) are released into the circulation; these are potent anticoagulants. The macrophage system likely is unable to clear the blood of FDPs because of lack of fibronectin. The clearance of particulate matter or fibrin clumps is mediated by the adhesive properties of fibronectin.

Treatment of DIC attempts to remove the underlying pathology, restore an appropriate balance between coagulation and fibrinolysis, and maintain organ viability. Organ viability is treated primarily by adequate fluid replacement to ensure adequate circulating blood volume so that optimal tissue perfusion can be maintained.

Practice Examination

1. Anemia refers to a deficiency of:

   a. blood plasma.
   b. erythrocytes.
   c. platelets.
   d. hemoglobin.
   e. Both b and d are correct.

2. Morphological classification of anemia is based on all of the following except:

   a. size.
   b. color.
   c. shape.
   d. cause.

3. Tissue hypoxia causes:

   a. arterioles, capillaries, and venules to constrict.
   b. the heart to contract less forcefully.
   c. the rate and depth of breathing to increase.
   d. Both a and b are correct.
   e. a, b, and c are correct.

Match the etiology of the anemia with its morphologic appearance.

4. ____ vitamin B_{12} deficiency
5. ____ iron deficiency
6. ____ folic acid deficiency
7. ____ impaired synthesis of beta chain of hemoglobin

a. macrocytic-normochromic
b. microcytic-hypochromic
c. normocytic-normochromic

8. Which symptoms are consistent with aplastic anemia but not with pernicious anemia?

   a. hemorrhage into the tissues
   b. pallor
   c. fatigue
   d. hypoxia
   e. neuropathy

9. The cause of macrocytic-normochromic anemia is:

   a. iron deficiency.
   b. deficiency of vitamin B_{12} and folic acid.
   c. an enzyme deficiency.
   d. inheritance of abnormal hemoglobin structure.
   e. None of the above is correct.

10. An individual having chronic gastritis and tingling in the fingers requires which of the following for treatment?

    a. oral B_{12}
    b. B_{12} by intramuscular injection
    c. ferrous fumarate by intramuscular injection
    d. oral folate
    e. transfusions

11. Secondary (relative) polycythemia may be caused by:

    a. dehydration.
    b. chronic obstructive pulmonary disease.
    c. living at high altitudes.
    d. Both b and c are correct.
    e. a, b, and c are correct.

12. The symptoms of polycythemia vera are essentially caused by:

    a. fewer erythrocytes than normal.
    b. decreased blood volume.
    c. increased blood viscosity.
    d. increased rate of blood flow.

Match the leukocytic alteration with its cause.

13. ____ eosinophilia
14. ____ leukopenia

a. pregnancy
b. allergic disorders
c. radiation
d. early stage of infection
e. surgical stress

15. Leukocytosis is found in all of the following except:

    a. inflammatory responses.
    b. allergic responses.
    c. bacterial infections.
    d. bone marrow depression.

16. What is the most notable characteristic of infectious mononucleosis?

    a. It has a short incubation period of less than one week.
    b. It usually affects preteens.
    c. Atypical lymphocytes account for some of the lymphocytosis.
    d. Lymphocytosis persists for less than one week.

17. Which likely does not play a role in leukemia?

    a. radiation
    b. Down syndrome
    c. polycythemia vera
    d. chloramphenicol
    e. diet

18. CML is characterized by its:

    a. acute onset.
    b. high incidence in children.
    c. presence of the Philadelphia chromosome.
    d. survival time of days to months.

19. Clinical manifestations of multiple myeloma include all of the following except:

    a. bone pain.
    b. decreased serum calcium.
    c. m-protein.
    d. renal damage.
    e. pathological fractures.

Match the characteristic with the malignant lymphoma.

20. ____ Epstein-Barr virus

21. ____ Reed-Sternberg cell

22. ____ more frequent extranodal involvement

a. Hodgkin

b. non-Hodgkin

23. A thrombocytopenia with a platelet count below 50,000/mm^3 likely will cause:

   a. hemorrhage from minor trauma.
   b. spontaneous bleeding.
   c. death.
   d. polycythemia.

24. Thromboembolic disease can be caused by all of the following except:

   a. injured vessel walls.
   b. tissue damage that releases excessive tissue thromboplastin.
   c. obstructed blood flow.
   d. deficient dietary intake of vitamin K.
   e. polycythemia.

25. DIC is associated with:

   a. endothelial damage.
   b. activation of factor X.
   c. release of tissue thromboplastin.
   d. Both a and c are correct.
   e. a, b, and c are correct.

Case Study 1

Ann is a healthy 26-year-old white female. Since the beginning of this current golf season, Ann has noted increased shortness of breath and low levels of energy and enthusiasm. These symptoms seem worse during her menses. Today, while playing poorly in a golf tournament at a high, mountainous course, she became lightheaded and was taken by her golfing partner to the emergency clinic of a multi-specialty medical group.

The attending physician's notes indicated a temperature of 98° F, an elevated heart rate and respiratory rate, and low blood pressure. Ann states that heavy menstrual flow has been a problem for 10 to 12 years and she takes 1000 mg of aspirin every three to four hours for six days during menstruation. During the summer months while playing golf, she also takes aspirin to avoid "stiffness in my joints."

Laboratory values are:

Hemoglobin = 8g/dl
Hematocrit = 32%
Erythrocyte count = 3.1×10^6/mm^3
RBC smear showed microcytic and hypochromic cells.
Reticulocyte count = 1.5%
Other laboratory values were within normal limits.

Considering the circumstances and the preliminary work-up, what type of anemia is most likely for Ann? Which clinical sign shows her body is attempting to compensate for anemia?

Case Study 2

L.L., a nine-year-old male, was brought to his dentist for a regular preschool check-up. The dentist and mother were having a chatty conversation when L.L.'s mother stated that her son recently had stopped showing interest in sports and complained of fatigue. During the dental examination, the dentist noted gingival bleeding whenever the tissue was lightly probed. Three nontender lymph nodes were palpable in the submandibular nodes. No other abnormalities were noted. The dentist advised the mother to take L.L. to the medical clinic next door.

The physical examination by the nurse practitioner showed L.L.'s skin to be pale with ecchymoses and petechiae of the trunk. The spleen and liver were not palpable and the remaining examination was unremarkable. A sample of blood was withdrawn.

The CBC revealed:

Hemoglobin = 9.2 g/dl
Hematocrit = 30%
RBCs = $3 \times 10^6/mm^3$
WBCs = $16 \times 10^3/mm^3$
Neutrophils = $8 \times 10^3/mm^3$
Basophils = $250/mm^3$
Eosinophils = $445/mm^3$
Monocytes = $1900/mm^3$
Lymphocytes = $4500/mm^3$
Blasts = much higher than normal
Platelets = $30 \times 10^3/mm^3$

Considering the examinations and CBC, what would the nurse practitioner likely conclude and do?

CHAPTER

20

Alterations of Hematologic Function in Children

Foundational Objective

a. Identify the postnatal changes occurring in the blood throughout childhood. Review page 527; refer to Table 18-7.

Memory Check!

- Blood cell counts tend to rise above adult levels at birth and then decline gradually throughout childhood. The immediate rise in values is the result of accelerated hematopoiesis during fetal life, the trauma of birth, and cutting of the umbilical cord. The presence of large numbers of immature erythrocytes and leukocytes in peripheral blood is found in the neonate. Within the first two weeks to three months of life, up to one year, normal values for adults are approached. Platelet counts in full-term neonates are comparable to those of adults and remain so throughout infancy and childhood. Average blood volume in the full-term neonate is slightly above that of older children and adults, 85 ml/kg of body weight compared with 75 ml/kg. Blood decreases proportionately during the first few months.

Objectives

After studying this chapter, the learner will be able to:

1. Describe the etiology of childhood iron deficiency anemia and identify appropriate diagnostic and treatment measures.
Study page 568; refer to Table 20-1.

Iron deficiency anemia is the most common childhood anemia and is caused by poor dietary iron intake, occult blood, or both. Early exposure to cow's milk protein often causes hemorrhagic bowel inflammation and occult blood loss in the infant. The onset of menstruation in females also is a contributor. Poor socioeconomic status can be a significant causal factor. The highest incidence of iron deficiency anemia occurs at six months to two years of age and peaks again in adolescence during rapid growth periods.

There are few symptoms in infants and young children until moderate anemia develops. General irritability, activity intolerance, and weakness are indicators of anemia. When hemoglobin falls below 5 g/dl, specific indicators may occur. Iron stores are best measured by serum ferritin and total iron-binding capacity. Treatment for iron deficiency anemia is iron supplements; oral supplements are preferred.

2. Compare and contrast the two major causes of hemolytic disease of the newborn.
Study pages 568-570; refer to Figure 20-1.

The two major causes of **hemolytic disease of the newborn** (HDN) are **blood type incompatibil-**

ity and **Rh factor incompatibility**. Blood type incompatibility is a mild form of hemolytic disease. Rh incompatibility is potentially much more severe. Blood type incompatibility in the mother occurs when maternal antibodies to fetal erythrocytes are formed because of a prior incompatible pregnancy, other antigenetic factors, or exposure of the mother to fetal erythrocytes during pregnancy. Incompatibility in the infant occurs when sufficient antibody, usually IgG, crosses the placenta from the mother to the infant or when maternal antibodies attach to and damage fetal erythrocytes. ABO incompatibility occurs in 20 to 25 percent of pregnancies, with only one in ten cases producing HDN. Usual causes are a type O mother with a type A or B fetus, a type A mother with a type B fetus, or a type B mother with a type A fetus. Hemolysis in the newborn is usually limited, resolves after birth, and requires limited treatment; however, mild hemolysis may contribute to hyperbilirubinemia.

Rh incompatibility occurs in less than 10 percent of pregnancies and rarely is a problem during the first pregnancy; the first pregnancy initiates sensitization. Rh incompatibility becomes a greater problem with subsequent pregnancies. It should be noted that HDN caused by Rh incompatibility occurs in only 5 percent of pregnancies after five or more pregnancies. In the most severe form, Rh incompatibility can lead to severe anemia, edema, central nervous system damage, and fetal death. It may also contribute to severe hyperbilirubinemia.

Blood typing in mothers and infants reveals those at risk. Indirect Coombs' test reveals antibodies in mothers, and direct Coombs' test reveals antibodies bound to fetal erythrocytes. In utero testing through the umbilical vein is now available. Immunoprophylaxis with Rh immunoglobulin (RhoGAM) for at-risk mothers has been very successful.

3. Describe childhood sickle cell disease and identify its most common forms of presentation.
Study pages 570-573; refer to Figures 20-2 and 20-3 and Table 20-2.

Sickle cell disease is an inherited, autosomal recessive disorder most common in the United States among African Americans. The disease is characterized by the presence of **hemoglobin S** (HbS) within the erythrocytes. This hemoglobin becomes elongated and sickle-shaped whenever it is deoxygenated or dehydrated.

The parent's medical history and clinical findings may generate an index of suspicion about the child. The sickle solubility test and hemoglobin electrophoresis are used to assist diagnosis. Prenatal chorionic villus sampling is now available.

Acute complications or crises occur in sickle cell disease and may be provoked by infection, exposure to cold, low PO_2, acidosis, or localized hypoxemia. Infections are frequent in childhood and may generate various degrees of other triggers.

Vasoocclusive crises result from a "log-jam" effect produced by stiff, sickled erythrocytes in the microcirculation. Symptoms include symmetric swelling of the hands and feet, which may be the first clinical manifestation in infancy. In older children, swollen painful joints, priapism, severe abdominal pain from infarctions of abdominal organs, and strokes may occur. Other complications include sickle cell retinopathy, renal necrosis, and necrosis of the femoral head.

Sequestration crises occur only in the young child. Large amounts of blood may pool in the liver and spleen which can contain as much as one-fifth of the blood volume and, thus, precipitate shock. Up to a 50 percent mortality rate has been reported with these crises.

Aplastic crises may occur because of the decreased survival of sickled erythrocytes, which is 10 to 20 days, and may lead to aplastic anemia if compensatory mechanisms are not intact. Most sickle cell deaths are due to overwhelming infection and sepsis.

4. Describe the thalassemias.
Study pages 573-574.

The alpha- and beta-thalassemias are inherited autosomal recessive disorders that cause an impaired rate of synthesis of one of the two chains —alpha or beta—of adult hemoglobin. Beta-thalassemia is more common than alpha-thalassemia.

Beta-thalassemia has slowed or defective synthesis of the beta globin chain and is prevalent among Greeks, Italians, some Arabs, and Sephardic Jews. Alpha-thalassemia, wherein the alpha chain is affected, is most common among Chinese, Vietnamese, Cambodians, and Laotians. Both thalassemias are common among African Americans. The effects range from mild microcytosis to death in utero, and the pathophysiology depends on the number of defective genes and mode of inheritance.

The fundamental defect in beta-thalassemia is the uncoupling of alpha and beta chain synthesis.

The free alpha chains are unstable and easily precipitated in the cell. Most erythroblasts that contain precipitates are destroyed by mononuclear phagocytes in the marrow, resulting in ineffective erythropoiesis and anemia. Individuals with beta-thalassemia minor, the mild form, are usually asymptomatic. Persons with beta-thalassemia major, the severe form, may become quite ill. Anemia is severe and results in significant cardiovascular overload with high output congestive heart failure. Today, blood transfusion can increase life span by a decade or two. Death is usually caused by hemochromatosis.

There are four forms of **alpha-thalassemia**, with each dependent on the number of defective genes. The severity is variable. Individuals who inherit the mildest form of alpha-thalassemia, the alpha trait, usually are symptom free or have mild microcytosis. Alpha-thalassemia major causes hydrops fetalis and fulminant intrauterine congestive heart failure. The fetus has a grossly enlarged heart and liver. Diagnosis usually is made post mortem. In children with thalassemia major, cardiovascular compromise causes death by five to six years of age if untreated.

Individuals who are carriers or have thalassemia minor generally have few symptoms and require no specific treatment. For thalassemia major, therapies to support and prolong life are necessary. There is no cure for either condition.

5. Describe childhood hemophilias and their complications.
Study pages 574-576; refer to Tables 20-3 and 20-4.

Hemophilia or spontaneous bleeding is rare in the first year of life, although significant bleeding may occur during circumcision. However, this is an unusual complication, as hemostasis in these infants is achieved through the extrinsic pathway that does not require factors VIII, IX, or XI, which are responsible for 90 to 95 percent of bleeding if they are absent. **Hematoma** formation is a more common problem during the first year of life and may be due to injections, firm holding, or the many accidents that occur in the development of movement in children. These accidents may also precipitate bleeding in the joints. Spontaneous hematuria and epistaxis are bothersome but rarely serious. Life-threatening intracranial and cervical bleeding may result from normal childhood injury. The administration of blood products to replace deficient or absent factors has enhanced the physical capabilities of individuals suffering hemophilic defects.

6. Describe the pathophysiology of idiopathic thrombocytopenic purpura and identify its most likely etiology.
Study pages 576-577.

Idiopathic thrombocytopenic purpura (ITP) is the most common thrombocytopenic purpura of childhood. Antiplatelet antibodies attach to platelets that are then sequestered in the spleen where they are destroyed by mononuclear phagocytes.

Classic symptoms of bruising and petechiae are usually preceded from one to four weeks by a viral illness that may cause sensitization of the platelets which triggers an antibody response; high levels of IgG have been found on the platelets of affected children.

The prognosis is excellent. The acute phase lasts one to two weeks, although thrombocytopenia may persist longer. Complete recovery occurs in approximately 75 percent of individuals at three months after onset, with 90 percent of afflicted children recovering by 9 to 12 months. Although serious complications are few, severe intracranial bleeding does occur in about 1 percent of cases and can be devastating.

7. Describe proposed causative factors and common manifestations for childhood leukemias.
Study pages 577-579.

Leukemia, in its various forms, is the most common childhood malignancy; it comprises 33 percent of the neoplasms of children. Acute lymphoblastic leukemia (ALL) represents 80 to 85 percent of all childhood leukemias. Peak incidence of ALL occurs between two and six years of age and is twice as common in white children as in nonwhite children. The etiology of leukemia is probably multifactorial, with genetic predisposition, environment, and viruses playing a role. Exposure to high levels of radiation also has become an established etiological factor.

The appearance of symptoms may be rapid or slow but generally reflects the effects of bone marrow failure. Findings include decreased red blood cells and platelets and changes in white blood cells. Pallor, fatigue, petechiae, purpura, and fever are generally present. Fever may be due to a hypermetabolic state brought on by the rapid production and destruction of leukemic cells or because of a secondary infection due to neutropenia. Renal failure may ensue because of high uric acid levels that produce precipitates of urates in the renal tubules. Other symptoms, such as bone and joint pain, may be due to infiltration of leukemic cells into other organs. The central nervous system is a common site of extramedullary infiltration, although few children have this problem at diagnosis; it occurs later in the course of the disease.

8. Distinguish between non-Hodgkin lymphoma and Hodgkin disease.
Study pages 579-580.

Non-Hodgkin lymphoma (NHL) and Hodgkin disease comprise approximately 11 percent of all childhood cancer; NHL is the most common. Either group of disease is rare before the age of five years, and the relative incidence increases throughout childhood. Males are affected more often than females. At particular risk are children with inherited or acquired immunodeficiency syndromes. A viral etiology is suggested; a strong correlation between the Epstein-Barr virus and lymphoma exists.

Childhood **non-Hodgkin lymphoma** is a diffuse rather than nodular disease. Disease sites commonly involve extranodal sites such as brain, lung, bone, and skin. Rapidly enlarging lymphoid tissue and painless lymphadenopathy are common with abdominal sites. Symptoms often include abdominal pain and vomiting, but a palpable mass is not always present. An anterior mediastinal mass, with or without pleural effusion, may be present. If the mass is large, respiratory compromise, tracheal compression, and superior vena cava syndrome may arise. CNS involvement is common.

Most children with NHL are cured. Optimal treatment is evolving, but combination chemotherapy with or without radiation therapy is successful.

Besides a viral etiology for **Hodgkin disease** in children, genetic susceptibility has been suggested as a cause. Hodgkin disease incidence gradually rises through the age of 11. There is a marked increase through adolescence that continues into the thirties.

Painless lymphadenopathy in the lower cervical chain, with or without fever, is the most common symptom. Mediastinal involvement can lead to airway obstruction. Extranodal primary involvement is rare in Hodgkin disease.

Treatment for Hodgkin disease includes chemotherapy and radiation therapy. The survival rate for children with Hodgkin disease is high; 70 to 90 percent is common.

Practice Examination

True/False

1. ____ Early initiation of iron-rich cow's milk in an infant's diet is an excellent preventive measure against iron deficiency anemia.

2. ____ Although a frequent problem, ABO incompatibility seldom results in significant disease.

3. ____ Sequestration crisis is a serious complication of sickle cell disease unique to childhood.

4. ____ Rh incompatibility is a problem only of an Rh-positive woman bearing an Rh-negative fetus during a second pregnancy.

5. ____ Since hemostasis in the newborn is chiefly attained through the extrinsic pathway, serious bleeding in the newborn period is usually not a problem in hemophiliacs.

6. ____ Idiopathic thrombocytopenic purpura is a genetically transmitted disease.

7. ____ Leukemias are multifactorial diseases with genetic disposition, environment, and bacterial infections playing a role in their etiology.

8. Which is the most frequent blood disorder of infancy and childhood?

   a. iron deficiency anemia
   b. pernicious anemia
   c. folate deficiency anemia
   d. sideroblastic anemia

9. Maternal-fetal blood incompatibility may exist in which condition?

   a. Rh-positive mother, Rh-negative fetus
   b. Rh-negative mother, Rh-positive fetus
   c. Rh-negative father, Rh-positive mother
   d. Rh-negative father, Rh-negative mother

10. Beta-thalassemia is:

    a. common among Italians.
    b. an X-linked recessive disorder.
    c. an autosomal recessive disorder.
    d. Both a and b are correct.
    e. Both a and c are correct.

11. Which statement is correct?

    a. Sickle cell disease is an autosomal dominant disorder.
    b. Sickle cell disease is an X-linked recessive disorder.
    c. Sickle cell disease is an X-linked dominant disorder.
    d. Sickle cell disease is an autosomal recessive disorder.

12. Idiopathic thrombocytopenic purpura involves antibodies against:

    a. neutrophils.
    b. eosinophils.
    c. platelets.
    d. basophils.

13. Which are factors associated with iron deficiency anemia?

    a. rapid growth
    b. low socioeconomic status
    c. cow's milk for infants
    d. Both a and c are correct.
    e. a, b, and c are correct.

14. What is the most likely cause of idiopathic thrombocytopenic purpura?

    a. stress and fatigue
    b. genetic predisposition
    c. prolonged occult bleeding
    d. viral sensitization
    e. Both b and c are correct.

15. Hodgkin disease has:

a. extensive extranodal involvement.
b. rare extranodal involvement.
c. painless cervical lymphadenopathy.
d. Both a and c are correct.
e. Both b and c are correct.

16. In sickle cell disease, vasoocclusive crisis is the result of:

a. damage to platelets due to IgG.
b. "plugging" of peripheral blood vessels by "stiff" sickled erythrocytes.
c. ingestion of sulfa drugs.
d. sequestration of large numbers of erythrocytes in the spleen.

17. Which factor may play a part in the development of childhood leukemia?

a. genetic predisposition
b. environmental factors
c. viral infections
d. radiation
e. All of the above are correct.

18. Which statement is true about acute lymphocytic leukemia?

a. It is the most common childhood leukemia.
b. It usually occurs between two and six years of age.
c. It is uniformly fatal.
d. It is easily predicted through genetic testing.
e. Both a and b are correct.

Match the circumstance with the alteration.

19. ____ leukocyte counts approaching 100,000/mm^3
20. ____ low platelet counts
21. ____ lack of coagulation factors VIII, IX, and XI
22. ____ may present early as symmetric, painful swelling of hands and feet
23. ____ may cause severe hemolysis in the newborn period
24. ____ may result in aplastic crises
25. ____ may result in fetal death

a. leukemia
b. ITP
c. sickle cell disease
d. Rh incompatibility
e. hemophilia

Case Study

Steven D. is a 10-year-old white male seeking medical attention because of possible physical abuse observed by his gym teacher. The teacher noticed severe bruising over much of his upper body when his shirt "rode up" during an exercise. Steven emphatically states that he has never been abused by anyone. He denies any accidents and didn't tell anyone about his bruises because he thought they might "get me into trouble." His mother cannot explain the bruises either and did not see them before today because her son does all of his own hygiene and is quite modest about revealing his body even to family members. Steven's physical examination is benign except for multiple, irregular dark purple bruises over most of his torso and lower extremities. His complete blood count is well within normal limits except for a low platelet count of 18,000/mm^3.

What is Steven's diagnosis?

CHAPTER 21

Structure and Function of the Cardiovascular and Lymphatic Systems

Objectives

After review of this chapter, the learner will be able to:

1. **Describe the function of the circulatory system; distinguish between pulmonary and systemic circulation.**
   Review page 585; refer to Figure 21-1.

2. **Describe the heart wall and the chambers, fibrous skeleton, valves, and great vessels of the heart; trace the blood flow through the heart.**
   Review pages 585-589; refer to Figures 21-2 through 21-8.

3. **Describe the coronary arteries, veins, and lymphatic vessels.**
   Review pages 589-592; refer to Figure 21-9.

4. **Describe the initiation of and conduction sequence of electrical impulses through the heart; identify the autonomic innervation and its effects on the heart.**
   Review pages 592-597; refer to Figures 21-10 through 21-12.

5. **Identify the structure and characteristics of myocardial cells.**
   Review pages 597-600; refer to Figures 21-13 through 21-16.

6. **Use the Frank-Starling law and Laplace's law to demonstrate interrelationships that affect cardiac function.**
   Review pages 601-605; refer to Figures 21-17 through 21-19.

7. **Contrast the structure and function of arteries, capillaries, and veins.**
   Review pages 605-610; refer to Figures 21-20 through 21-24.

8. **Describe the determinants of blood flow.**
   Review pages 610-614; refer to Figures 21-25 through 21-29.

9. **Identify the factors that regulate arterial and venous blood pressure.**
   Review pages 614-617; refer to Figures 21-30 and 21-31 and Table 21-2.

10. **Describe the normal structure and function of the lymphatic system.**
    Review page 618; refer to Figures 21-32 through 21-34.

11. **Note the changes that aging causes in the cardiovascular system.**
    Review page 604.

Practice Examination

1. Oxygenated blood flows through the:

   a. superior vena cava.
   b. pulmonary veins.
   c. pulmonary arteries.
   d. coronary veins.
   e. None of the above is correct.

2. The hepatic vein:

   a. carries blood from the vena cava to the liver.
   b. carries blood from the liver to the vena cava.
   c. carries blood from the aorta to the liver.
   d. carries blood from the liver to the aorta.

3. The position of the heart in the mediastinum is:

   a. inferior to the diaphragm and between the lungs.
   b. between the lungs, superior to the diaphragm.
   c. posterior to the trachea, anterior to the esophagus.
   d. posterior to the lungs and anterior to the diaphragm.

4. The pericardial space is found between the:

   a. myocardium and parietal pericardium.
   b. endocardium and visceral pericardium.
   c. visceral and parietal pericardium.
   d. visceral and epicardial pericardium.

5. In the normal cardiac cycle, which of the following occurs? (*More than one answer may be correct.*)

   a. The right atrium and right ventricles contract simultaneously.
   b. The two atria contract simultaneously while the two ventricles relax.
   c. The two ventricles contract simultaneously while the two atria relax.
   d. Both the ventricles and atria contract simultaneously to increase cardiac output.

6. The QRS complex of the EKG represents:

   a. atrial depolarization.
   b. ventricular depolarization.
   c. atrial contraction.
   d. ventricular repolarization.
   e. atrial repolarization.

7. A person having a heart rate of 100, a systolic blood pressure of 200, and a stroke volume of 40 would have an average cardiac output of:

   a. 0.5 milliliters.
   b. 5 liters.
   c. 4 milliliters.
   d 8000 milliliters.
   e. None of the above is correct.

8. During atrial systole, the:

   a. AV valves are open.
   b. atria are filling.
   c. ventricles are emptying.
   d. semilunar valves are open.

9. Which does not significantly affect heart rate?

   a. sympathetic nerves
   b. parasympathetic nerves
   c. atrioventricular valves
   d. acetylcholine

10. One cardiac cycle:

    a. has a duration that changes if the heart rate changes.
    b. usually requires less than one second to complete.
    c. is equal to stroke volume times heart rate.
    d. pumps approximately 5 liters of blood.
    e. Both a and b are correct.

11. Compared with arteries, veins:

    a. have a larger diameter.
    b. are thick-coated.
    c. recoil quickly after distension.
    d. Both a and b are correct.

12. Normal systolic pressure within the left ventricle is in the range of:

    a. 100-140 mm Hg.
    b. 15-30 mm Hg.
    c. 0-10 mm Hg.
    d. None of the above is correct.

13. Backflow of blood from the arteries into the relaxing ventricles is prevented by the:

    a. venous valves.
    b. pericardial fluid.
    c. semilunar valves.
    d. atrioventricular valves.

14. Another name for the mitral valve is the:

    a. aortic semilunar valve.
    b. pulmonary semilunar valve.
    c. tricuspid valve.
    d. bicuspid valve.

15. The Frank-Starling law of the heart concerns the relationship between:

    a. the length of the cardiac muscle fiber and the strength of contraction.
    b. stroke volume and arterial resistance.
    c. rapidity of nerve conduction and stroke volume.
    d. systolic rate and cardiac output.

16. How does cardiac muscle differ from skeletal muscle? (*More than one answer may be correct.*)

    a. It is arranged in parallel units.
    b. It is arranged in branching networks.
    c. It is multinucleated.
    d. It is single nucleated.
    e. It is more accessible to sodium and potassium ions.

17. Blood pressure is measured by the:

    a. pressure exerted on the ventricular walls during systole.
    b. pressure exerted by the blood on the wall of any blood vessel.
    c. pressure exerted on arteries by the blood.
    d. product of the stroke volume times heart rate.

18. Identify the correct sequence of the portions of the pulmonary circulation.

1. pulmonary veins	a. 1, 5, 3, 2, 4
2. pulmonary arteries	b. 4, 2, 3, 1, 5
3. lungs	c. 4, 1, 3, 2, 5
4. right ventricle	d. 5, 2, 3, 1, 4
5. left atrium	e. 5, 1, 3, 2, 4

19. The heartbeat is initiated by the:

    a. coronary sinus.
    b. atrioventricular bundle.
    c. right ventricle.
    d. SA node.
    e. AV node.

20. If the sympathetic nervous system stimulation of the heart predominates over parasympathetic nervous system stimulation, the heart will:

    a. increase its rate.
    b. contract with greater force and at a slower rate.
    c. decrease its rate and force of contraction.
    d. contract with less force and at a higher rate.

21. When fluids exhibit a turbulent flow:

    a. resistance increases.
    b. it is a sign of greater blood viscosity.
    c. the fluids have greater velocity than with laminar flow.
    d. there is greater hydrostatic pressure than if the fluids had laminar flow.

22. Identify the normal sequence of an electrical impulse through the heart's conduction system.

1. atrioventricular bundle	a. 4, 1, 2, 5, 3
2. AV node	b. 4, 2, 5, 1, 3
3. Purkinje fibers	c. 2, 4, 1, 5, 3
4. SA node	d. 4, 2, 1, 5, 3
5. right and left bundle branches	

23. Which factor might increase resistance to the flow of blood through the blood vessels?

a. an increased inner radius or diameter of blood vessels
b. decreased numbers of capillaries
c. decreased blood viscosity
d. decreased numbers of red blood cells

24. Depolarization of cardiac muscle cells occurs because of:

a. the cell's interior becoming more negatively charged.
b. the cell's interior becoming less negatively charged.
c. impermeability of the cell membrane to sodium.
d. impermeability of the cell membrane to potassium.

25. Which statement is true?

a. Lymphatic walls consist of multiple layers of flattened endothelial cells.
b. Lymph from the entire body, except the upper right quadrant, eventually drains into the thoracic duct.
c. The thoracic duct has approximately the same diameter as the great veins.
d. Lymph contains more proteins than does blood plasma.
e. The lymphatic system, like the circulatory system, is a closed circuit.

CHAPTER

22

Alterations of Cardiovascular Function

Foundational Objectives

a. Describe the flow of blood through the heart and identify the coronary vessels. Refer to Figures 21-5 and 21-9.

Memory Check!

- The pumping action of the heart consists of contraction and relaxation of the myocardial layer of the heart wall. During relaxation, termed diastole, blood fills the chambers. The contraction that follows, termed systole, forces the blood from the chamber into the pulmonary or systemic circulation. During diastole, blood from the veins of the systemic circulation enters the thin-walled right atrium from the superior vena cava and the inferior vena cava. Venous blood from the coronary circulation enters the right atrium through the coronary sinus. The right atrium fills and its fluid pressure pushes open the right atrioventricular or tricuspid valve. Blood fills the right ventricle. The same sequence of events occurs a fraction of a second earlier in the left heart. The four pulmonary veins, two from the right lung and two from the left lung, carry oxygenated blood from the pulmonary circulation to the left atrium. As the left atrium fills, its fluid pressure pushes the cusps of the mitral valve open and blood flows into the left ventricle. Blood circulates from the left ventricle and returns to the right atrium because of a progressive fall in pressure from the left ventricle to the right atrium of approximately 120 mm Hg. Blood always flows from a higher pressure area toward a lower pressure area.
- The blood within the heart chambers does not supply oxygen and other nutrients to the cells of the heart. Like all other organs, heart structures are nourished by vessels of the systemic circulation. The coronary circulation consists of coronary arteries and cardiac veins. The right and left coronary arteries traverse the epicardium and branch several times. The left coronary artery arises from a single opening behind the left cusp of the aortic semilunar valve. It divides into two branches, the left anterior descending artery and the circumflex artery. The left anterior descending artery delivers blood to portions of the left and right ventricles and much of the interventricular septum. The circumflex artery supplies blood to the left atrium and the lateral wall of the left ventricle. The circumflex artery often branches to the posterior surfaces of the left atrium and left ventricle. The right coronary artery originates from an opening behind the right aortic cusp. Three major branches of the right coronary artery supply blood to the right atrium, upper right ventricle, and both ventricles.
- Collateral arteries are connections or anastomoses between two branches of the same coronary artery or connections of branches of the right coronary artery with branches of the left. They are particularly common within the interventricular and interatrial septa, at the apex of the heart, over the anterior surface of the right ventricle, and around the sinus node. The heart has an extensive capillary network with about one capillary per muscle cell. Blood travels from the arteries to the arterioles, then into the capillaries, where exchange of oxygen and other nutrients takes place.
- Blood from the coronary arteries drains into the cardiac veins which travel alongside the arteries. The cardiac veins feed into the great cardiac vein and then into the coronary sinus located between the atria and ventricles. The coronary sinus empties into the right atrium.

b. Describe the conduction system of the heart. Review pages 592-597; refer to Figures 21-10 through 21-12.

Memory Check!

- Continuous, rhythmic repetition of the cardiac cycle or systole and diastole depends on the continuous, rhythmic transmission of electrical impulses. As an electrical impulse passes from cell to cell in the myocardium, muscular contraction or systole occurs. After the action potential passes, the fibers relax and return to their resting length; this relaxation is diastole.
- The myocardium differs from other muscle tissues; it contains its own intrinsic conduction system. It can generate and transmit action potentials without stimulation from the nervous system. These cells are concentrated at certain sites in the myocardium called nodes. Although the heart is innervated by both sympathetic and parasympathetic fibers, neural impulses are not needed to maintain the cardiac cycle.
- Normally, electrical impulses arise in the sinoatrial node or SA node, often called the pacemaker of the heart. There are numerous autonomic nerve endings within the node which enable the node to respond to the nervous system. In the resting adult, the SA node generates about 75 action potentials per minute. Each action potential travels rapidly from cell to cell and through special pathways in the atrial myocardium which causes both atria to contract. Atrial contraction initiates systole. Transmission of the action potential from the atrial to the ventricular myocardium occurs through muscle fibers of the conduction system. The action potential travels first to the atrioventricular node or AV node, then to the atrioventricular bundle, then to the common bundle, and finally through the bundle branches of the interventricular septum to Purkinje fibers in the heart wall.
- The extensive network of Purkinje fibers enables the rapid spread of the impulse to the ventricular apices.
- Electrical activation of the muscle cells, or depolarization, is caused by the movement of electrically charged solutes, primarily sodium and potassium, across cardiac cell membranes. Deactivation, or repolarization, occurs by ion movement in the opposite direction. Movement of ions into and out of the cell creates an electrical or voltage difference across the cell membrane. This difference or potential of charged ions causes the impulse to flow within cells and from cell to cell.
- Sympathetic neural stimulation of the myocardium and coronary vessels depends on the presence of adrenergic receptors that are able to bind specifically with neurotransmitters of the sympathetic nervous system. Norepinephrine binding to receptors increases the rate of impulse generation and conduction and also the strength of myocardial contraction during systole. Also, coronary arterioles dilate to supply the heart with more oxygen and nutrients. These effects enable the heart to pump more blood. Parasympathetic or vagus nerve activity decreases the heart rate. The vagus nerve releases acetylcholine.

c. Describe the interrelationships between myocardial stretch and chamber wall dimensions and the contractible force of the heart. Review pages 601-605; refer to Figures 21-17 through 21-19.

Memory Check!

- Cardiac muscle, like other muscle, increases its strength of contraction within certain limits when it is stretched. The Frank-Starling law of the heart states that there is a direct relationship between the volume of blood in the heart and stretch or length of cardiac fibers at the end of diastole and the force of contraction during the next systole. The greater the stretch from preload blood volume, the stronger the contraction.
- Laplace's law states the relationships between wall thickness, pressure, and wall tension. Wall tension is related directly to the product of intraventricular pressure and internal radius and inversely to the wall thickness. Stated another way, the pressure or contractible force is directly related to wall thickness and wall tension and indirectly related to the radius. The thicker the wall and greater the wall tension and smaller the radius, the greater the force of contraction.

d. Establish the determinants of blood flow. Review pages 610-614; refer to Figures 21-25 through 21-29.

Memory Check!

- Blood flow is determined primarily by two factors: pressure and resistance. Pressure in a liquid system is the force exerted on the liquid per unit area. Fluid moves from the arterial "side" of the capillaries, which is a region of greater pressure, to the venous side, which is a region of lesser pressure. Resistance opposes force. In the cardiovascular system, most opposition to blood flow is because of the diameter and length of the blood vessels themselves.

- The relationship between blood flow, pressure, and resistance can be stated as Q equals P divided by R, where Q is blood flow, P is the pressure difference, and R is resistance.

- Resistance to fluid flow considers the length of the tube or vessel, the viscosity of the fluid, and the radius of the lumen. According to Poiseuille's formula, the resistance equals viscosity of blood times length of vessel divided by the fourth power of the lumen's radius.

- Because this equation was derived using straight, rigid tubes with steady, streamlined flow, it cannot be applied exactly to the vascular system. Nevertheless, it is a useful model for vascular resistance assessment. Small changes in the lumen's radius lead to large changes in vascular resistance. Because vessel length is relatively constant, length is not as important as lumen size in determining flow through a single vessel. However, blood flowing through the distributing arteries encounters more resistance than blood flowing through the capillary bed. In the capillary bed, flow is distributed among many short, tiny branches.

- If R equals viscosity times length divided by the fourth power of radius is substituted into the formula Q equals P divided by R, a helpful summary of likely factors affecting blood flow rate can be expressed. Now, blood flow equals pressure times radius to the fourth power divided by the viscosity times the length. The higher the pressure and greater the vessel radius and the less the viscosity of blood and length of vessel, the greater the flow of blood.

e. Establish the determinants of blood pressure. Review pages 614-617; refer to Figures 21-30 and 21-31 and Table 21-2.

Memory Check!

- The mean arterial pressure, which is the average pressure in the arteries throughout the cardiac cycle, depends on the elastic properties of the arterial walls and the mean volume of blood in the arterial system. The main determinants of venous blood pressure are the volume of fluid within the veins and the compliance or distensibility of their vessel walls. The venous system accommodates approximately 60 percent of the total blood volume at any given moment with a venous pressure averaging less than 10 mm Hg. Conversely, the arteries accommodate about 15 percent of the total blood volume with a pressure of about 100 mm Hg. Some important relationships are:
- Mean blood pressure equals cardiac output times peripheral resistance.
- Cardiac output equals heart rate times stroke volume.
- Peripheral resistance equals blood viscosity times vessel length divided by vessel radius raised to the fourth power.
- Blood pressure equals heart rate times stroke volume times viscosity times length divided by the radius to the fourth power. The higher the heart rate, stroke volume, blood viscosity, and vessel length and the less the vessel radius to the fourth power, the greater the blood pressure.

Objectives

After studying this chapter, the learner will be able to:

1. **Distinguish between arteriosclerosis and atherosclerosis; describe the development of atheromatous plaque and its manifestations.**
   Study pages 627-629; refer to Figures 22-1 and 22-2 and Table 22-1.

Arteriosclerosis is a chronic disease of the arterial system characterized by abnormal thickening and hardening of the vessel walls. Smooth muscle cells and collagen fibers migrate into the tunica intima, causing it to stiffen and thicken; this decreases the artery's ability to change lumen size.

Atherosclerosis is a form of arteriosclerosis in which the thickening of vessel walls is caused by hardening of soft deposits of intraarterial fat and fibrin that reduce lumen size. Atherosclerosis can take several forms depending on the anatomic vessel location, the individual's age and genetic and physiologic status, and the risk factors to which each individual may have been exposed. It is the leading contributor to coronary artery and cerebrovascular disease.

Lipid deposition is an early event in atherogenesis and occurs with excessive influx and deposition of cholesterol into the arterial wall. The lesions of atherosclerosis occur primarily within the tunica intima or the innermost layer. These lesions include the fatty streak, fibrous plaque, and the complicated lesion. The early **fatty streak** is a flat, yellow, lipid-filled smooth muscle cell that causes no obstruction of the affected vessel.

Fibrous plaque is the characteristic lesion of advancing atherosclerosis and consists of lipid-laden smooth muscle cells surrounded by collagen, elastic fibers, and a mucoprotein matrix. The lesion is elevated and protrudes into the lumen of the artery. The growing mass fixes to the inner wall of the tunica intima and may invade the muscular tunica media. Fibrous plaques likely develop from fatty streaks. The core of the fibrous plaque consists of lipids and debris from cellular necrosis caused by insufficient blood supply. If the lesion progresses sufficiently, it occludes the arterial lumen at arterial bifurcations, curves, or regions where the arteries taper.

Complicated lesions occur as the fibrous plaques are altered by hemorrhage, calcification, cellular necrosis, and blood clots throughout the intimal layer. As the altered complex structure becomes rigid, it causes extensive vascular occlusion.

Atherosclerotic lesions generally cause no symptoms until 60 percent or more of the tissue's arterial blood supply is occluded. If plaque formation occurs slowly, collateral arteries may develop to provide tissues with adequate blood supply. Atherosclerosis may have many different manifestations. High blood pressure develops if atherosclerosis elevates systemic vascular resistance. Cerebral or myocardial ischemia is a life-threatening manifestation of atherosclerosis that occurrs in the vessels of the brain or heart.

Dietary modifications are always the first treatment for atherosclerosis. Daily cholesterol intake must be reduced to 250 to 300 mg. Drugs that decrease lipidemia are prescribed if serum lipoproteins are not reduced by dietary modification or if lipid levels are dangerously elevated in an individual, requiring a lengthy time for significant dietary change and weight reduction.

2. **Distinguish between primary, secondary, complicated, and malignant hypertension.**
   Study pages 629-634; refer to Figures 22-3 and 22-4 and Tables 22-2 and 22-3.

Adult hypertension begins when the systolic pressure exceeds 140 mm Hg and the diastolic pressure exceeds 90 mm Hg. Increasing pressures in both systolic and diastolic pressure categorize hypertension from stage 1 (mild) to stage 4 (severe).

Hypertension is caused by increases in cardiac output, total peripheral resistance, or both. Cardiac output is increased by any condition that increases heart rate or stroke volume, whereas peripheral resistance is increased by any factor that increases blood viscosity or reduces vessel diameter.

Primary hypertension, which is also called essential or idiopathic hypertension, has a combination of genetic and environmental factors likely responsible for its development. Primary hypertension affects 92 to 95 percent of hypertensive individuals.

The **hemodynamic hypothesis** of onset attributes the onset of hypertension to fluid overload.

According to this hypothesis, early primary hypertension consists of a series of cardiovascular adjustments to an increase in blood volume. First, cardiac output increases to handle the increased volume of blood circulating through the heart. As the systemic arteries sense the volume increase, their autoregulatory mechanisms try to slow things down by causing vasoconstriction. Because blood volume remains high, the increase in total peripheral resistance caused by the vasoconstriction leads to hypertension.

The **autoregulatory hypothesis** proposes that, although primary hypertension begins with increased cardiac output, it is maintained by an alteration of vascular autoregulation. The defect consists of the failure of autoregulatory mechanisms to return toward baseline following water and sodium excretion by the kidneys.

Another hypothesis about the onset of primary hypertension is that **neurally stimulated vasoconstriction** is the initiating event. Herein, the cardiovascular control centers in the brain overstimulate the sympathetic branch of the autonomic nervous system, which causes vasoconstriction. Because the sympathetic nervous system innervates both the heart and the vessels, sympathetic overstimulation increases cardiac output as well as peripheral resistance.

Sodium retention may initiate primary hypertension by an inherited defect of sodium excretion in the kidneys. The defect in renal sodium excretion is aggravated by dietary sodium intake of more than 50 mEq/day. Another mechanism of sodium retention is believed to be an interruption of the sodium-potassium pump. In individuals with this defect, a hormone is thought to inhibit sodium excretion from cells. This undiscovered **humoral sodium-transport inhibitor** not only would cause intracellular sodium to accumulate but also seems to cause increases of intracellular calcium. The presence of extra calcium in vascular smooth muscle cells increases vascular vasoconstriction and increases peripheral resistance.

Secondary hypertension is caused by any systemic disease process that raises peripheral vascular resistance or cardiac output. Fortunately, if the cause is identified and removed before permanent structural changes occur, blood pressure can return to normal.

Complicated hypertension is sustained primary hypertension that causes pathologic effects in addition to hemodynamic alterations and fluid and electrolyte imbalances. Complicated hypertension compromises the structure and function of vessels, the heart, kidneys, eyes, and the brain. Vascular complications include the formation, dissection, and rupture of aneurysms or outpouchings in vessel walls as well as gangrene resulting from vessel occlusion. Possible renal complications include parenchymal damage, renal arteriosclerosis, and renal insufficiency or failure.

Cardiovascular complications include left ventricular hypertrophy, angina pectoris, congestive heart failure or left heart failure, coronary artery disease, myocardial infarction, and sudden death. Complications specific to the retina include retinal vascular sclerosis, exudation, and hemorrhage. Cerebrovascular complications are similar to those of other arterial beds and include transient ischemia, stroke, cerebral thrombosis, aneurysm, and hemorrhage.

Malignant hypertension is a rapidly progressive hypertension in which diastolic pressure is usually above 140 mm Hg. It can cause profound cerebral edema that disrupts cerebral function and causes loss of consciousness. High hydrostatic pressures in the capillaries cause vascular fluid to move into the interstitial space. If blood pressure is not reduced, cerebral edema and dysfunction increase until death occurs.

The early stages of hypertension have no clinical manifestations; thus, hypertension is called a silent disease. Some hypertensive individuals never have signs, symptoms, or complications; others become very ill and their hypertension can cause death. Others have anatomic and physiologic damage caused by past hypertensive disease even if current blood pressure is within normal ranges. Most of the clinical manifestations of hypertensive disease are caused by complications that damage organs and tissues other than the vascular system. Besides elevated blood pressure, the signs and symptoms are specific for the organs or tissues affected. Heart disease, renal insufficiency, central nervous system dysfunction, impaired vision, impaired mobility, vascular occlusion, or edema can be caused by sustained hypertension.

Hypertension is usually managed with both pharmacologic and nonpharmacologic methods. Treatment begins with reducing or eliminating risk factors. The usual recommendations are to restrict sodium intake, increase physical training, and discontinue cigarettes.

Four groups of drugs are used to manage hypertension: diuretics, angiotensin inhibitors, vascular smooth muscle relaxants, and adrenergic blockers. Diuretics and B-blockers are initially used because they reduce morbidity and mortality. If the response is inadequate, others are added.

3. Define and identify the causes of orthostatic or postural hypotension.
Study pages 634-636.

Orthostatic or **postural hypotension** is a drop in both systolic and diastolic arterial blood pressure on standing from a reclining position. The normal or compensatory vasoconstrictor response to standing is replaced by a marked vasodilation and blood pooling in the muscle vasculature and in the splanchnic and renal beds. Acute orthostatic hypotension may be the result of (1) anatomic variation, (2) altered body chemistry, (3) antihypertensive and antidepressant therapy, (4) prolonged immobility caused by illness, (5) starvation, (6) physical exhaustion, (7) fluid volume depletion, and (8) venous pooling.

Chronic orthostatic hypotension may be secondary to a specific disease. The diseases that may cause secondary orthostatic hypotension are adrenal insufficiency, diabetes mellitus, intracranial tumors, cerebral infarcts, and peripheral neuropathies.

4. Define aneurysm and list the types.
Study pages 636-637; refer to Figures 22-5 through 22-7.

An **aneurysm** is a localized dilation or outpouching of a vessel wall or cardiac chamber. The tension on the wall increases as the vessel becomes thinner, so the possibility of rupture increases. This is an example of the law of Laplace. The stretching produces infarct expansion, a weak and thin layer of necrotic muscle, and fibrous tissue that bulges with each systole. With time, the aneurysm can leak, cause pressure on surrounding organs, impair blood flow, or rupture.

The aorta is particularly susceptible to aneurysm formation because of the constant stress on its vessel wall and the absence of penetrating vasa vasorum in its adventitial layer. Three-fourths of all aneurysms occur in the abdominal aorta.

True aneurysms are fusiform and circumfunctional in nature and involve all three layers of the arterial wall; there is weakening of the vessel wall. **False aneurysms** or **saccular aneurysms** are usually the result of trauma. These aneurysms are caused by a break in the wall or a dissection of the layers of the arterial wall; blood is contained at the point of aneurysm by the adventitial layer.

Treatment of aneurysms is nearly always surgical. Leaking cerebral aneurysms are treated with clot-stabilizing drugs and a number of clinical measures designed to reduce intracranial pressure and promote hemodynamic stability before surgical intervention.

5. Distinguish between a thrombus and an embolus.
Study pages 637-638; refer to Table 22-4.

A **thrombus** is a blood clot that remains attached to a vessel wall. Thrombi tend to develop wherever intravascular conditions promote activation of the coagulation cascade. In the arteries, activation of the coagulation cascade is usually caused by roughening of the tunica intima by atherosclerosis. Infectious agents also roughen the normally smooth lining of the artery, which causes platelets to adhere readily. Pooling of arterial blood within an aneurysm can stimulate thrombus formation. In the veins, thrombus formation is more often associated with inflammation. Thrombi also form on heart valves if there is inflammation of the endocardium or rheumatic heart disease.

A thrombus poses two threats to the circulation. First, the thrombus may be large enough to occlude the artery and cause ischemia in the tissue supplied by the artery. Alternatively, the thrombus may dislodge and travel through the vascular system until it occludes flow into a distal systemic or pulmonic vascular bed.

Pharmacologic treatment includes the administration of heparin, warfarin, and streptokinase. A balloon-tipped catheter can be used to remove or compress a thrombus.

Embolism is the obstruction of a vessel by an **embolus** or a bolus of matter that circulates in the bloodstream. The embolus may be a dislodged thrombus, an air bubble, or an aggregate of fat, bacteria, or cancer cells. An embolus travels in the bloodstream until it reaches a vessel through which it cannot pass; an embolus will eventually lodge in a systemic or pulmonary vessel. Pulmonary emboli originate mostly from the deep veins of the legs or in the heart. Systemic emboli most commonly originate in the left heart and are associated with thrombi after myocardial infarction, valvular disease, left heart failure, endocarditis, and dysrhythmias.

Embolism of a coronary or cerebral artery is an

immediate threat to life if the embolus severely obstructs these important vessels. Occlusion of a coronary artery will cause a myocardial infarction, whereas occlusion of a cerebral artery will cause a stroke or CVA.

6. **Distinguish between arterial and venous occlusive disease.**
   Study pages 638-640; refer to Figures 22-8 and 22-9.

Thromboangiitis obliterans, or Buerger disease, tends to occur in young men who are heavy cigarette smokers. It is an inflammatory disease of the peripheral arteries. Inflammation, thrombus formation, and vasospasm can eventually occlude and obliterate portions of small and medium-sized arteries in the feet and sometimes in the hands. The pathogenesis of thromboangiitis obliterans is unknown.

The chief symptom of thromboangiitis obliterans is pain and tenderness of the affected part. Clinical manifestations are caused by sluggish blood flow and include rubor caused by dilated capillaries under the skin and cyanosis caused by blood that remains in the capillaries after its oxygen has diffused into the interstitium.

The most important part of treatment is cessation of cigarette smoking. Vasodilators may alleviate vasospasm. If vasospasm persists, sympathectomy may be performed and gangrene necessitates amputation.

Raynaud phenomenon and **Raynaud disease** are characterized by attacks of vasospasm in the small arteries and arterioles of the fingers and, less commonly, the toes. Raynaud phenomenon is secondary to systemic diseases such as collagen vascular disease, pulmonary hypertension, thoracic outlet syndrome, myxedema trauma, serum sickness, or long-term exposure to environmental conditions like cold or vibrating machinery in the workplace. Raynaud disease is a primary vasospastic disorder of unknown origin tending to affect young women. It consists of vasospastic attacks triggered by brief exposure to cold or by emotional stress. Genetic predisposition may play a role in its development.

The vasospastic attacks of either disorder cause changes in skin color and sensation because of ischemia. Vasospasm occurs with varying frequency and severity and causes pallor, numbness, and the sensation of cold in the digits. Also, sluggish blood flow resulting from ischemia may cause the skin to appear cyanotic. Rubor follows as vasospasm ends and the capillaries become engorged with oxygenated blood.

Treatment for Raynaud phenomenon consists of removing the stimulus or treating the primary disease process. Treatment of Raynaud disease is limited to prevention or alleviation of vasospasm itself. Cold, emotional stress, and cigarette smoking are avoided. Exercises that build centrifugal force in the extremities are also helpful in the early stages of vasospasm for either entity.

A **varicose vein** is a vein in which blood has pooled. Varicose veins are distended, tortuous, and palpable. Varicose veins in the legs are caused by trauma to the saphenous veins that damages one or more valves or by venous distention from a combination of standing for long periods and the action of gravity on blood within the legs. If a valve is damaged and permits backflow, a section of the vein is subjected to the pressure exerted by a larger volume of blood under the influence of gravity. The vein swells as it becomes engorged and surrounding tissue becomes edematous because increased hydrostatic pressure pushes plasma through the stretched vessel wall.

Varicose veins and valvular incompetence can progress to **chronic venous insufficiency** (CVI). This condition is characterized by chronic pooling of blood in the veins of the lower extremities and leads to hyperpigmentation of the skin over the feet and ankles. Edema of the feet and ankles may progress proximally to the knees. Any trauma or pressure lowers the oxygen supply by further reducing blood flow into the area. Cell death occurs and necrotic tissue develops into **venous stasis ulcers**. Persistent ulceration develops because the high metabolic demands of healing tissue cannot be met by the existing compromised circulation.

Venous thrombi are more common than arterial thrombi because flow and pressure are lower in the veins than in the arteries. With aging, the deep veins in the lower extremities become especially susceptible to thrombus formation. This is notable in individuals with long-term bed rest or those wearing constrictive clothing.

The inflammatory response triggered by the clotting cascade causes extreme tenderness, swelling, and redness in the area of thrombus formation. With venous occlusion, the skin is discolored rather than pale, edema is prominent, and pain is most marked at the site of occlusion. Treatment of varicose veins and chronic venous insufficiency begins conservatively. If conservative treatment is ineffective, saphenous vein stripping may be performed.

Superior vena cava syndrome (SVCS) is a progressive occlusion of the superior vena cava (SVC) that leads to venous distention in the upper extremities and head. The leading cause of SVCS is bronchogenic cancer, followed by lymphomas and metastasis of other cancers. The SVC is a relatively low-pressure vessel that lies in the closed thoracic compartment; therefore, tissue expansion within the thoracic compartment can easily compress the SVC.

Clinical manifestations of SVCS include edema and venous distension in the upper extremities and face including the ocular beds. Cerebral and central nervous system edema may cause headache, visual disturbance, or impaired consciousness. Respiratory distress may be present because of edema of the bronchial structures or compression of the bronchus by a carcinoma.

SVCS is generally not a vascular emergency but rather is an oncologic problem. Treatment consists of radiotherapy for the neoplasm and the administration of diuretics, steroids, and anticoagulants.

7. Characterize coronary artery disease; distinguish between myocardial ischemia and myocardial infarction and list complications of each.
Study pages 640-649; refer to Figures 22-10 through 22-15 and Tables 22-5 and 22-6.

Coronary artery disease, myocardial ischemia, and **myocardial infarction** all impair the pumping ability of the heart by depriving the heart muscle of oxygen and nutrients. **Coronary artery disease** (CAD) diminishes the myocardial blood supply until deprivation impairs myocardial metabolism. The myocardial cells remain alive but are unable to function normally. Persistent ischemia or the complete occlusion of a coronary artery causes infarction or death of the deprived myocardial cells and tissues.

In the United States, coronary artery disease is responsible for nearly 50 percent of all deaths and one-third of deaths in persons between 35 and 65 years of age. The risk factors for CAD are classified as either modifiable or nonmodifiable. The nonmodifiable risk factors are variables that cannot be altered by persons wishing to decrease their risk of cardiovascular disease. These include advanced age, male gender until age 60, genetic predisposition, and diabetes mellitus type I. The modifiable risk factors include hyperlipidemia, hypertension, cigarette smoking, diabetes mellitus type II, obesity, sedentary lifestyle, postmenopausal hormone therapy, and heavy alcohol consumption.

The most common cause of **myocardial ischemia** is atherosclerosis. The growing mass of plaque, platelets, fibrin, and cellular debris can eventually narrow the coronary artery lumen enough to impede blood flow. Platelet aggregations are known to release a prostaglandin that is a potent vasoconstrictor capable of causing spasm of the coronary arteries. This prostaglandin, thromboxane A_2, also promotes platelet aggregation, so a vicious positive feedback cycle of vasoconstriction and platelet buildup occurs in the vessel walls.

Imbalances between blood supply and myocardial demand cause myocardial ischemia. Supply is reduced by increased resistance in coronary vessels, hypotension, decreased blood volume, valvular incompetence, or anemia. Demand is increased by high systolic blood pressure, increased ventricular volume, left ventricular hypertrophy, increased heart rate, and hyperviscosity of the blood. Ischemia occurs whenever demand exceeds supply.

Myocardial cells become ischemic within ten seconds of coronary occlusion. After several minutes, the heart cells lose their ability to contract. Anaerobic processes take over and lactic acid accumulates. Cardiac cells remain viable for approximately 20 minutes under ischemic conditions. If blood flow is restored, aerobic metabolism resumes, and contractility is restored. If the coronary arteries cannot compensate for lack of oxygen, **myocardial infarction** occurs.

The number and severity of postinfarction complications depend on the location and extent of necrosis, the individual's physiologic condition before the infarction, and the therapeutic intervention. Dysrhythmias or arrhythmias, which are disturbances of cardiac rhythm, are the most common complication of acute myocardial infarction and affect more than 90 percent of individuals. Sudden death resulting from cardiac arrest is often caused by dysrhythmias, particularly ventricular fibrillation. Acute myocardial infarction is usually accompanied by left ventricular failure characterized by pulmonary congestion, reduced myocardial contractility, and abnormal heart wall motion. Inflammation of the pericardium, or pericarditis, is a frequent complication of acute myocardial infarction. Dressler's postinfarction pericarditis syndrome is thought to be an antigen-antibody response to the necrotic myocardium. Pain, fever, friction rub, pleural effusion, and arthralgias may

Myocardial Ischemia/Infarction

Stable Angina	Unstable Angina	Prinzmetal Angina	Infarction
		Cause	
Temporary ischemia, exertion	Advanced ischemia, occurs at rest	Vasospasm, occurs at night and at rest	Irreversible ischemia, cellular necrosis with repair or scarring
		Electrocardiography	
Normal, transient ST depression and T wave inversion	Normal, transient ST depression and T wave inversion	Transient ST elevation	Irreversible abnormal, pronounced Q waves
		Plasma Enzyme Levels	
Negative	Negative	Negative	CPK-MB fraction, LDH, and SGOT or AST elevation
		Pain Relief and Treatment	
Rest and nitroglycerin, beta blockers, calcium antagonists	Rest and nitroglycerin ineffective, beta blockers, calcium antagonists	Nitroglycerin, beta blockers, calcium antagonists	Narcotics, anticoagulant therapy, thrombolytic agents, beta blockers, surgery

Note: The first symptom of myocardial ischemia or infarction is usually sudden, severe chest pain. The pain of infarction is more severe and persistent than the pain of ischemia; it may be heavy and crushing and radiating to neck, jaw, back, shoulder, or left arm.

accompany this syndrome. Transient ischemic attacks or an outright cerebrovascular accident may result from thromboemboli that have broken loose from coronary arteries or cardiac valves to occlude cerebral vessels. Pulmonary emboli are especially common. Rupture of the wall of the infarcted ventricle may be a consequence of aneurysm formation because of decreased muscle mass at the infarcted site.

8. Characterize the terms associated with pericardial disease.
Study pages 649-653; refer to Figures 22-16 through 22-18.

Pericardial disease is often a localized manifestation of another disorder. Infection, trauma or surgery, neoplasms, or metabolic, immunologic, or vascular disorders can elicit a pericardial response. Pericarditis, pericardial effusion, or constrictive pericarditis are the consequences of the response.

Acute pericarditis, although idiopathic, is commonly caused by infection, connective tissue disease, or radiation therapy. The pericardial membranes become inflamed and roughened, and an exudate may develop.

Symptoms include sudden onset of severe chest pain that worsens with respiratory movements. Individuals with acute pericarditis may also report dysphagia, restlessness, irritability, anxiety, weakness, and malaise. Friction rub or a short, scratchy, grating sensation similar to the sound of sandpaper may be heard at the cardiac apex and left sternal border and is pathognomonic for pericarditis. Treatment for uncomplicated acute pericarditis consists of relieving symptoms.

Pericardial effusion is the accumulation of fluid in the pericardial cavity and is possible with all forms of pericarditis. The fluid may be a transudate or an exudate. Pericardial effusion indicates an underlying disorder. If the fluid creates sufficient pressure to cause cardiac compression, it becomes a serious condition known as **tamponade**. The danger of tamponade is that pressure exerted by the pericardial fluid will eventually equal diastolic pressure within the heart chambers. The first structures to be affected by tamponade are the right atrium and ventricle as diastolic pressures are normally lowest. Subsequent decreased atrial filling leads to decreased ventricular filling, decreased stroke volume, and reduced cardiac output. Life-threatening circulatory collapse may develop.

The most significant clinical finding in tamponade is pulsus paradoxus. In this circumstance, arterial blood pressure during expiration exceeds arterial pressure during inspiration by more than 10 mm Hg. There is impairment of diastolic filling of the left ventricle plus reduction of blood volume within all cardiac chambers.

Treatment of pericardial effusion or tamponade generally consists of aspiration of the excessive pericardial fluid. Persistent pain is treated with analgesics, antiinflammatory agents, or steroids. Surgery may be required if the tamponade cause is trauma or aneurysm.

Constrictive pericarditis is either idiopathic or associated with radiation exposure, rheumatoid arthritis, uremia, or coronary artery bypass graft. In constrictive pericarditis, fibrous scarring with occasional calcification of the pericardium causes the visceral and parietal pericardial layers to adhere; thus, there is obliteration of the pericardial cavity. Like tamponade, constrictive pericarditis compresses the heart and eventually reduces cardiac output. Unlike tamponade, however, constrictive pericarditis always develops gradually.

Symptoms are exercise intolerance, dyspnea on exertion, fatigue, anorexia, weight loss, edema, distention of the jugular vein, and hepatic congestion. Chest x-ray films frequently show prominent pulmonary vessels and calcification of the pericardium.

Initial treatment for constrictive pericarditis involves digitalis glycosides, diuretics, and sodium restriction. Surgical removal of the pericardium may be indicated since its removal does not compromise cardiac function.

9. Compare the cardiomyopathies.

Study page 653; refer to Figure 22-19 and Tables 22-7 and 22-8.

The **cardiomyopathies** are a diverse group of diseases that primarily affect the myocardium itself and are not secondary to the usual cardiovascular disorders such as coronary artery disease, hypertension, or valvular dysfunction. They may be secondary to infectious disease, exposure to toxins, systemic connective tissue disease, infiltrative and proliferative disorders, or nutritional deficiencies; most cases of cardiomyopathy are idiopathic.

Characteristics of Cardiomyopathies

	Dilated	Hypertrophic	Restrictive
Hemodynamic changes			
Cardiac output	Decreased	Normal	Normal or decreased
Stroke volume	Decreased	Normal or increased	Normal or decreased
Ventricular filling pressure	Increased	Normal or increased	Increased
Structural changes	Chamber size increased, decreased mitral valve competence	Chamber size normal or decreased, decreased mitral valve competence	Chamber size decreased, decreased mitral valve competence

10. Identify the causes and manifestations of valvular dysfunction.
Study pages 654-658; refer to Figures 22-20 through 22-23 and Table 22-9.

In **valvular stenosis,** the valve orifice is constricted or narrowed. This impedes the forward flow of blood and increases the workload of the cardiac chamber "in front" of or before the diseased valve. Increased volume and pressure cause the myocardium to work harder and myocardial hypertrophy develops.

In **valvular regurgitation**, known also as insufficiency or incompetence, the valve leaflets or cusps fail to close completely. This permits blood flow to continue even when the valve should be closed. During systole, some blood leaks back into the atrial "upstream" chamber. This increases the workload of both atrium and ventricle. Increased volume leads to chamber dilatation; increased workload leads to hypertrophy. Although all four heart valves may be affected, those of the left heart are more commonly affected than those of the right heart.

Valvular Stenosis and Regurgitation

Valvular Disorders	Causes	Manifestations
Aortic stenosis	Rheumatic heart disease, congenital malformation, calcification degeneration	Decreased stroke volume, left ventricular failure, dyspnea, angina, systolic murmur
Mitral stenosis	Acute rheumatic heart fever, bacterial endocarditis	Decreased stroke volume, right ventricular failure, chest pain, orthopnea, pulmonary hypertension, dysrhythmia, palpitations, induced thrombi, ascites, diastolic murmurs
Aortic regurgitation	Bacterial endocarditis, hypertension, connective disease disorders	Congestive left heart failure, dyspnea, throbbing peripheral pulse, palpitations, chest pain, diastolic and systolic murmurs
Mitral regurgitation	Rheumatic heart disease, mitral valve prolapse, CAD, infective endocarditis, connective tissue disorders	Left heart failure, pulmonary hypertension, dyspnea, hemoptysis, palpitations, murmur throughout systole
Tricuspid regurgitation	Congenital, high blood pressure in pulmonary circulation or right ventricle	Right heart failure, peripheral edema, ascites, hepatomegaly, murmur throughout systole

11. Distinguish between rheumatic heart disease and infective endocarditis.
Study pages 658-663; refer to Figures 22-24 and 22-25 and Table 22-10.

Rheumatic Heart Disease and Infective Endocarditis

Cause	Pathophysiology	Manifestations	Treatment
RHD			
Sequel to pharyngeal infection with group A beta-hemolytic streptococci, immune response to streptococcal cell membrane antigens	Carditis of all three layers of heart wall, endocardial inflammation and vegetative growth on valves, valvular stenosis, Aschoff bodies	Fever, lymphadenopathy, acute migratory polyarthritis, chorea, erythema marginatum or truncal rash, history of streptococcal pharyngeal infection, high antistreptolysin O titer, ECG abnormalities	Oral penicillin or erythromycin, salicylates, surgical repair of damaged valves
Infective Endocarditis			
Streptococci or staphylococci, viruses, fungi, rickettsiae	Prior endothelial damage to valves, mitral valve prolapse, prosthetic valves, septal defects, blood-borne microbial colonization to damaged valve, adhered microbes multiply and form endocardial vegetations	Fever, cardiac murmur, petechial lesions of skin and mucosa, positive blood cultures, ECG abnormalities	Long-term antimicrobial therapy—penicillin and streptomycin, prophylactic antibiotics for procedures increasing risk of transient bacteremia

12. Characterize dysrhythmias of the heart.
Study page 663; refer to Tables 22-11 and 22-12.

Dysrhythmias or arrhythmias can be caused by either an abnormal rate of impulse generation or an abnormal conduction of impulses. Dysrhythmias can impair the pumping of the heart and cause heart failure. One kind of dysrhythmia is a **heart block**. In AV node block, impulses are prevented from reaching the ventricular myocardium; the ventricles contract at a slower rate than normal.

Bradycardia is a slow heart rhythm below 60 beats per minute. Bradycardia can result from vagal hyperactivity. Pacemakers can assist in blocks and bradycardia.

Tachycardia is a very rapid heart rhythm over 100 beats per minute. Tachycardia results with improper autonomic control mechanisms of the heart, lung disease, shock, and fever.

Sinus dysrhythmia is a variation in heart rate during breathing. The causes of sinus dysrhythmia are unknown. This phenomenon is common in young people and infrequently requires treatment.

Premature contractions or extrasystoles are contractions that occur before the next expected contraction. Premature contractions may occur with hyperkalemia or hypercalcemia. Frequent premature contractions can lead to fibrillation during which cardiac muscle fibers contract out of sequence with each other. In fibrillation, the affected heart chambers do not effectively pump blood, so tissue and organ perfusion is impaired. **Ventricular fibrillation** is a life-threatening condition as the ventricle cannot fill or eject blood to vital tissues since contractions are so rapid. If fibrillation is not corrected immediately by defibrillation or some other method, death may occur within minutes.

13. Discuss altered contractility and ratio of oxygen supply and demand as mechanisms for heart failure.
Study pages 663-670; refer to Figures 22-26 and 22-27.

According to the Frank-Starling law of the heart, contractility is optimal within a certain range of myocardial cell lengths; the more the myocardium is stretched, the harder it contracts. Normally, an increase of diastolic stretch results in a larger systolic ejection force and a larger stroke volume. Increases of preload increase myocardial oxygen consumption by requiring a greater force of contraction to accomplish systole. The increased force of cardiac contraction is accompanied by increased metabolic demand in the myocardium and more oxygen is required to support myocardial metabolism. Unfortunately, increased myocardial stretch decreases myocardial capillary perfusion by mechanically narrowing coronary capillary lumina. Also, if preload increases beyond the ventricle's ability to empty, the coronary artery blood supply will drop as the ejection fraction decreases. These two factors will cause the overworked and overstretched myocardium to become hypoxic.

Afterload is the force or pressure against which a cardiac chamber must eject blood during systole. Increased afterload is associated with increased systemic vascular resistance or pulmonary vascular resistance such as occurs in systemic or pulmonary hypertension. To maintain cardiac output, the ventricles must eject the same amount of blood during the same amount of time into an area of higher resistance. Therefore, the ventricular myocardium must use greater force during ejection and consume more oxygen with each contraction. To maintain blood pressure, the ventricles must contract with more force to raise the ejection fraction. The ventricular myocardium will also require more oxygen as the force of contraction increases. The myocardial need for oxygen is affected by heart rate, force of contraction, and metabolic rate.

14. Compare the pathophysiology, manifestations, and treatment of right and left heart failure.
Study pages 671-675; refer to Figures 22-28 through 22-31.

Right Heart Failure

Right Heart Failure (Cor Pulmonale)	Manifestations of Right Heart Failure
Decreased right ventricular emptying (Decreased volume to lungs)	Fatigue
↓	Ascites
Increased volume and pressure in right ventricle	Gastrointestinal disorders
↓	Liver and spleen engorgement
Increased volume and pressure in right atrium	Cyanosis
↓	Distended jugular veins
Increased volume and pressure in the great veins	Elevated venous pressure
↓	Dependent edema
Increased volume in the systemic venous circulation	
↓	
Increased volume in distensible organs	
↓	
Increased capillary pressure	
↓	
Peripheral edema and serous effusion	

Note: Treatment for right heart failure begins with treatment of the underlying left heart failure or pulmonary disease. Diuretics and restricted water and sodium intake are used to reduce venous blood volume or preload. Myocardial contractility is enhanced with digoxin or other cardiotonic medications.

Left Heart Failure

Left Heart Failure (Congestive Heart Failure)	Manifestations of Left Heart Failure
Decreased left ventricular emptying (Less perfusion to body tissues) ↓ Increased volume and pressure in left ventricle ↓ Increased volume and pressure in left atrium ↓ Increased volume in pulmonary veins ↓ Increased volume in pulmonary capillary bed ↓ Fluid transudation from capillaries to alveoli ↓ Alveolar space fluid ↓ Pulmonary edema	Exertional and noctural dyspnea Blood-tinged sputum Orthopnea Cough Cyanosis Elevated pulmonary capillary pressure

Note: Treatment for left heart failure is to correct the underlying cause. Valvular dysfunction may require surgery. Vasodilators can improve coronary artery perfusion. The hypotension associated with left ventricular failure is usually treated with a cardiotonic antihypotensive. Oxygen is administered continuously to increase the supply of oxygen to the myocardium. Diuretics are given to decrease pulmonary edema and blood volume, and sodium and fluid intake are restricted. Morphine sulfate dilates the pulmonary and systemic vessels, which decreases pulmonary and systemic capillary hydrostatic pressure. Also, morphine sulfate is an analgesic and an opiate, which improves the emotional state of the individual and may limit the cerebrally mediated release of epinephrine.

15. Distinguish between impaired cardiac function and excessive cardiac demands as causes of heart failure.
Study pages 675-676; refer to Figures 22-32 and 22-33.

Causes of Heart Failure

Impaired Cardiac Function	Excessive Cardiac Demands

Myocardial disease
  Coronary artery disease
  Myocardial infarction
  Myocarditis
  Cardiomyopathies
Valvular heart disease
  Stenotic valves
  Regurgitant valves
Severe pericardial effusion
Pericarditis
Congenital heart defects
	Increased pressure
	  Systemic hypertension
	  Pulmonary hypertension
	
	Increased volume
	  Excessive intravenous fluid
	
	Increased perfusion
	  Thyrotoxicosis
	  Anemia
	  Septicemia

16. Classify the different types of shock by etiology.
Study pages 676-682; refer to Figures 22-34 through 22-38 and Table 22-13.

Shock is a condition in which the cardiovascular system fails to perfuse the tissues adequately. This failure results in widespread impairment of cellular metabolism. Any factor that alters heart function, blood volume, or blood pressure can cause shock.

Ultimately, shock, irrespective of its cause, progresses to organ failure and death unless compensatory mechanisms or clinical intervention reverse the process. Shock causes many diverse signs and symptoms. The individual may feel sick, weak, cold, hot, nauseated, dizzy, confused, afraid, thirsty, and short of breath. Blood pressure, cardiac output, and urinary output are usually decreased. Respiratory rate is usually increased.

Types of Shock

Type	Causes
Cardiogenic (heart failure)	Myocardial ischemia, myocardial infarction, congestive heart failure, myocardial or pericardial infections, drug toxicity
Hypovolemic (insufficient intravascular fluid volume)	Loss of whole blood plasma or extracellular fluid, fluid sequestration
Neurogenic (neural alterations of vascular smooth muscle tone)	Loss of sympathetic motor tone to vascular smooth muscle with vasodilation
Anaphylactic (immunologic alterations)	Hypersensitivity leads to vasodilation and peripheral pooling
Septic (infectious processes)	Bacteremia, endotoxins, interleukins (IL), tumor necrosis factor (TNF), platelet-activating factor (PAF), and myocardial depressant substance (MDS) all promote the inflammatory process and vasodilation, reduced cardiac output and tissue perfusion, impaired cellular metabolism

17. Briefly diagram the common events found in all types of shock and relate the events to the signs and symptoms of shock.
Refer to Figures 22-34 through 22-38.

Events, Signs, and Symptoms of Shock

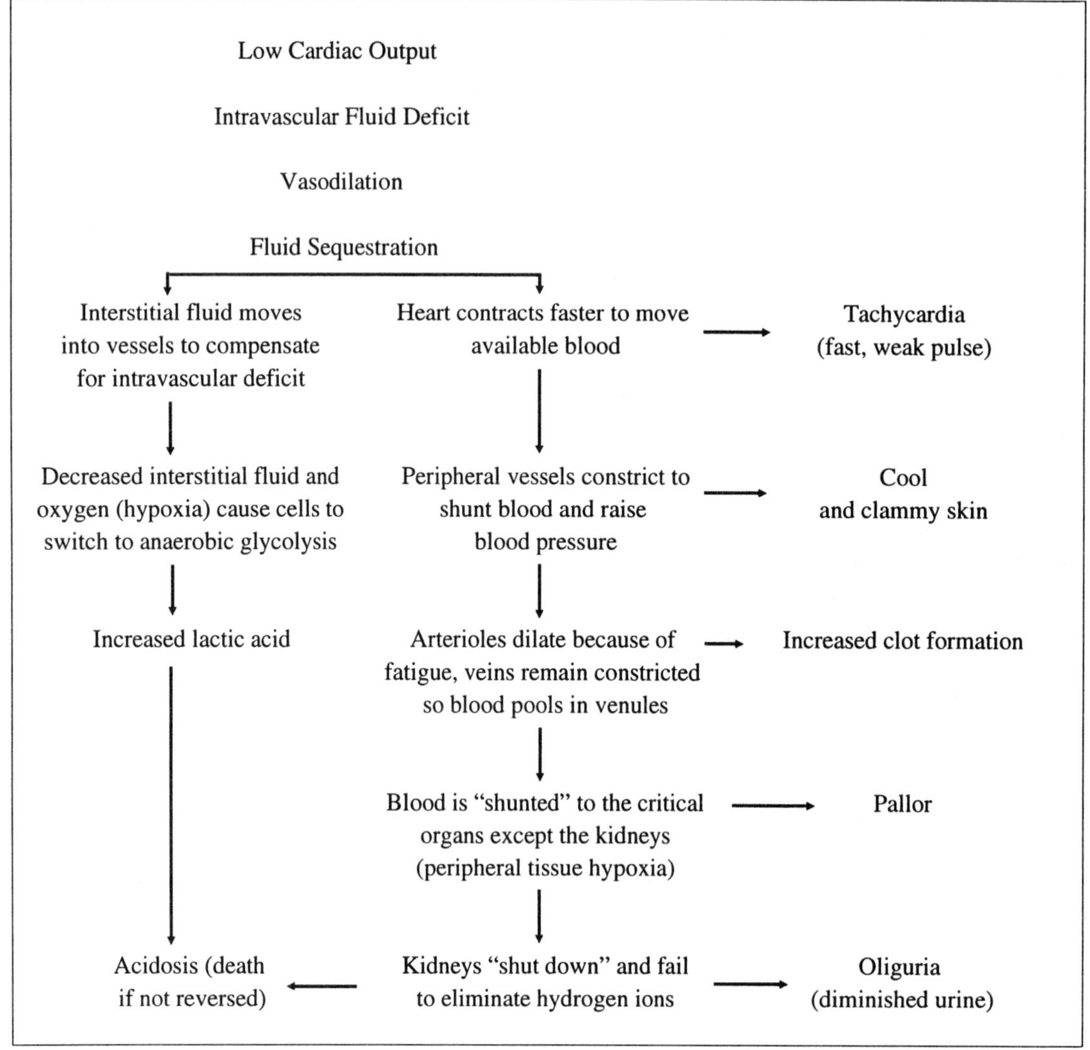

18. Illustrate the pathogenic sequence of multiple organ dysfunction syndrome (MODS) because of shock.
Study pages 682-687; refer to Figures 22-39 and 22-40 and Table 22-14.

Sepsis and septic shock are the most common causes of MODS. Severe trauma, burns, and respiratory or renal failure also contribute to MODS. The following diagram is illustrative of the pathogenesis of MODS:

Pathogenesis of Multisystem Organ Failure

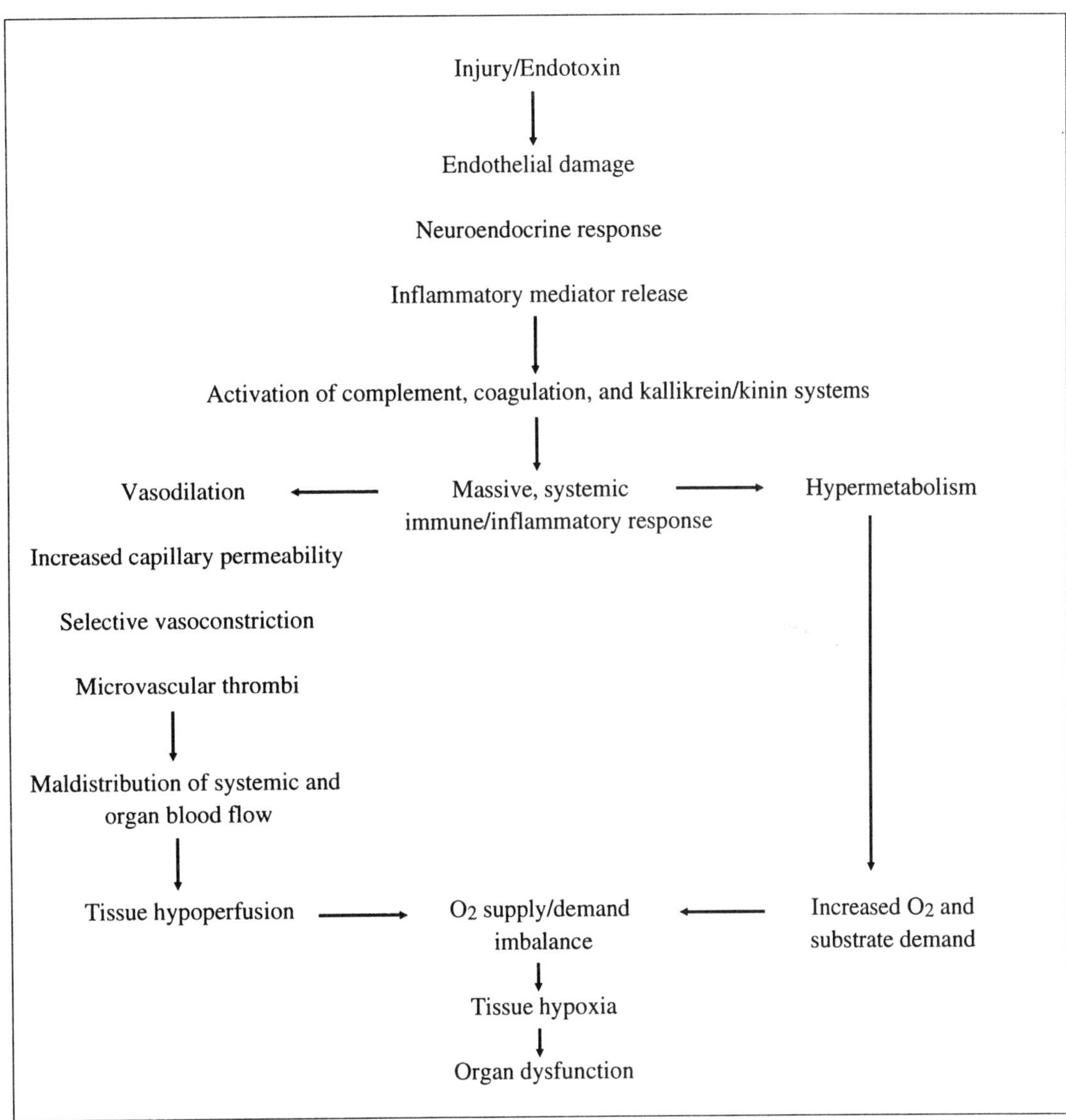

19. Characterize impaired cellular metabolism because of shock.
Study pages 685-687; refer to Figure 22-40.

The final outcome of any type of shock is impaired cellular metabolism and cellular lysis. The following diagram is illustrative of these events:

Shock's Impairment of Cellular Metabolism

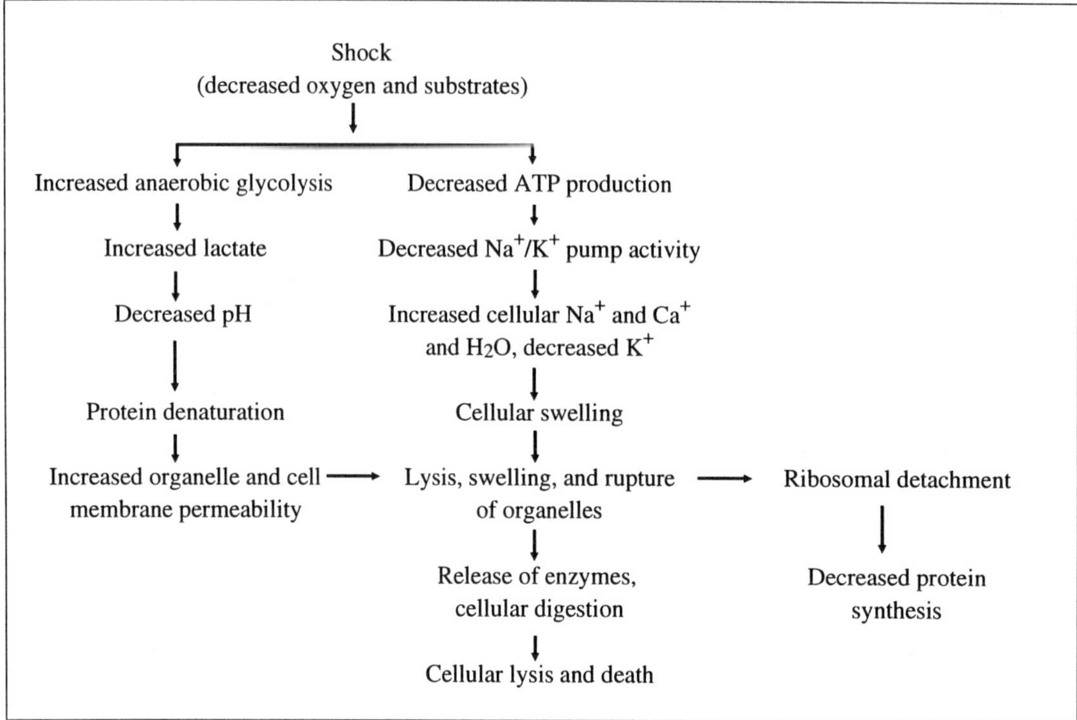

Practice Examination

1. Arteriosclerosis raises the systolic blood pressure by:

   a. increasing arterial distensibility and vessel lumen radius or diameter.
   b. increasing arterial distensibility and decreasing vessel lumen radius or diameter.
   c. decreasing arterial distensibility and increasing vessel lumen radius or diameter.
   d. decreasing arterial distensibility and lumen diameter.
   e. None of the above is correct.

2. Events in the development of atherosclerotic plaque include all of the following except:

   a. accumulation of LDL (low-density lipoprotein).
   b. smooth muscle proliferation.
   c. calcification.
   d. decreased elasticity.
   e. complement activation.

3. G.P. is a 50-year-old male who was referred for evaluation of blood pressure. If he has a high diastolic blood pressure, which reading belongs to G.P.?

   a. 140/82 mm Hg
   b. 160/72 mm Hg
   c. 130/95 mm Hg
   d. 95/68 mm Hg
   e. 140/72 mm Hg

4. The complications of uncontrolled hypertension include all of the following except:

   a. cerebrovascular accidents.
   b. anemia.
   c. renal injury.
   d. cardiac hypertrophy.
   e. All of the above are complications.

5. Primary hypertension:

   a. is essentially idiopathic.
   b. can be caused by renal disease.
   c. can be caused by hormone imbalance.
   d. results from arterial coarctation.
   e. b, c, and d are correct.

6. Orthostatic hypotension is caused by all of the following except:

   a. increased age.
   b. increased blood volume.
   c. autonomic nervous system dysfunction.
   d. bed rest.
   e. severe varicose veins.

7. Localized outpouching of a vessel wall or heart chamber is a/an:

   a. thrombus.
   b. embolus.
   c. thromboembolus.
   d. aneurysm.
   e. vegetation.

8. Which is a possible cause of varicose veins?

   a. gravitational forces on blood
   b. long periods of standing
   c. trauma to the saphenous veins
   d. Both b and c are correct.
   e. a, b, and c are correct.

9. A 76-year-old male came to the emergency room after experiencing chest pain while shoveling snow. Laboratory tests revealed essentially normal blood levels of SGOT or AST, CPK, and LDH enzymes. The chest pain was relieved following bed rest and nitroglycerin therapy. The most probable diagnosis is:

   a. myocardial infarct.
   b. emphysema.
   c. angina pectoris.
   d. hepatic cirrhosis.
   e. acute pancreatitis.

10. Complications of an infarcted myocardium likely could include which of the following? (*More than one answer may be correct.*)

   a. emphysema
   b. heart failure
   c. endocarditis
   d. death
   e. systemic thromboembolism

11. In pericardial effusion:

   a. fibrotic lesions obliterate the pericardial cavity.
   b. there is associated rheumatoid arthritis.
   c. tamponade compresses the right heart before affecting other structures.
   d. arterial blood pressure during expiration exceeds that during inspiration.
   e. Both c and d are correct.

12. Chamber volume increase is observed in ____ cardiomyopathy.

   a. dilated
   b. hypertrophic
   c. restrictive
   d. Both a and b are correct.
   e. a, b, and c are correct.

Match the valvular dysfunction with its characteristic.

13. ____ aortic stenosis	a. right ventricular hypertrophy
14. ____ tricuspid regurgitation	b. left ventricular hypertrophy
15. ____ mitral stenosis	c. right atrial hypertrophy
16. ____ mitral regurgitation	d. left atrial hypertrophy
	e. left atrial/right ventricular hypertrophy
	f. right and left ventricular/left atrial hypertrophy
	g. hypertrophy of all chambers

17. Which statement is true regarding rheumatic heart disease? (*More than one answer may be correct.*)

    a. It is caused by staphylococcal infections.
    b. It is caused by hypersensitivity/immunity to streptococci.
    c. It damages the tricuspid valve most often.
    d. It usually damages a mitral valve.

18. Which is not an expected finding in acute rheumatic fever?

    a. elevated ESR (erythrocyte sedimentation rate)
    b. elevated ASO titer (antistreptolysin O)
    c. leukopenia
    d. fever

19. Bacterial (or infective) endocarditis differs from rheumatic heart disease because of which of the following? (*More than one answer may be correct.*)

    a. Bacterial endocarditis is an infection of the heart, endocardium, and valves.
    b. It always follows rheumatic fever.
    c. It may occur following dental or bladder catheterization procedures.
    d. It commonly involves the vena cava valve.
    e. It is caused by a type III hypersensitivity.

20. Patients with only left heart failure would exhibit which of the following? (*More than one answer may be correct.*)

    a. hepatomegaly
    b. dyspnea
    c. ankle swelling
    d. pulmonary edema
    e. peripheral edema

21. In congestive heart failure, the pump or myocardium itself fails because of which of the following? (*More than one answer may be correct.*)

    a. loss of contractile force of the heart
    b. hypertension
    c. cardiac dysrhythmias
    d. intermittent claudication from occlusive vascular disease

22. Shock is a complex pathophysiological process involving all of the following except:

    a. decreased blood perfusion to kidneys.
    b. acidosis.
    c. rapid heart rate.
    d. hypertension.
    e. anaerobic glycolysis.

23. Most septic shock is the result of:

    a. anesthetics.
    b. gram-negative bacteremia.
    c. massive loss of body fluid.
    d. emotional stress causing collapse of blood vessel tone.
    e. pump failure.

24. Which statement is incorrect concerning hypertension?

    a. Malignant hypertension is characterized by a diastolic pressure of over 140 mm Hg.
    b. More than 90% of cases are of the essential or primary type.
    c. Headache is the most reliable symptom.
    d. When left untreated, the major risks include CVAs and cardiac hypertrophy.

25. A 53-year-old male was admitted to the emergency room after experiencing shortness of breath, weakness, cardiac dysrhythmias, and chest pain which did not subside following nitroglycerin therapy. Laboratory tests revealed the patient had an elevated serum CPK and SGOT or AST level. EKG tracings revealed a prominent Q wave and an elevated ST segment. The most probable diagnosis is:

    a. a transient ischemic attack.
    b. an acute myocardial infarct.
    c. an attack of unstable angina pectoris.
    d. Prinzmetal angina.
    e. coronary artery vasospasm.

Case Study

W.S., a 51-year-old white male, was assisting in the launching of his best friend's water-ski boat from a faulty boat trailer when he began to experience chest discomfort. At first, he believed his discomfort was because of the extreme July heat. Gradually, the discomfort became a crushing pain in his sternal area that radiated into his left arm and lower jaw. His friend suspected an ensuing heart attack and convinced W.S. to check into an emergency room. During the drive down a canyon with steep, winding curves, W.S. collapsed.

On arrival at the emergency room, W.S. was unconscious. His skin was cool, clammy, and very pale. His blood pressure was very low and his pulse was weak and irregular. Established resuscitation procedures were followed. After W.S.'s return to consciousness, an electrocardiogram showed evidence of myocardial injury and blood was drawn to check enzyme and electrolyte levels. When history was obtained, W.S. stated he is a harassed advertising executive and denied significant illnesses. However, he was being treated for primary hypertension. He acknowledged smoking three packs of cigarettes a day for 30 years. His father died of a heart attack at the age of 47.

W.S.'s subsequent electrocardiograms and serum levels of CPK, LDH, and SGOT or AST verified anterior myocardial infarction.

Knowing the diagnosis, identify W.S.'s risk factors, the early causes and precipitating events of his infarction, and the justification for using anticoagulant therapy.

CHAPTER

23

Alterations of Cardiovascular Function in Children

Foundational Objective

a. Describe the chambers, valves, and great vessels of the heart. Review pages 585-589; refer to Figures 21-3 through 21-5.

Memory Check!

- The heart has four chambers, the left and right atria and the right and left ventricles. The atria are smaller than the ventricles and have thinner walls. Their walls are thin because they are low-pressure chambers that serve as conduits for blood rather than as pumps that must forcefully eject blood. The ventricles propel blood all the way through the pulmonary or systemic circulation and so must pump against pressure throughout these systems. Pressure is greatest in the systemic circulation, which is driven by the left ventricle.

- The right ventricle ejects large volumes of blood through a very small valve into the low-pressure pulmonary system. The left ventricle is larger and ejects blood through a relatively large valve into the high-pressure systemic circulation.

- The atria are separated by the interatrial septum and the ventricles by the interventricular septum. Indentation of the endocardium for valves occurs to separate the atria from the ventricles and the ventricles from the aorta and pulmonary arteries. One-way blood flow through the heart is ensured by the four heart valves, the atrioventricular (mitral and tricuspid) and the semilunar (pulmonary and aortic). The valve openings are guarded by flaps of tissue called leaflets or cusps which are attached to the papillary muscles by the chordae tendineae cordis. The papillary muscles are extensions of the myocardium that pull the cusps together and downward at the onset of ventricular contraction, thus preventing their backward expulsion.

- The right heart atrium receives venous blood from the systemic circulation through the superior and inferior venae cavae. The pulmonary artery leaves the right ventricle and its branches enter the pulmonary circulation. Oxygen and carbon dioxide exchange occurs and four pulmonary veins carry oxygenated blood from the lungs to the left side of the heart. The oxygenated blood moves through the left atrium and ventricle into the aorta, which delivers blood to systemic vessels to supply the body.

Objectives

After studying this chapter, the learner will be able to:

1. **Relate left heart failure to congenital heart disease in children; describe the manifestations of left heart failure.**
Study pages 696-697; refer to Table 23-1.

Left heart failure is a common complication of many congenital heart defects. The most common causes of left heart failure in infancy are pressure and volume overloads secondary to congenital disease.

Dyspnea on exertion is manifested in infants as difficulty with feeding. When the infant tries to suck and swallow, breathing is interrupted and the child becomes exhausted. Poor feeding and failure to thrive are primary indicators of left heart failure in infants. The infant's respiratory rate may be greater than 40 breaths per minute. In severe left heart failure, tachypnea may be accompanied by retractions, grunting, nasal flaring, wheezing, coughing, and rales. Hepatomegaly is typically attributable to systemic venous congestion caused by right ventricular failure. In left heart failure in infants, the liver has a dull, rounded edge that is felt more than 3 cm below the costal margin and may be tender. Fluid retention in infants is usually manifested by weight gain without any increase in caloric intake.

2. **Describe the pathophysiology related to Kawasaki disease.**
Study pages 697-698.

Kawasaki disease is an acute, self-limiting vasculitis that may result in cardiac sequelae. Eighty percent of cases occur in children younger than five years of age; a peak incidence is in toddlerhood. Currently, it is the leading cause of pediatric acquired heart disorders in the United States. This disease tends to cluster in miniepidemics and may be related to an infectious process with an autoimmune component. The disease process progresses through four clinical stages:

Stage 1 - onset to 12 days: Small venules, arterioles, and the heart become inflamed.

Stage 2 - 12 to 25 days: Inflammation of larger vessels occurs and coronary artery aneurysms appear.

Stage 3 - 26 to 40 days: Medium-sized arteries begin granulation, and inflammation subsides in the microcirculation.

Stage 4 - day 40 and beyond: The vessels develop scarring, thickening of the intima, calcification, and formation of thrombi; arteritis is most frequent in the coronaries but may occur in a variety of arteries; 10 to 20 percent of children develop aneurysms in this process.

Diagnosis is made by evaluating six major findings, five of which must be present for diagnosis. These findings include (1) fever greater than 104° F, (2) bilateral conjunctivitis, (3) erythema of the oral mucosa, (4) erythema with desquamation of the palms and soles, (5) polymorphous erythematous rash, and (6) cervical lymphadenopathy. These may be accompanied by arthritis and abdominal pain. Later complications include coronary thrombosis. Echocardiography may monitor the disease in the coronary arteries. Treatment is nonspecific and supportive.

3. **Describe susceptibility and manifestations of primary hypertension in children.**
Study pages 698-700; refer to Figure 23-1 and Table 23-2.

In the past, most hypertension in children was considered to be secondary to other diseases. **Primary hypertension** is now known to exist in children. Autopsies on infants have shown fatty streaks, the earliest lesions of atherosclerosis, in the intimal lining of blood vessels. Hypertension-causing arterial disease can begin very early in life.

Obesity is a risk factor for hypertension in children. Hypertension in black children is associated with body mass and renal mechanisms; in white children, it is associated with obesity and neurohumoral factors. Research indicates that height and weight are more important than age in determining normal pressure in children. In all children, genetic correlates are strong. High cholesterol levels may be a significant risk factor for hypertension because high cholesterol levels are associated with atherosclerosis. Smoking doubles the risk of hypertension and other cardiovascular diseases at any age. A child who is consistently at the 95th percentile of hypertensive levels likely is at risk for adult hypertension and cardiovascular disease.

Diagnosis of primary hypertension in children is difficult since early stages may be asymptomatic and blood pressures vary from child to child and change as the child grows. The preventive efficacy of antihypertensive therapy during childhood is debatable and some clinicians prefer to control or eliminate risk factors.

4. Identify the most common congenital defects that obstruct outflow and describe their pathophysiology.

Study pages 702-705; refer to Figures 23-4 through 23-6.

Coarctation of the aorta is caused by a narrowing of the aorta anywhere between the origin of the aortic arch and the abdominal bifurcation. This defect may be considered in terms of its proximity to the ductus arteriosus. A narrowing near the ductus arteriosus results in increased blood flow to the head and upper extremities and decreased blood flow to the lower extremities. There are signs of left heart failure in infants. Surgical correction includes resection of the affected site on the aorta with various grafts and closure of the ductus.

Aortic stenosis is a narrowing or stricture of the aortic valve, causing resistance to blood flow in the left ventricle, decreased cardiac output, left ventricular hypertrophy, and pulmonary vascular congestion.

Children show signs of exercise intolerance, chest pain, and dizziness when standing for long periods. There is a characteristic murmur. Individuals are at risk for bacterial endocarditis, coronary insufficiency, and ventricular dysfunction.

Aortic valvotomy is a palliative procedure. A valve replacement may be required as a subsequent procedure.

Pulmonic stenosis is caused by the restriction or thickening of the leaflets of the pulmonary valve. Outflow is restricted from the right ventricle, resulting in increased afterload, and, if severe, may cause right ventricular hypertrophy and dilation. If pressures are high enough, the foramen ovale may reopen, resulting in a right-to-left shunt and cyanosis. Mild cases result in little or no symptomatology, while severe cases may require surgical correction.

5. Describe the defects with increased pulmonary blood flow and their pathophysiology and treatment.

Study pages 705-706; refer to Figures 23-7 and 23-8.

Atrioventricular canal defect consists of a low atrial septal defect that is continuous with a high ventricular septal defect and clefts of the mitral and tricuspid valves. A large central atrioventricular defect allows blood to flow between all four chambers of the heart. The directions of flow are determined by pulmonary and systemic resistance, left and right ventricular pressures, and the compliance of each chamber. Flow is generally from left to right.

There is usually moderate to severe left heart failure and a characteristic murmur. There may be little to mild cyanosis; the cyanosis increases with crying.

Complete surgical repair can be performed in infants. If the mitral valve defect is severe, a valve replacement may be needed.

Patent ductus arteriosus (PDA) results from the failure of the ductus arteriosus to close within the first weeks of life. Continued patency permits blood to flow from the higher-pressure aorta to the lower-pressure pulmonary artery, causing a left-to-right shunt to develop. Clinical manifestations are usually without cyanosis and include a "machinery" murmur and pulmonary vascular obstuctive disease in later life. Treatment is usually by surgical ligation.

6. Describe the defects with decreased pulmonary blood flow and their pathophysiology and treatment.

Study pages 706-708; refer to Figures 23-9 and 23-10.

Tetralogy of Fallot is a syndrome of four defects. The associated defects that comprise tetralogy are (1) a ventricular septal defect (VSD), (2) an overriding aorta that straddles the VSD, (3) pulmonic stenosis, and (4) right ventricular hypertrophy. The pathophysiology associated with tetralogy may be varied and is dependent on the degree of pulmonary stenosis as well as the size of the VSD and pulmonary and systemic pressures. The shunt may be either left-to-right or right-to-left. In any event, these defects result in hypoxia in the systemic circulation while the body attempts to compensate by increasing red cell production and increasing blood flow to the lungs through collateral bronchial vessels. Cyanotic episodes may also be accompanied by syncope or seizures due to hypoxia. Surgical treatment is usually accomplished by various surgical procedures.

Tricuspid atresia is the failure of the tricuspid valve to develop. Thus, there is no communication from right atrium to right ventricle. Blood flows through an atrial septal defect or a patent foramen ovale to the left heart and through a ventricular septal defect to the right ventricle and then to the lungs. It is often associated with pulmonic stenosis and transposition of the great arteries. There is complete mixing of unoxygenated and oxygenated blood in the left heart.

Cyanosis is usually seen in the newborn period. There may be tachycardia and dyspnea. Older children exhibit chronic hypoxemia with clubbing. Individuals are at risk for bacterial endocarditis, brain abscess, and stroke.

Palliative treatment is the placement of a shunt to increase blood flow to the lungs. Corrective repair consists of a surgical connection between the right atrium and the pulmonary artery.

7. **Describe defects that permit mixing of pulmonary and systemic blood.**
   Study pages 708-711; refer to Figures 23-11 through 23-14.

Complete transposition of the great vessels results in the effective switching of the aorta and pulmonary arteries so the pulmonary artery leaves the left ventricle and the aorta leaves the right ventricle. This creates two separate circulatory systems with no communication between them. Children with minimum communication are severely cyanotic. If large septal defects exist, cyanosis may be less but symptoms of left heart failure occur. Cardiomegaly develops a few weeks after birth. Switching procedures to make the left ventricle the systemic pump may be the best alternative of the various surgical corrections.

Total anomalous pulmonary venous connection (TAPVC) is a disorder in which the pulmonary circulation enters the right atrium instead of the left. TAPVC has four different variations with the same resultant pathophysiology, all of which are associated with atrial septal defects (ASD). The most common forms of this anomaly are (1) drainage of the pulmonary veins into the superior vena cava and right atrium, (2) drainage into the right atrium through the coronary sinus, and (3) drainage into the right atrium through the inferior vena cava. TAPVC in any form results in a mixture of oxygenated and unoxygenated blood being pumped to the systemic circulation. The shunt is usually right-to-left. The amount of cyanosis generated by this anomaly is dependent on the mixture of unoxygenated and oxygenated blood. Thus, the greater the pulmonary blood flow, the less the cyanosis. Congestive heart failure is a frequent complication. Most infants die by two months of age without surgical correction.

Truncus arteriosus is failure of normal septation and division of the embryonic vessel trunk into the pulmonary artery and the aorta; the resulting single vessel overrides both ventricles. Blood from both ventricles mixes in the common great artery and causes desaturation and hypoxemia. Blood ejected from the heart flows to the lower-pressure pulmonary arteries and causes increased pulmonary blood flow and reduced systemic blood flow.

Most infants have moderate to severe left heart failure and variable cyanosis, poor growth, and activity intolerance. There is a characteristic murmur, and children are at risk for brain abscess and bacterial endocarditis.

Corrective surgery involves closing the defect so that the truncus arteriosus receives the outflow from the left ventricle, excising the pulmonary arteries from the aorta, and attaching them to the right ventricle by a homograft.

Hypoplastic left heart syndrome is underdevelopment of the left heart which results in a hypoplastic left ventricle and aortic atresia. Most blood from the left atrium flows across the patent foramen ovale to the right atrium, to the right ventricle, and out the pulmonary artery.

There is mild cyanosis and signs of left heart failure until the patent ductus arteriosus closes. Then, there is progressive deterioration with cyanosis and decreased cardiac output which leads to cardiovascular collapse. Without intervention, it is usually fatal in the first months of life.

A several-stage surgical repair approach is used for correction of this condition. Some believe that heart transplantation in the newborn period is the best option for these infants.

Practice Examination

True/False

1. ____ Shunts are usually independent of systemic or pulmonary pressures and are due solely to defects within the heart.

2. ____ A patent ductus arteriosus or VSD is sometimes helpful when it is associated with other cardiac defects.

3. ____ VSDs always require surgical closure.

4. ____ In ASD or VSD, murmurs indicate defects.

5. ____ Cyanosis is not a major finding in transposition of the great vessels due to the fact that the blood is free to travel normally to the lungs.

Fill-in-the-Blank

6. Abnormal blood flow within the heart is usually referred to as a __________.

7. In VSD, the shunt is generally __________-to-__________.

8. Cyanotic defects usually shunt __________-to-__________.

9. Cyanosis due to cardiac defects is usually due to mixture of __________ and __________ blood.

10. Some cardiac defects are not obvious at birth due to the fact that systemic and pulmonary pressures are nearly __________ at that point.

11. The patent ductus arteriosus has a __________-to-__________ shunt.

12. The ductus arteriosus should be totally closed within the __________ of life.

13. Thickening or restriction of the valve from the right ventricle is known as __________.

14. Defects that obstruct outflow from the ventricles tend to cause increased __________ which may lead to __________.

15. Narrowing of the great vessel leading to the systemic circulation is known as __________.

Match the description with the alteration.

16. ____ associated with dyspnea when feeding
17. ____ likely associated with an infectious etiology and an autoimmune response
18. ____ vasculitis associated with aneurysm
19. ____ if mild, often self-correcting
20. ____ "blue spells"
21. ____ ASD, overriding aorta, pulmonic stenosis, right ventricular hypertrophy
22. ____ common complication of congenital heart defects
23. ____ immediate cyanosis and distress after birth
24. ____ two separate circulatory systems
25. ____ may be associated with coronary thrombosis

a. Kawasaki disease
b. VSD
c. tetralogy of Fallot
d. transposition of the great vessels
e. left heart failure

Case Study

David M. is a seven-year-old boy requiring a routine physical examination at the nurse practitioner's office. David's past medical and family history is not unusual. His activity level is normal and his mother assumes that he is quite healthy.

David's physical examination is normal until the cardiovascular system is evaluated. Then, he is noted to have a systolic murmur. There are also bounding pulses in the arms and severely decreased pulses in the legs. A pediatric cardiology consultation is requested.

What cardiac defect causes such a striking discrepancy in blood flow to the upper and lower extremities?

CHAPTER 24

Structure and Function of the Pulmonary System

Objectives

After review of this chapter, the learner will be able to:

1. **Identify the sequence of structures of the pulmonary system as air moves into and out of the lungs; list the defense mechanisms of the pulmonary system.**
   Review pages 716-722; refer to Figures 24-1 through 24-7 and Table 24-1.

2. **Describe lung volumes and capacities.**
   Review pages 722-724; refer to Figures 24-9 and 24-10 and Table 24-2.

3. **Relate changes in the thoracic volume to muscular contractions, alveolar surface tension, elastic properties of the lungs and chest wall, and conducting airway resistance.**
   Review pages 724-726; refer to Figures 24-11 and 24-12.

4. **Describe the neurochemical control of ventilation.**
   Review pages 726-729; refer to Figure 24-13.

5. **Identify the factors in the transport of oxygen to the cells of the body and describe oxyhemoglobin association and disassociation; identify the factors in the transport of carbon dioxide from the cells.**
   Review pages 729-735; refer to Figures 24-14, 24-15, and 24-17.

6. **Identify the normal values for arterial and venous blood gases.**
   Refer to Figure 24-16.

7. **Note the pulmonary changes that occur with normal aging.**
   Refer to Figure 24-18.

Practice Examination

1. Considering the sequence of structures through which air enters the pulmonary system, the pharnyx is to the trachea as the:

   a. bronchioles are to the segmental bronchi.
   b. alveoli are to the alveolar ducts.
   c. alveolar ducts are to respiratory bronchioles.
   d. respiratory bronchioles are to the alveolar ducts.
   e. All of the above are correct.

2. The cilia of the bronchial wall:

   a. ingest bacteria.
   b. trigger the sneeze reflex.
   c. trap and remove bacteria.
   d. propel mucus and trapped bacteria toward the oropharynx.
   e. Both a and c are correct.

3. As the terminal bronchioles are approached:

   a. the epithelium becomes thicker.
   b. mucus-producing glands increase.
   c. the epithelium becomes thinner.
   d. cartilaginous support increases.
   e. the smooth muscle layer thickens.

4. The left bronchus:

   a. is shorter and wider than the right.
   b. is symmetrical to the right.
   c. has a course more vertical than the right's.
   d. is more angled than the right.
   e. has more bronchial wall layers.

5. The respiratory unit consists of:

   a. cilia.
   b. bronchiolar arteries and veins.
   c. goblet cells and alveoli.
   d. respiratory bronchioles and alveoli.
   e. All of the above are correct.

6. Alveoli are excellent gas exchange units because of:

   a. their large surface area.
   b. a very thin epithelial layer.
   c. extensive vascularization.
   d. Both b and c are correct.
   e. a, b, and c are correct.

7. Surfactant:

   a. facilitates O_2 exchange.
   b. produces nutrients for the alveoli.
   c. permits air exchange between alveolar ducts.
   d. facilitates alveolar expansion during inspiration.
   e. All of the above are correct.

8. During expiration, which relationship is true?

   a. As the lung volume decreases, the number of molecules of the gas increases.
   b. As the lung pressure increases, the number of molecules of the gas increases.
   c. As the lung volume decreases, the pressure increases.
   d. As the partial pressure increases, less gas will dissolve in a liquid.

9. When the diaphragm and external intercostal contract:

   a. the intrathoracic volume increases.
   b. the intrathoracic pressure increases.
   c. the intrathoracic volume decreases.
   d. None of the above is correct.

Match the term with the description or example.

10. ____ inspiratory reserve volume

11. ____ vital capacity

a. amount of air remaining in lungs after a forced expiration

b. taking an extra-deep breath of air just before diving

c. includes sum of tidal, expiratory reserve, and inspiratory reserve volumes

d. the extra air pushed out during a forced exhalation

12. Oxygen diffusion from the alveolus to the alveolar capillary occurs because:

   a. the pO_2 is less in the capillary than in the alveolus.
   b. the pO_2 is greater in the atmosphere than in the arterial blood.
   c. oxygen diffuses faster than CO_2.
   d. the pO_2 is higher in the capillary than in the alveolus.

13. A shift to the right in the oxyhemoglobin dissociation curve:

   a. prevents oxygen release at the cellular level.
   b. causes oxygen to bind tighter to hemoglobin.
   c. improves oxygen release and increases oxygen movement into the cells.
   d. Both a and b are correct.
   e. None of the above is correct.

14. In which sequence does pO_2 progressively decrease?

   a. blood in aorta, atmospheric air, body tissues
   b. body tissues, arterial blood, alveolar air
   c. body tissues, alveolar air, arterial blood
   d. atmospheric air, aortic blood, body tissues

15. Most O_2 is carried in the blood ____; most CO_2 is carried ____.

   a. dissolved in plasma / associated with salt or an acid
   b. bound to hemoglobin / associated with bicarbonate/carbonic acid
   c. combined with albumin / associated with carbonic acid and hemoglobin
   d. bound to hemoglobin / bound to albumin

16. Alveoli are well-suited for diffusion of respiratory gases because:

   a. they are small and thus have a small total surface area.
   b. vascularization is minimal, allowing greater air circulation.
   c. they contain four thick layers, preventing air leakage.
   d. they contain surfactant which helps prevent alveolar collapse.

17. Which ordinarily brings about the greatest increase in the rate of respiration?

    a. excess carbon dioxide
    b. increased O_2
    c. increased arterial pH
    d. sudden rise in blood pressure

18. Given that the oxygen content of blood equals (1.34 ml of O_2 per gram of hemoglobin) times arterial oxygen saturation percent, if hemoglobin concentration is 15 g/dl and arterial saturation is 98%, what is the arterial oxygen content?

    a. 13.2 ml/dl of blood
    b. 19.7 ml/dl of blood
    c. 14.7 ml/dl of blood
    d. None of the above is correct.

19. The major muscles of inspiration are the:

    a. diaphragm.
    b. sternocleidomastoid.
    c. external intercostals.
    d. internal intercostals.
    e. Both a and c are correct.

20. Stretch receptors:

    a. are sensitive to volume changes in the lung.
    b. are located in bronchial smooth muscles.
    c. decrease ventilatory rate when stimulated.
    d. prevent lung overinflation when stimulated.
    e. All of the above are correct.

21. Which increase the respiratory rate?

    a. increased pCO_2, decreased pH, decreased pO_2
    b. increased pCO_2, increased pH, decreased pO_2
    c. decreased pCO_2, decreased pH, increased pO_2
    d. decreased pCO_2, decreased pH, decreased pO_2

22. The dorsal respiratory group (DRG) of neurons:

    a. sets the automatic rhythm of respiration.
    b. modifies the rhythm of respiration.
    c. is active when increased ventilation is required.
    d. None of the above is correct.

Match the normal range of blood gases with its arterial or venous state.

23. ____	pCO_2 of 40 mm Hg	a. arterial blood
24. ____	oxygen saturation of 70%	b. mixed venous blood
25. ____	oxygen content of blood of 19-20 ml/dl	

CHAPTER 25

Alterations of Pulmonary Function

Foundational Objectives

a. Compare the structures of the lower airway as the generations of division move toward the alveoli. Refer to Figures 24-4 through 24-7.

Memory Check!

- The trachea and mainstem bronchi are composed mainly of cartilage with a lining of mucous membrane. When the bronchi enter the lungs, they branch further. Instead of cartilaginous rings, smooth muscle encircles the bronchi with cartilage interspersed among the muscle bundles. By the time the bronchioles are reached, supportive cartilage is no longer present. The bronchioles are capable of constriction because of their layer of smooth muscle. Smooth muscle becomes thinner in the terminal bronchioles. The epithelium changes from pseudostratified and ciliated columnar in the bronchi to nonciliated cuboidal in the terminal bronchioles and finally to squamous in alveoli. Macrophages must remove any debris that reaches the respiratory bronchioles and alveoli because of the absence of cilia.

b. Define the measurements of lung volume. Review pages 723-724; refer to Figure 24-10 and Table 24-2.

Memory Check!

- Tidal volume (TV) is the amount of gas inspired and expired during normal breathing. Inspiratory reserve volume (IRV) is the amount of gas that can be inspired in addition to the tidal volume. Expiratory reserve volume (ERV) is the amount of gas that can be expired after a passive or relaxed expiration. Residual volume (RV) is the volume of gas that cannot be expired and is always present in the lungs.
- Total lung capacity (TLC) is the total gas volume in the lung when the lung is maximally inflated. It includes RV, ERV, TV, and IRV. Vital capacity (VC) is the maximum amount of gas that can be expired from the lung. It includes IRV, TV, and ERV. Functional residual capacity (FRC) is the amount of gas remaining in the lung at the end of a passive expiration or RV and ERV. Inspiratory capacity (IC) is the amount of gas that can be inspired after a passive expiration from FRC. It includes TV and IRV. The lung capacities are always the sum of two or more volumes. Normal values for volumes and capacities are based on age, sex, and height.

(Continued)

Memory Check! (cont)

- With each breath, a portion of the tidal volume remains in the conducting airways. This is the anatomical dead space. In certain disease conditions, some of the respiratory bronchioles and alveoli receive adequate ventilation but do not participate in gas exchange because they are not perfused by the pulmonary circulation. The volume of gas in unperfused alveoli is known as alveolar dead space.

c. Describe the diaphragmatic movements in inspiration and expiration; indicate other factors involved in the mechanism of breathing. Review pages 724-726; refer to Figures 24-11 and 24-12.

Memory Check!

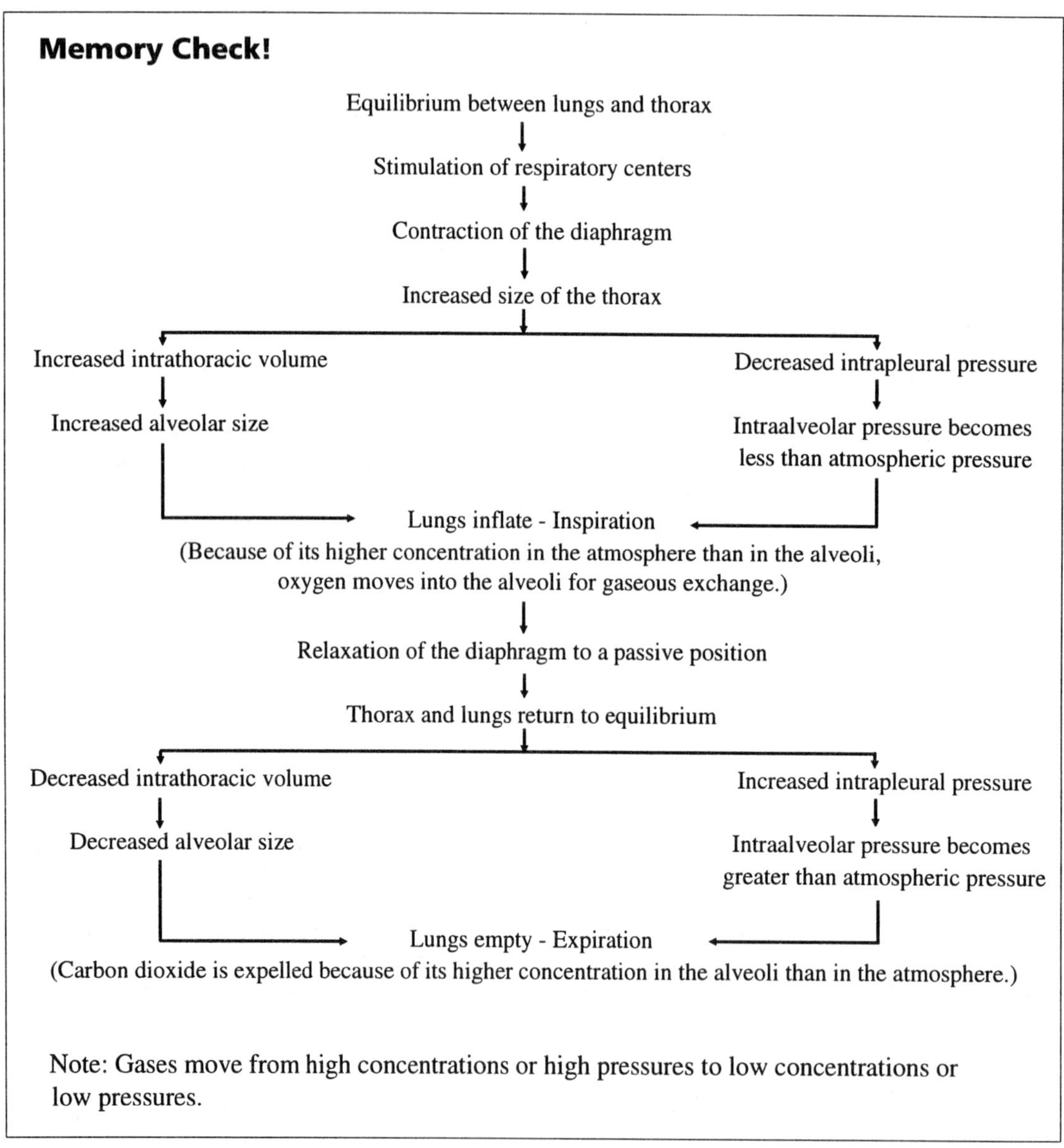

Note: Gases move from high concentrations or high pressures to low concentrations or low pressures.

Memory Check!

- Other factors involved in the mechanics of breathing include alveolar surface tension, elasticity of the lungs and chest wall, and resistance to air flow through the conducting airways. Surface tension occurs at any gas-liquid interface and is the tendency for liquid molecules exposed to air to adhere to one another. This phenomenon decreases the surface area exposed to the air. According to the law of Laplace, the pressure (P) required to inflate a sphere is equal to two times the surface tension (T) divided by the radius (r) of the sphere, or $P = 2T/r$. As the surface tension increases and the radius of the sphere or alveolus becomes smaller, more pressure is required to inflate it.
- Surfactant in the alveoli has a detergent-like effect that separates the liquid molecules, thus decreasing alveolar surface tension. Surfactant reverses the law of Laplace. The alveoli are much easier to inflate at low lung volumes after expiration than at high volumes after inspiration. The decrease in the surface tension caused by surfactant also is responsible for keeping the alveoli free of fluid. In the absence of surfactant, the surface tension tends to attract fluid into the alveoli.
- The lung and chest wall have elastic properties that permit expansion during inspiration and relaxation to original dimension during expiration. During inspiration, the diaphragm and intercostal muscles contract, air flows into the lungs, and the chest wall expands. Muscular effort is needed to overcome the resistance of the lungs to expansion. During expiration, the muscles relax and the elastic recoil of the lungs causes the thorax to decrease in volume until balance between the chest wall and lung recoil forces is reached.
- Compliance is the measure of lung and chest wall distensibility. It represents the relative ease with which these structures can be stretched. Compliance is, therefore, the reciprocal of elasticity. An increase in compliance indicates that the lungs and/or chest wall are abnormally easy to inflate and have lost some elastic recoil. A decrease indicates that the lungs and/or chest wall are abnormally stiff or difficult to inflate.
- Airway resistance is determined by the length, radius, and cross-sectional area of the airways and density, viscosity, and velocity of the gas. Resistance (R) is computed by dividing change in pressure (P) by rate of flow (F), or $R = P/F$. Resistance is inversely proportional to the fourth power of the radius; thus, anything decreasing the radius of the airways increases airway resistance.

Objectives

After studying this chapter, the learner will be able to:

1. Define the terms used in describing the signs and symptoms of pulmonary disease. Study pages 740-741; refer to Figure 25-1.

Dyspnea is the subjective sensation of uncomfortable breathing. It is often described as breathlessness, air hunger, shortness of breath, or labored breathing. Dyspnea occurs if increased airway resistance or decreased compliance causes respiratory effort greater than appropriate for the ventilation achieved. The signs of dyspnea include flaring of the nostrils, use of accessory muscles of respiration, and retraction of the intercostal spaces.

Orthopnea is experienced in the horizontal position. This position redistributes body water and causes the abdominal contents to exert pressure on the diaphragm, which decreases its efficiency of contraction and causes dyspnea.

Paroxysmal nocturnal dyspnea is seen in individuals with left ventricular failure who wake up at night gasping for air and have to sit up or stand to relieve the dyspnea. This dyspnea results from redistribution of body water into the lungs while the individual is recumbent.

Strenuous exercise or metabolic acidosis induces **Kussmaul respiration** or **hyperpnea.** Kussmaul respiration is characterized by a slightly increased ventilatory rate, effortless tidal volumes, and no expiratory pause.

Cheyne-Stokes respirations are characterized by alternating periods of deep and shallow breathing. Apnea, cessation of breathing lasting from 15 to 60 seconds, is followed by increased ventilation after which ventilation decreases again to apnea.

Cheyne-Stokes respirations occur in any condition that slows the blood flow to the brain stem or slows impulses to the respiratory centers of the brain stem.

Hypoventilation is inadequate alveolar ventilation in relation to metabolic demands. It is caused by alterations in pulmonary mechanics or in the neurologic control of breathing. With hypoventilation, CO_2 removal does not keep up with production and CO_2 rises in the blood, causing **hypercapnia.**

Hyperventilation is alveolar ventilation that exceeds metabolic demands. The lungs remove CO_2 at a faster rate than it is produced, which results in **hypocapnia** or low levels of CO_2 in the blood.

Coughing is a protective reflex that cleanses the lower airways by an explosive expiration that removes inhaled particles, accumulated mucus, or foreign bodies. Stimulating the irritant receptors in the airway initiates the cough.

Hemoptysis is coughing up blood or bloody secretions. Hemoptysis indicates a localized infection or inflammation that has damaged the bronchi or the lung parenchyma.

Cyanosis is a bluish discoloration of the skin and mucous membranes caused by increasing amounts of desaturated or reduced hemoglobin in the blood. Cyanosis can result from decreased arterial oxygenation or decreased cardiac output.

Pain is caused by pulmonary disorders that originate in the pleurae, airways, or chest wall. Infection and inflammation of the parietal pleura cause pain when the pleura stretches during inspiration. Pain that is pronounced after coughing occurs in individuals with infection and inflammation of the trachea and/or bronchi. Pain in the chest wall occurs with excessive coughing which makes the muscles sore.

Clubbing is the selective bulbous enlargement of the end of a finger or toe. Its pathogenesis is unknown but is associated with diseases that interfere with oxygenation.

An **abnormal sputum** is seen with different pulmonary disorders. Changes in the amount and consistency of sputum provide information about the progression of disease and the effectiveness of therapy.

2. **Characterize lung conditions that are caused by pulmonary disease or injury.** Study pages 742-749; refer to Figures 25-2 through 25-6 and Tables 25-1 and 25-2.

Conditions Caused by Pulmonary Disease or Injury

Condition	Pathology	Cause
Hypoxemia	Reduced oxygenation of arterial blood	Decreased oxygen content of inspired gas, hypoventilation diffusion abnormalities in emphysema, abnormal ventilation/perfusion ratios in bronchitis, right-to-left shunts in RDS or atelectasis
Pulmonary edema	Excess water in lungs	Heart disease increases pulmonary capillary hydrostatic pressure so fluid moves into interstitium; ARDS or inhalation of toxic gases injures capillaries and increases permeability; blockage of lymphatic vessels by CHF, edema, or tumors
Aspiration	Passage of fluid and solids into lungs, obstruction of airway, localized inflammation, noncompliance, edema, collapse	Decreased levels of consciousness, CNS abnormalities

(Continued)

Conditions Caused by Pulmonary Disease or Injury (cont'd)

Condition	Pathology	Cause
Atelectasis	Collapse of lung tissue	External pressure from tumor or fluid or air in pleural space, abdominal distension, bronchi obstruction, inhalation of concentrated oxygen or anesthetics
Bronchiectasis	Persistent abnormal dilation of bronchi	Obstruction of airway, atelectasis, infection, cystic fibrosis, tuberculosis, weakness of bronchial wall
Bronchiolitis	Inflammatory obstruction of bronchioles	Chronic bronchitis, infection, inhalation of toxic gases
Pneumothorax	Air or gas in pleural space collapses the lung partially or totally	Rupture of pleura or chest wall
Pleural effusion	Fluid in the pleural space collapses the lung partially or totally	Fluid from blood or lymphatic vessels from CHF, hypoproteinemia, infections or malignancies cause mast cell release of capillary permeability mediators, trauma that damages blood vessels
Empyema	Pus in pleural space	Bacterial pneumonia
Pleurisy	Inflammation of the pleura, exudate of lymph, fibrin, and cells cause a friction rub	Respiratory infection
Abscess	Circumscribed area of suppuration of lung parenchyma	Aspiration pneumonia
Fibrosis	Fibrous or connective tissue in lung	Scar tissue following ARDS, tuberculosis, or inhalation of dust or asbestos
Chest wall restriction	Compromised ventilation	Grossly obese, lateral bending and rotation of spine, arthritis of spine, depression of the sternum, neuromuscular disease
Flail chest	Compromised ventilation	Fracture of ribs or sternum
Toxic gas exposure	Inflammation of airways, alveolar and capillary damage, pulmonary edema	Inhalation of smoke, ammonia, hydrogen chloride, sulfur dioxide, chlorine, phosgene, and nitrogen dioxide; prolonged levels of high concentrations of oxygen
Pneumoconiosis	Fibrous tissue or nodules in lungs	Silicosis—inhalation of silica, anthracosis—inhalation of coal dust, asbestosis—inhalation of asbestos
Allergic alveolitis	Lung inflammation or pneumonitis	Inhalation of allergens—grains, silage, bird droppings, feathers, cork dust, animal pelts, molds, mushroom compost

3. In a diagrammatic scheme, interrelate the pathogenic factors in adult respiratory distress syndrome.
Study pages 749-751; refer to Figure 25-7.

(See box below.)

4. Compare and contrast the obstructive pulmonary diseases.
Study pages 751-756; refer to Figures 25-8 through 25-12 and Table 25-3.

Obstructive pulmonary disease is characterized by difficult expiration. More force or the use of accessory muscles of expiration is required to expire a given volume of air. The most common obstructive diseases are asthma, chronic bronchitis, and emphysema. Since many individuals have both chronic bronchitis and emphysema, these diseases are grouped together and are called chronic obstructive pulmonary disease (COPD). Asthma is more acute and intermittent than COPD, but it also can be chronic. (See box on page 213 of *Workbook*.)

ARDS Pathophysiology

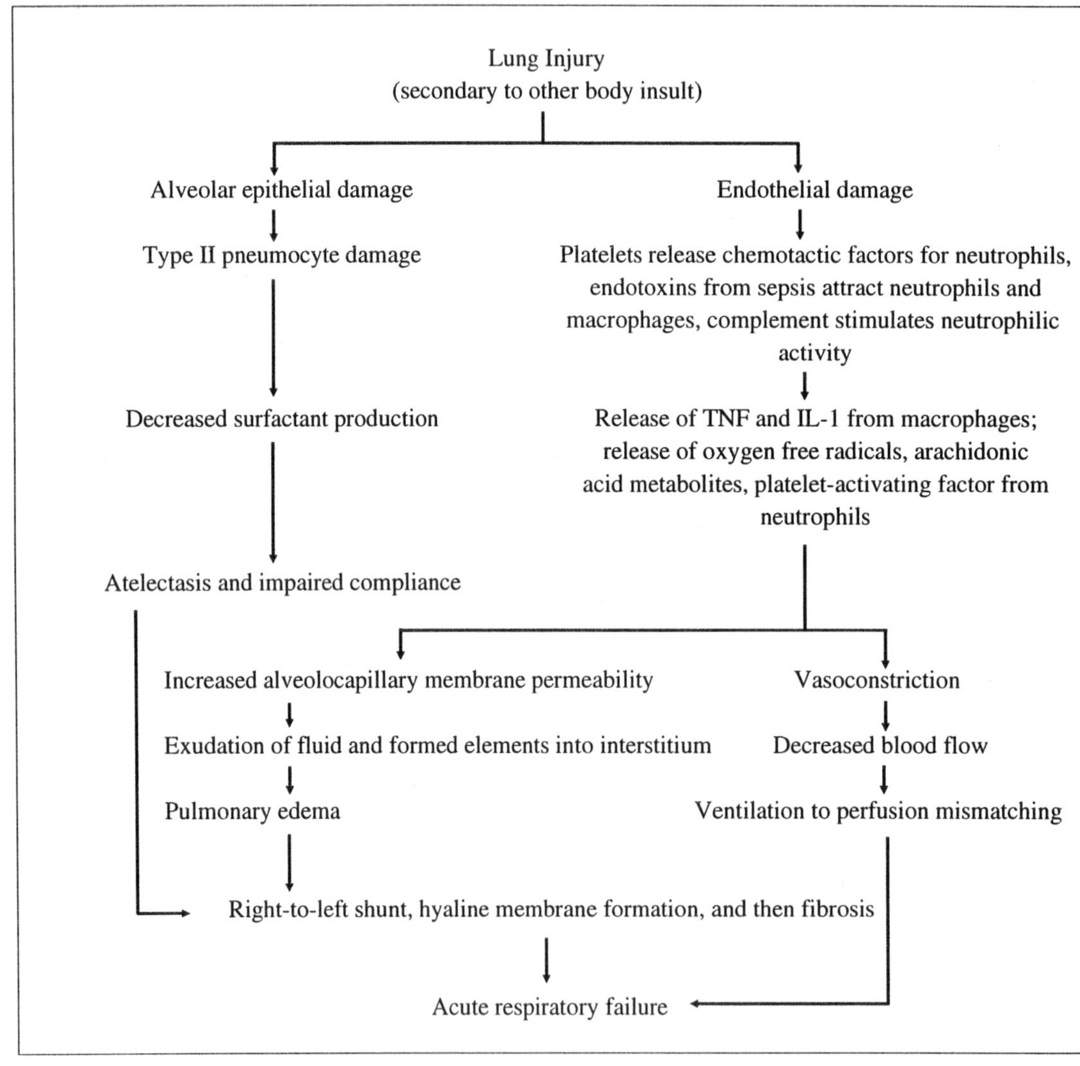

Obstructive Pulmonary Diseases

	Asthma	Emphysema	Chronic Bronchitis
Cause of airway obstruction	Thick mucus, mucosal edema, smooth muscle spasm	Enlargement and destruction of alveoli, loss of elasticity, trapping of air	Inflammation and thickening of mucous membrane, ciliary impairment, accumulation of mucus and pus
Precipitating causes	Extrinsic: Environmental antigens or allergens, IgE-mast cell complex releases inflammatory mediators Intrinsic: Respiratory infections, drugs, air pollutants, cold and dry air, exercise and emotional stress (parasympathetic dominance causes bronchospasm)	Alpha-1-antitrypsin deficiency, cigarette smoke	Cigarette smoke, air pollutants, infections
Manifestations	Dyspnea, wheezing, nonproductive cough early but later mucoid, prolonged expiration, tachycardia, tachypnea, acidosis	Marked dyspnea, no cough early but later, tachypnea with prolonged expiration, uses accessory muscles for ventilation, barrel chest, normal or elevated hematocrit, late cor pulmonale	Exercise intolerance, late dyspnea, wheezing, productive cough, marked hypoxemia leading to polycythemia and cyanosis, early cor pulmonale, CHF
Treatment	Antiinflammatory agents, bronchodilators	Prophylactic antibiotics, relief of dyspnea, cautious oxygen administration	Bronchodilators, expectorants, postural drainage, percussion, antiinflammatory agents

5. Define pneumonia and describe its causes, manifestations, and treatment.
Study pages 756-760; refer to Figure 25-13.

Pneumonia is an acute infection of the lung caused by bacteria, bacteria-like microbes, or viruses. The most common causal microbes are the following:

Gram-Positive Bacteria	Gram-Negative Bacteria	Nonbacterial Organisms
Streptococcus pneumoniae	*Escherichia coli*	*Pneumocystis carinii*
Staphylococcus aureus	*Pseudomonas aeruginosa*	*Mycoplasma pneumoniae*
Streptococcus pyogenes	*Klebsiella pneumoniae*	Fungi
	Proteus	Viruses
	Bacteroides species	
	Haemophilus species	
	Legionella species	

mucociliary clearance, and phagocytosis by alveolar macrophages, normally prevent infection by these pathogens. The body's immune system and various components of the inflammatory response further aid healthy individuals to prevent disease. In susceptible individuals, the invading pathogen is not contained. Instead, it multiplies and re-

Fungi infrequently cause pneumonia, but **fungal pneumonia** can be caused in immunosuppressed individuals by *Candida, Mucor,* and *Aspergillus.* The most common cause of **community-acquired pneumonia** is *Streptococcus pneumoniae. Mycoplasma pneumoniae* is the next most common cause of community-acquired pneumonia. *Staphylococcus aureus* and *Klebsiella pneumoniae* cause some community-acquired disease, usually in individuals with other health problems such as COPD or alcoholism or in individuals with a primary viral illness.

Most **nosocomial** or **hospital-acquired pneumonias** are caused by gram-negative bacteria such as *Escherichia coli, Klebsiella pneumoniae,* and *Pseudomonas aeruginosa.* When the gram-positive organism *Staphylococcus aureus* infects hospitalized individuals, it causes a more serious infection. These staphylococcal infections also are more likely to result in lung necrosis, abscesses, or empyema.

The *Legionella* species are widely distributed in water environments and are present in cooling systems, condensers, shower heads, and water reservoirs. Infections may occur in outbreaks or sporadically.

Pathogenic microorganisms can reach the lung by inspiration, by aspiration of oropharyngeal secretions, or via the circulation. This last source is usually by systemic infection, sepsis, or contaminated needles of intravenous drug users. The lungs' defense mechanisms, namely, the cough reflex, leases damaging toxins and stimulates full-scale inflammatory and immune responses. The immune response and the endotoxins released by some microorganisms damage bronchial mucous membranes and alveolocapillary membranes. Inflammation and edema cause the acinus and terminal bronchioles to fill with infectious debris and exudate; ventilation-perfusion abnormalities follow. If the pneumonia is caused by *Staphylococcus* or gram-negative bacteria, necrosis of lung parenchyma may also occur.

Streptococcus pneumoniae organisms cause most **bacterial pneumonias**. In this bacterial infection, the involved lobe undergoes consolidation or solidification of the tissue as it fills with exudate. A stage of red hepatization follows in which alveoli fill with blood cells, fibrin, edematous fluid, and pneumococci. This gives the lung tissue a red appearance. Next is a stage of gray hepatization in which affected tissues become gray because of fibrin deposition over the pleural surfaces and the presence of fibrin and leukocytes in the consolidated alveoli.

Viral pneumonia is usually mild and self-limiting, but it can set the stage for a secondary bacterial infection by providing an ideal environment for bacterial growth and by damaging ciliated epithelial cells. Viral pneumonia can be a primary infection or a complication of another viral illness such as chickenpox or measles. Viral pneumonia is usually caused by influenza viruses.

Most cases of pneumonia are preceded by an upper respiratory viral infection. Individuals then develop fever, chills, productive or dry cough, malaise, pleural pain, and sometimes dyspnea and hemoptysis. The white blood count is usually elevated, but it may be low if the individual is debilitated. Chest radiographs reveal infiltrates that may involve a single lobe of the lung (lobar pneumonia) or may be more diffuse (bronchopneumonia). Purulent sputum is expectorated by individuals with bacterial pneumonia, while viral pneumonia and pneumonia caused by *Mycoplasma pneumoniae* characteristically show scant sputum production.

Antibiotics are used to treat bacterial and mycoplasmal pneumonia. Viral pneumonia is treated with supportive therapy unless secondary bacterial infection is present.

6. Describe the pathogenesis of tuberculosis.
Study pages 759-760.

Tuberculosis is an infection caused by *Mycobacterium tuberculosis*, which is an acid-fast bacillus that usually affects the lungs but may invade other body systems. In the last decade, the number of reported tuberculosis cases has increased. A major reason for this trend is the epidemic of acquired immunodeficiency syndrome (AIDS). Individuals with AIDS are highly susceptible to respiratory infections including tuberculosis. A second important reason is the growing number of drug-resistant strains of tuberculosis bacillus that have developed because a large number of individuals do not consistently take their medications. This allows resistant strains to develop and spread. Emigration of infected individuals from high-prevalence countries, transmission in crowded institutional settings, substance abuse, and lack of access to medical care have also contributed to the growing problem.

Tuberculosis is transmitted from person to person in airborne droplets. Once the bacilli are inspired into the lung, they multiply and cause nonspecific lung inflammation. Some bacilli migrate through the lymphatics and become lodged in the lymph nodes where they encounter lymphocytes and initiate an immune response.

Neutrophils and alveolar macrophages wall off the colonies of bacilli and form a granulomatous lesion called a tubercle. Infected tissues within the tubercle die and form a cheeselike material; this is called **caseation necrosis**. Collagenous scar tissue then grows around the tubercle, which prevents further multiplication of bacilli.

Once the bacilli are isolated in tubercles and immunity develops, tuberculosis may remain dormant for life. However, if the immune system is impaired or if live bacilli escape into the bronchi, active disease occurs and may spread through the blood and lymphatics to other organs. Endogenous reactivation of dormant bacilli in the elderly may be caused by poor nutritional status, insulin-dependent diabetes, long-term corticosteroid therapy, and other debilitating diseases.

In many infected individuals, tuberculosis is asymptomatic. In others, symptoms develop so gradually that they are not noticed until the disease is well advanced. Common clinical manifestations include fatigue, weight loss, lethargy, loss of appetite, and a low-grade fever that usually occurs in the afternoon. A cough with purulent sputum develops slowly and becomes more frequent after weeks or months. "Night sweats" and general anxiety are often present. A positive tuberculin skin test indicates that an individual has been infected and has produced antibodies against the bacillus. Chest radiographs and culturing the bacillus from the sputum aid in the diagnosis of tuberculosis. Six grades of tuberculosis are possible; the grades aid in evaluation and the determination of appropriate therapy.

Treatment consists of antibiotic therapy to control active or dormant tuberculosis and prevent transmission. Today, with the increased numbers of immunosuppressed and susceptible individuals and drug-resistant bacilli, the recommended treatment for those at high risk is a combination of four drugs: isoniazid, rifampin, pyrazinamide, and ethambutol. Treatment continues until sputum cultures show that the active bacilli have been eliminated.

7. Compare and contrast pulmonary embolism, pulmonary hypertension, and cor pulmonale.
Study text pages 760-763; refer to Figures 25-14 and 25-15.

Blood flow through the lungs can be disrupted by a number of disorders that occlude the vessels, increase pulmonary vascular resistance, or destroy the vascular bed. Major disruptive disorders include pulmonary embolism, pulmonary hypertension, and cor pulmonale. (See box on page 216 of *Workbook.*)

Pulmonary Vascular Disease

	Embolism	Hypertension	Cor Pulmonale
Cause	Blood-borne substances from venous stasis, vessel injury, or hypercoagulation lodge in a branch of pulmonary artery and obstruct blood flow	Pulmonary arterial pressure is elevated by increased left atrial pressure, pulmonary blood flow, or vascular resistance secondary to lung disease	Right heart failure because of primary pulmonary disease and long-standing pulmonary hypertension
Manifestations	Earlier evidence of deep vein thrombosis of legs or pelvis, tachypnea, dyspnea, chest pain, hypotension, shock, possible radiographic wedge shape bordering the pleura	Fatigue, chest discomfort, tachypnea, dyspnea with exercise, a radiograph or electrocardiogram that shows right ventricular hypertrophy	Chest pain, second heart sound or closure of pulmonic valve is accentuated, tricuspid valve murmur, radiograph and electrocardiogram show right ventricular enlargement
Treatment	Avoid venous stasis, anticoagulant therapy, fibrinolytic agent if life-threatening	Supplemental oxygen, digitalis, and diuretics are palliative while lung transplantation is therapeutic	Same as pulmonary hypertension

8. Describe laryngeal cancer.
Study pages 763-764; refer to Figure 25-17.

The risk for **laryngeal cancer** is increased by and related to the amount of tobacco smoked; the risk is heightened when smoking is combined with alcohol consumption. Carcinoma of the glottis is more common than that of the epiglottis, aryepiglottic folds, arytenoids, and false cords. Squamous cell carcinoma is the most common cell type.

Progressive hoarseness is the most significant symptom and can result in voice loss. Dyspnea is rare with supraglottic tumors but can be severe in subglottic tumors. Laryngeal pain or a sore throat is likely with supraglottic lesions.

Radiation therapy has shown good results for early carcinoma of the vocal cords. Partial laryngectomies are the preferred treatment for small glottic malignancies. Total laryngectomy is required when lesions are extensive and involve the cartilage.

9. Describe the four major histologic types of lung cancer.
Study pages 764-768; refer to Figures 25-18 and 25-19 and Tables 25-4 and 25-5.

Lung cancers or **bronchogenic carcinomas** arise from the epithelium of the respiratory tract. Lung cancer and malignant melanoma are the only major cancers whose incidence is rapidly increasing in the United States. The most common cause of lung cancer is cigarette smoking; heavy smokers have about 25 times greater chance of developing lung cancer than nonsmokers. Cigarette smoke contains several organ-specific carcinogens for organs or tissues other than lung tissue; smoking has been causally related to carcinogenesis of the larynx, oral cavity, esophagus, and urinary bladder. Genetic predisposition to developing lung cancer also plays a role in lung cancer pathophysiology. (See box on page 217 of *Workbook*.)

Characteristics of Lung Cancer

Type/ Frequency	Growth Rate	Metastasis	Manifestations/ Treatment
Adenocarcinoma; 35%	Moderate	Early	Pleural effusion; surgical treatment
Squamous cell; 30%	Slow	Late	Cough, sputum production, airway obstruction; surgical treatment
Small cell (oat cell) carcinoma; 20-25%	Very rapid	Very early and widespread	Airway obstruction, excessive ACTH secretion with its signs and symptoms; chemotherapy and radiation to thorax and CNS
Large cell carcinoma; 10-15%	Rapid	Early and widespread	Pain, pleural effusion, cough, sputum production, hemoptysis, airway obstruction; surgical treatment

Note: The current accepted system for the staging of lung cancer is the TNM classification. In this system, T denotes the extent of the primary tumor, N indicates the nodal involvement, and M describes the extent of metastasis.

Practice Examination

Match the pulmonary condition with the characteristic.

1. ____ Kussmaul respiration
2. ____ hemoptysis
3. ____ cyanosis
4. ____ Cheyne-Stokes respiration
5. ____ pleural space atelectasis
6. ____ bronchiectasis
7. ____ pneumoconiosis
8. ____ flail chest
9. ____ pneumothorax
10. ____ abscess

a. inadequate alveolar ventilation

b. ventilation exceeding metabolic demand

c. coughing blood or bloody secretions

d. abnormal dilation of bronchi

e. fibrous tissue or nodules in lungs

f. fractured ribs or sternum

g. increased ventilatory rate, effortless tidal volume, and no expiratory pause

h. decreased arterial oxygenation

i. alveolar collapse

j. pleural space air

k. pleural space pus

l. apnea, increased ventilations, then apnea again

m. aspiration pneumonia

11. High altitudes may produce hypoxemia by:

    a. right-to-left shunts.
    b. hypoventilation.
    c. decreased oxygen inspiration.
    d. diffusion abnormalities.
    e. All of the above are correct.

12. In ARDS, increased alveolocapillary membrane permeability is due to:

    a. PAF.
    b. oxygen free radicals.
    c. TNF.
    d. Both a and c are correct.
    e. a, b, and c are correct.

13. Type II pneumocyte damage causes:

    a. increased alveolocapillary permeability.
    b. chemotaxis for neutrophils.
    c. exudation of fluid from capillaries into interstitium.
    d. decreased surfactant production.
    e. All of the above are correct.

14. Pulmonary edema may be caused by abnormal:

    a. capillary hydrostatic pressure.
    b. capillary oncotic pressure.
    c. capillary permeability.
    d. Both a and c are correct.
    e. a, b, and c are correct.

15. In bronchial asthma:

    a. bronchial muscles contract.
    b. bronchial muscles relax.
    c. mucous secretions decrease.
    d. imbalances within the CNS develop.

16. Intrinsic asthma is precipitated by which of the following? (*More than one answer may be correct.*)

    a. IgE
    b. airborne pollens
    c. animal danders
    d. emotional stress

17. In emphysema:

    a. there is increased area for gaseous exchange.
    b. there are prolonged inspirations.
    c. the bronchioles are primarily involved.
    d. there is increased diaphragm movement.
    e. None of the above is correct.

18. Chronic bronchitis (*more than one answer may be correct*):

    a. is caused by lack of surfactant.
    b. is caused by air pollutants.
    c. exhibits a productive cough.
    d. causes collapsed alveoli.

19. Which is inconsistent with pneumonia?

    a. chest pain, cough, and rales
    b. only involves interstitial lung tissue
    c. may be caused by mycoplasmas
    d. can be lobar pneumonia or bronchopneumonia

20. Tuberculosis (*more than one answer may be correct*):

    a. is caused by an aerobic bacillus.
    b. may affect other organs.
    c. involves a type III hypersensitivity.
    d. antibodies may be detected by a skin test.

21. Pulmonary emboli usually (*more than one answer may be correct*):

    a. obstruct blood supply to lung parenchyma.
    b. have origins from thrombi in the legs.
    c. occlude pulmonary vein branches.
    d. occlude pulmonary artery branches.

22. Pulmonary hypertension:

    a. is seen in elevated left arterial pressure.
    b. involves deep vein thrombosis.
    c. shows right ventricular hypertrophy.
    d. Both a and c are correct.
    e. a, b, and c are correct.

23. Cor pulmonale:

    a. occurs in response to long-standing pulmonary hypertension.
    b. is right heart failure.
    c. is manifested by altered tricuspid and pulmonic valve sounds.
    d. Both b and c are correct.
    e. a, b, and c are correct.

24. A lung cancer characterized by many anaplastic figures and the production of hormones is most likely:

    a. squamous cell carcinoma.
    b. small cell carcinoma.
    c. large cell carcinoma.
    d. adenocarcinoma.
    e. bronchial adenoma.

25. The metastasis of lung squamous cell carcinoma is:

   a. late.
   b. very early and widespread.
   c. early.
   d. early and widespread.
   e. never seen.

Case Study

Mr. S. is a retired 69-year-old county attorney who was on a buying trip with his wife for old, classic cars in the high, mountainous country of Colorado when he became extremely short of breath. His alarmed wife took him to a multispecialty medical clinic for evaluation.

On admission to the clinic, Mr. S. was restless and dyspneic. His chest had an increased anteroposterior dimension.

His past history revealed a habit of smoking two packs of cigarettes a day for 45 years. During the past few years, Mr. S. had noticed a cough each morning on arising. Recently, while working in his flower garden, he had to stop at times to catch his breath. Even while watching television, he had experienced dyspnea.

A chest radiograph was taken and pulmonary function tests were done. The chest radiograph revealed a flat, low diaphragm with lung hyperinflation but clear fields. Pulmonary function tests showed decreased tidal volume and vital capacity, increased total lung capacity, and prolonged forced expiratory volume.

Which pulmonary disease is exhibited by Mr. S.'s symptoms? Justify your answer.

CHAPTER

26

Alterations of Pulmonary Function in Children

Foundational Objective

a. Identify differences between children and adults that affect the pulmonary system. Review pages 773 and 778-779; refer to Figure 26-5.

Memory Check!

- Premature infants have immature lungs, placing them at risk for respiratory failure. Both premature infants and newborns have limited abilities to form antibodies. This inability increases their vulnerability to respiratory infection, particularly viral pneumonia. Shorter and straighter eustachian tubes of young children increase the incidence of otitis media.
- Infants are particularly at anatomic and physiologic disadvantage because of (1) their relatively small alveolocapillary surface area; (2) narrow airways that increase resistance to airflow; (3) the horizontal insertion angle of their diaphragm, which increases the work of breathing; (4) the relatively large number of mucous glands per area of bronchial mucosa; and (5) a deficiency in the numbers of pores of Kahn and Lambert that promote atelectasis distal to obstructions. Also, premature infants have a weak, compliant chest wall and insufficient surfactant. One anatomic advantage of infants is the relatively small amount of smooth muscle in their airways; bronchospasm is less severe.

Objectives

After studying this chapter, the learner will be able to:

1. **Identify two different forms of croup syndrome and differentiate between them by respective etiologies, anatomic involvement, and seriousness.**
   Study pages 774-776; refer to Figures 26-1 through 26-3 and Table 26-1.

Croup syndrome is a very generic term that refers to a number of primarily infectious processes of different etiologies affecting the structures of the upper airway. These vary from relatively benign to acutely life-threatening and are usually easily differentiated by matching the symptoms with the probable anatomic site involved.

Epiglottitis is an acutely life-threatening emergency. The etiologic agent is usually the bacteria *Haemophilus influenzae* type b. Children aged two to seven years are affected, with the peak incidence at three and one-half years. The affected structures are the epiglottis and the very small glottic space.

Onset is rapid and respiratory distress tends to be severe and quickly progresses to respiratory arrest without appropriate intervention. The child will be quite restless and fearful because of air hunger and will generally have severe respiratory stridor and be unable to swallow, causing copious drooling. Symptoms are due to marked edema of the epiglottis secondary to infection. The swollen epiglottis (1) obstructs the esophagus which leads to dysphagia and (2) quickly begins to obstruct the larnyx, leading to stridor and distress. If the airway of a child who displays the symptoms of epiglottitis is examined, respiratory arrest may result due to laryngospasm. Total airway obstruction and arrest are imminently probable.

Treatment consists of establishing an emergency airway by intubation or tracheotomy in instances of increasing larngneal obstruction. Appropriate antibiotics are necessary to treat the underlying bacterial infection. Administering oxygen, aerosolized epinephrine, and nebulized glucocorticoids will relieve inflammation and obstruction.

Laryngotracheobronchitis is generally a more common and benign form of croup syndrome than epiglottitis. The etiologic agent is usually parainfluenza virus. The affected age range is usually six months to three years, and recurrences are common.

Classic symptoms are generally preceded by two to three days of "cold" symptoms such as rhinorrhea and low-grade fever that progress to a high-pitched cough, muffled voice, and inspiratory stridor that is variable in intensity but often worse at night. Obstruction is caused by swelling of the subglottic tissues, and spasm of the vocal cords occurs as the inflammation extends. Treatment is with intravenous fluid therapy, oxygen supplementation, air humidification or cool mist, and inhaled epinephrine to temporarily decrease airway edema.

2. **Identify the most common forms of aspiration syndrome in infants and children.**
   Study pages 776-777.

Foreign body aspiration is common and frequently life-threatening in children. Offending objects are often toys or bits of food. Cough, hoarseness and dyspnea are common with a foreign body in the larynx. Similar symptoms with blood-streaked sputum are associated with bronchus obstruction. Complications include pneumonia, atelectasis, bronchiectasis, and lung abscesses if treatment is delayed. Lodged objects require endoscopic removal.

Foreign substance aspiration, such as baby powder or gastric fluid, may cause severe airway and lung inflammation. The inflammation may result in chemical pneumonia and respiratory distress. Infants may aspirate amniotic fluid which may be contaminated with meconium or bacteria from the birth canal. Aspirated bacteria may result in serious bacterial pneumonia. Prevention primarily consists of appropriate suctioning of the infant's upper airway on delivery of the head.

3. **Describe SIDS.**
   Study page 777.

Sudden infant death syndrome (SIDS) refers to the sudden, unexpected death of any infant or young child in whom a postmortem examination fails to demonstrate a cause for death. The incidence is 1.5 to 2 per 1,000 live births. The highest incidence is between two and four months of age; it mostly occurs during sleep and with greater frequency during winter months.

The cause of SIDS is unknown; however, new information suggests that it involves an abnormal T lymphocyte-mediated inflammatory response in the lungs. The degranulation of eosinophils could cause pulmonary edema, fatal respiratory obstruction, and hypoxia.

There is no treatment because the death is sudden and unexplained. There is evidence that infants should not be placed in the prone position during the first six months of life.

4. **Describe the pathophysiologic processes, manifestations, and treatment of asthma.**
   Study pages 777-779; refer to Figure 26-4.

Asthma is a chronic illness of highly variable severity which tends to be punctuated with more or less frequent episodes of acute exacerbation. The pathophysiologic basis of asthma involves hyperresponsive lower airways responding in an obstructive manner to various triggers. The triggers include allergens, exercise, cold air, viruses and other infectious agents, aerosolized irritants such as pollutants, and cigarette smoke. Responses include spasm of the respiratory smooth muscle that encircles the airways, edema of the airway mucosa, mucus plugging of the airways, and cellular infiltration into the airways. Asthma attacks may have two phases. The early phase of the attack is caused by IgE mediation resulting from mast cell degranulation and histamine release in response to the triggering factor. The late phase follows in six to eight hours and is caused by inflammatory mediators released from cells attracted to the airways. Activity of the parasympathetic nervous system can cause bronchoconstriction. Clinical manifestations may include persistent cough, expiratory wheeze, and signs of respiratory distress. Nearly half of affected children seem to outgrow asthma by adolescence; half do not.

Treatment involves the administration of adrenergic and bronchodilator aerosols, inhaled corticosteroids, and hyposensitization therapy.

5. Describe the most common etiologic agents in respiratory tract infections and pneumonias in children.
Study page 779; refer to Table 26-2.

Pneumonia in the first three months of life is most frequently caused by gram-negative bacteria, group B streptococci, and *Chlamydia trachomatis* acquired from the mother during the birth process. Viruses predominate in later infancy and early childhood, particularly respiratory syncytial virus and parainfluenza 3. Most bacterial pneumonias in children are due to *S. pneumoniae* followed by *Staphylococcus* and *H. influenzae*. *Mycoplasma pneumoniae* dominates in five- to ten-year-old children and continues into adolescence, although the total incidence of pneumonia declines in this age group.

Bronchitis in children occurs with other conditions of upper and lower airways such as asthma, cystic fibrosis, croup, pneumonia, or mild upper tract infections. Viruses cause most attacks of chronic bronchitis. Recurring childhood bronchitis predisposes for later bronchial lesions that lead to obstruction.

Treatment for viral respiratory infection is palliative. Bacterial infections are treated with appropriate antibiotics.

6. Identify the most common etiologic agent in bronchiolitis; describe the pathophysiology and the usual clinical course of the disease.
Study pages 779-781.

The most common cause of **bronchiolitis** is respiratory syncytial virus. Viral infection causes necrosis of the bronchial epithelium and destruction of ciliated epithelial cells. The submucosa of the bronchi becomes edematous and plugged with mucus and cellular debris, and bronchospasm narrows airways. Atelectasis occurs in some areas of the lungs and hyperinflation in others. The usual manifestation is an infant who has been exposed to family members with cold symptoms who develops mild cold symptoms. Symptoms progress to coughing, expiratory wheeze, and signs of respiratory distress including tachypnea, costal retractions, nasal flaring, and even cyanosis. Although most infants improve over three to four days, many require oxygen therapy and air humidification.

7. Describe the pathophysiologic processes involved in respiratory distress syndrome of the newborn.
Study pages 781-782; refer to Figure 26-6.

Respiratory distress syndrome (RDS) of the newborn is a lack of adequate surfactant to reduce alveolar surface tension. The small, underdeveloped alveoli of preterm infants require very high pressures to inflate. Absence of surfactant compounds this problem, and each breath the infant takes requires as much pressure as the first. Widespread atelectasis occurs, causing respiratory distress and increased pulmonary vascular resistance. Increased pulmonary vascular resistance causes shunting of the blood away from the lungs and results in a right-to-left shunt which further compounds the problem of hypoxia and hypercapnia. Hypoxia and hypercapnia trigger vasoconstriction of the pulmonary vascular bed and exacerbate shunting. Prolonged anaerobic metabolism produces metabolic acidosis.

Tachypnea, expiratory grunting, intercostal and subcostal retractions, nasal flaring, skin duskiness, and low body temperature are clinical manifestations. Treatment is supportive with mechanical ventilation. Exogenous surfactant administration has contributed significantly to the treatment of RDS.

8. Describe bronchopulmonary dysplasia.
Study page 783; refer to Figure 26-7.

Bronchopulmonary dysplasia (BPD) is a severe form of lung damage associated with neonatal chronic lung disease. Risk factors include premature birth and immature lungs, oxygen toxicity, positive pressure ventilation, respiratory infection, antiprotease deficiency, genetic predisposition, and ductus arteriosus.

Clinically, the infants remain oxygen- and ventilator-dependent and have respiratory symptoms and radiographic abnormalities after 28 days of life. Episodes of atelectasis, hyperinflation, pneumothorax, and interstitium air are characteristic.

BPD can cause death within a few weeks or can continue for months or years. Treatment is designed to accelerate lung maturation, maintain normal oxygenation, prevent further lung damage, and promote lung repair.

9. Describe the pulmonary pathophysiology associated with cystic fibrosis and identify general modes of diagnostic testing and therapy.
Study pages 784-785.

Cystic fibrosis is an autosomal recessive, genetically transmitted, multisystem disease in which exocrine or mucus-producing glands secrete abnormally thick mucus that obstructs the gastrointestinal system and lungs. An obstructed gastrointestinal system leads to malabsorption of nutrients. Thick secretions obstruct the bronchioles in the lung and predispose the lungs to recurrent or chronic infection. Chronic inflammation leads to destruction of the airway walls and hyperplasia of goblet cells. Bronchiectasis, pneumonia, and widespread pulmonary fibrosis follow. End-stage disease is characterized by cor pulmonale, chronic hypoxia, and pulmonary hypertension.

Chronic cough, sputum production, and purulent mucus indicate lung involvement. Labored ventilation results in hypoxia, finger clubbing, and cyanosis. Pulmonary disorders are the most common causes of morbidity and mortality.

Genetic testing is available to detect carriers. Sweat chloride testing is a definitive diagnostic test. Treatment includes aggressive chest physiotherapy and judicious use of antibiotics to control infection.

Practice Examination

True/False

1. ____ Although the infant has several mechanical disadvantages because of an immature respiratory anatomy, this is well compensated for by the nearly limitless metabolic resources that allow for prolonged, strenuous effort.

2. ____ At birth, the infant has approximately 300 million small, immature alveoli that develop into 25 million fully mature alveoli by approximately eight years of age.

3. ____ Surfactant production begins at birth and accelerates as airway lumenal growth begins at approximately five years of age.

4. ____ Failure to produce surfactant at birth results in severe atelectasis and RDS.

5. ____ Cystic fibrosis is a disease process primarily due to hyperresponsive airways that are sensitive to certain environmental triggers.

6. ____ Bronchiolitis and asthma produce symptoms that are similar.

7. Epiglottitis is characterized by:

   a. gradual onset.
   b. severe stridor.
   c. drooling.
   d. All of the above are correct.
   e. Both b and c are correct.

8. Laryngotracheobronchitis is characterized by:

    a. mild to moderate stridor, often worse at night.
    b. antecedent "cold" symptoms.
    c. swelling of subglottic tissues.
    d. a "barking" cough.
    e. All of the above are correct.

9. The most common cause of bronchiolitis is:

    a. *H. influenzae*.
    b. exposure to allergens.
    c. parainfluenza virus.
    d. respiratory syncytial virus.

10. Factors associated with upper respiratory infections in children include:

    a. frequent exposure.
    b. immune function.
    c. hyperresponsive airways.
    d. Both a and c are correct.
    e. Both a and b are correct.

11. Amniotic fluid aspiration in newborns is best avoided by:

    a. cesarian section delivery.
    b. withholding feedings for two hours after birth.
    c. suctioning the infant's airways on delivery of the head.
    d. thoroughly suctioning the birth canal just prior to delivery.

12. Bronchiolitis peaks at approximately six months of age. This is unfortunate because the:

    a. infant's airways are short and narrow at this age.
    b. infant has a relatively compliant chest wall at this age.
    c. infant has a very finite capacity to support prolonged respiratory effort.
    d. All of the above are correct.

13. All of the following statements about foreign body aspiration are true except:

    a. it is a relatively common occurrence in childhood.
    b. the offending objects include food and toys.
    c. it is rarely accompanied by serious complications.
    d. it may cause pneumonias and lung abscess.
    e. Both b and c are correct.

14. Which statement is true concerning cystic fibrosis?

    a. It is a multisystem disease.
    b. Defect results in overproduction of viscous mucus.
    c. It is difficult to detect carriers through genetic testing.
    d. Infectious complications are frequent.
    e. a, b, and d are correct.

15. Which statement is true concerning asthma?

    a. Its triggers include allergy, viruses, and cold air.
    b. Once asymptomatic for a number of years, affected individuals may be assumed to be cured.
    c. It is characterized by hyperresponsive airways.
    d. Both a and c are correct.
    e. a, b, and c are correct.

16. Which statement is true concerning pneumonias?

    a. They are frequently due to viruses.
    b. They are frequently due to bacteria.
    c. Incidence decreases with advancing age toward adolescence.
    d. All of the above are correct.

Match the circumstance or cause with the alteration.

17. ____ expiratory wheezing	a. asthma
18. ____ autosomal recessive	b. cystic fibrosis
19. ____ may result in persistent fetal circulation	c. laryngotracheobronchitis
20. ____ may be an outcome of prematurity	d. upper respiratory tract infections
21. ____ acute life-threatening infection	e. epiglottitis
22. ____ parainfluenza virus	f. respiratory distress syndrome
23. ____ occurs six to eight times per year	
24. ____ occurs epidemically in fall and winter	
25. ____ inflammatory basis with hyperresponsive airways	

Case Study

Tyler C. is a two-month-old boy who saw his physician three days ago with a history of mild nasal congestion without fever, cough, vomiting, or other complaints. His parents stated, however, that they were just getting over "terrible winter colds" and hoped they had not given it to Tyler.

Tyler has returned today because his mother is concerned that he is coughing severely, not feeding well at all, and "breathes funny." He still has no significant fever but is somewhat lethargic with a high respiratory rate, moderate intercostal retractions, nasal flaring, and light expiratory wheeze. Tyler is admitted to the hospital for further treatment.

What do Tyler's signs and symptoms suggest, and what is causing his signs? Why is hospitalization necessary?

CHAPTER 27

Structure and Function of the Renal and Urologic Systems

Objectives

After review of this chapter, the learner will be able to:

1. **Describe or identify the organs of the urinary system and the gross anatomical features of the kidneys.**
   Review page 790; refer to Figures 27-1, 27-2, and 27-7.

2. **Describe the microscopic structure of the nephron.**
   Review pages 790-793; refer to Figures 27-3 through 27-6.

3. **Identify the determinants of renal blood flow.**
   Review pages 795-796; refer to Figures 27-8 and 27-9.

4. **Describe the process of glomerular filtration.**
   Review pages 797-799; refer to Figures 27-10 and 27-11 and Table 27-1.

5. **Describe the process of tubular reabsorption and tubular secretion.**
   Review pages 799-800; refer to Figure 27-12.

6. **Differentiate the substances reabsorbed and secreted by different segments of the nephron tubules.**
   Refer to Figure 27-10.

7. **Describe the purposes of the countercurrent exchange system; note the actions of diuretics.**
   Review pages 800-802; refer to Figure 27-13.

8. **Identify the effects of hormones activated or synthesized by the kidney.**
   Review pages 802-803.

9. **Identify the changes that occur in renal function with advancing age.**
   Review page 804.

Practice Examination

1. Which sequence of structures does urine pass through as it leaves the body?

   1. ureter
   2. renal pelvis
   3. urinary bladder
   4. major calyx
   5. urethra
   6. minor calyx

   a. 2, 4, 6, 1, 3, 5
   b. 4, 2, 6, 1, 3, 5
   c. 6, 4, 2, 1, 3, 5
   d. 2, 6, 4, 5, 3, 1
   e. 6, 4, 2, 5, 3, 1

2. The functional unit of the human kidney is the:

   a. nephron.
   b. collecting tubule (duct).
   c. major calyx.
   d. minor calyx.
   e. pyramid.

3. One feature of the renal blood circulation that makes it unique is that:

   a. blood flows from arterioles into venules.
   b. blood flows from venules into arterioles.
   c. there is a double set of venules.
   d. there are two sets of capillaries.

4. Which has the opposite effect on urine production from the others?

   a. decreased solutes in blood
   b. decreased blood pressure
   c. increased ambient temperature
   d. dehydration
   e. reducing water consumption

5. The glomerular filtration rate is regulated by:

   a. the autonomic nervous system.
   b. the renin-angiotensin system.
   c. artrial natriuretic factor.
   d. All of the above are correct.
   e. Both a and b are correct.

6. If the following hypothetical conditions exist in the nephron, what would be the net (effective) filtration pressure?
   Glomerular blood hydrostatic = 80 mm Hg
   Glomerular blood osmotic = 20 mm Hg
   Capsular hydrostatic = 30 mm Hg

   a. 40 mm Hg
   b. 30 mm Hg
   c. 20 mm Hg
   d. 10 mm Hg

7. The capillaries of the glomerulus differ from other capillary networks in the body because they:

   a. have a larger area of anastomosis.
   b. branch from and drain into arterioles.
   c. lack endothelium.
   d. force filtrate from the blood.

8. Which is not a function of the kidney?

   a. water volume control
   b. blood pressure control
   c. urine storage
   d. converts vitamin D to an active form

9. Potassium is secreted by the ______ and reabsorbed by the ______.

   a. Bowman's capsule / loop of Henle
   b. proximal convoluted tubule / distal convoluted tubule
   c. loop of Henle / collecting ducts
   d. distal convoluted tubule / proximal convoluted tubule
   e. collecting ducts / loop of Henle

10. ADH causes water to:

    a. diffuse into the ascending limb of the vasa recta.
    b. return to the systemic circulation.
    c. be reabsorbed at the proximal tubule.
    d. Both a and b are correct.
    e. a, b, and c are correct.

11. Water reabsorbed from the glomerular filtrate initially enters the:

    a. afferent arterioles.
    b. efferent arterioles.
    c. Bowman's capsule.
    d. glomerulus.
    e. vasa recta.

12. Plasma contains a much greater concentration of ______ than the glomerular filtrate.

    a. sodium
    b. protein
    c. urea
    d. creatinine

13. An increase in water permeability of the distal convoluted tubules and collecting duct is due to:

    a. a decrease in the production of antidiuretic hormone (ADH).
    b. an increase in production of ADH.
    c. a decrease in blood plasma osmolality.
    d. an increase in water content within tubular cells.
    e. None of the above is correct.

14. The descending loop of the nephron allows:

    a. sodium secretion.
    b. potassium secretion.
    c. hydrogen ion secretion.
    d. water reabsorption.

15. Which most accurately describes the pressures affecting net glomerular filtration?

    a. Blood osmotic opposes capsular hydrostatic and blood hydrostatic.
    b. Blood hydrostatic opposes capsular hydrostatic and blood oncotic.
    c. Capsular hydrostatic opposes blood osmotic and blood hydrostatic.
    d. None of the above is correct.

16. Tubular secretion of urea is accomplished in:

    a. the glomerulus.
    b. the urethra.
    c. the renal pelvis.
    d. the distal convoluted tubule.
    e. None of the above is correct.

17. Tubular reabsorption and tubular secretion differ in that:

    a. secretion adds material to the filtrate; reabsorption removes materials from the filtrate.
    b. secretion is a passive process; reabsorption is an active transport process.
    c. reabsorption tends to increase urine volume; secretion tends to decrease urine volume.
    d. secretion adds materials to the blood; reabsorption removes materials from the blood.

18. The kidneys (*more than one answer may be correct*):

    a. conserve H^+.
    b. conserve NH^+4.
    c. eliminate H^+.
    d. eliminate NH^+4.
    e. conserve HCO_3^-.

19. If a small person excretes about 1 liter of urine during a 24-hour period, estimate the total amount of glomerular filtrate formed.

    a. 4 liters
    b. 10 liters
    c. 18 liters
    d. 100 liters

20. Which should not appear in the glomerular filtrate (in any significant quantity) just after the process of glomerular filtration has been accomplished?

    a. protein
    b. urea
    c. glucose
    d. Both a and b are correct.

21. Loop of Henle is to vasa recta as convoluted tubules are to:

    a. afferent arterioles.
    b. peritubular capillaries.
    c. efferent arterioles.
    d. renal arteries.

22. The two "currents" used in the countercurrent exchange system are the:

    a. afferent and efferent arterioles.
    b. glomerulus and glomerular (Bowman's) capsule.
    c. ascending and descending limbs.
    d. proximal and distal tubules.
    e. All of the above are correct.

23. The countercurrent exchange system:

    a. prevents water reabsorption from the collecting duct.
    b. concentrates sodium in the renal cortex.
    c. facilitates osmosis.
    d. concentrates chloride in the renal cortex.
    e. None of the above is correct.

24. Natriuretic hormone:

    a. increases ADH secretion.
    b. is produced by the kidney.
    c. causes more urine output.
    d. causes less urine output.

25. A waste product of protein metabolism is:

    a. pepsinogen.
    b. trypsin.
    c. amino acid.
    d. urea.
    e. urine.

CHAPTER

28

Alterations of Renal and Urinary Tract Function

Foundational Objectives

a. Define the renal processes of filtration, reabsorption, and secretion. Refer to Figure 27-10.

Memory Check!

- Glomerular filtration is the first step in urine formation in which permeable substances from the blood are filtered at the endothelial-capsular membrane and the filtrate enters the proximal convoluted tubule.
- Tubular reabsorption retains substances needed by the body, including water, glucose, sodium, potassium, and bicarbonate. This process removes materials from the filtrate and returns them to the blood.
- Tubular secretion excretes chemicals not needed by the body, including hydrogen and some amino acids, urea, creatinine, and some drugs. Secretion adds material to the filtrate from the blood.

b. Identify the forces and factors determining net filtration pressure; explain cause and effect of decreased filtration pressure. Review page 797; refer to Table 27-1.

Memory Check!

- Net filtration pressure is equal to glomerular blood hydrostatic pressure minus capsular hydrostatic pressure plus blood oncotic pressure. Stated mathematically, the formula is NFP = GBHP - (CHP + BOP). The pressure promoting filtration into Bowman's space is 47 mm Hg due to GBHP, while the pressure resisting flow to Bowman's space is 35 mm Hg due to 10 mm Hg of pressure from Bowman's capsule HP and 25 mm Hg from BOP. This provides a small net filtration pressure of 12 mm Hg. This net filtration pressure can be reduced by renal vasoconstriction, hypotension, hypovolemia, or low cardiac output. Any of these circumstances will reduce glomerular filtration rate (GFR). The GFR is directly related to renal blood flow (RBF) which is regulated by intrinsic neural and hormonal autoregulation. The blood flow is determined by arteriovenous pressure differences across the vascular bed divided by the vascular resistance or, stated mathematically, RBF = PA - PV/R. As pressure increases and resistance decreases, renal blood flow increases. Sympathetic nerve activity stimulates renal arteriolar vasoconstriction and decreases both RBF and GFR.

(Continued)

Memory Check! (cont'd)

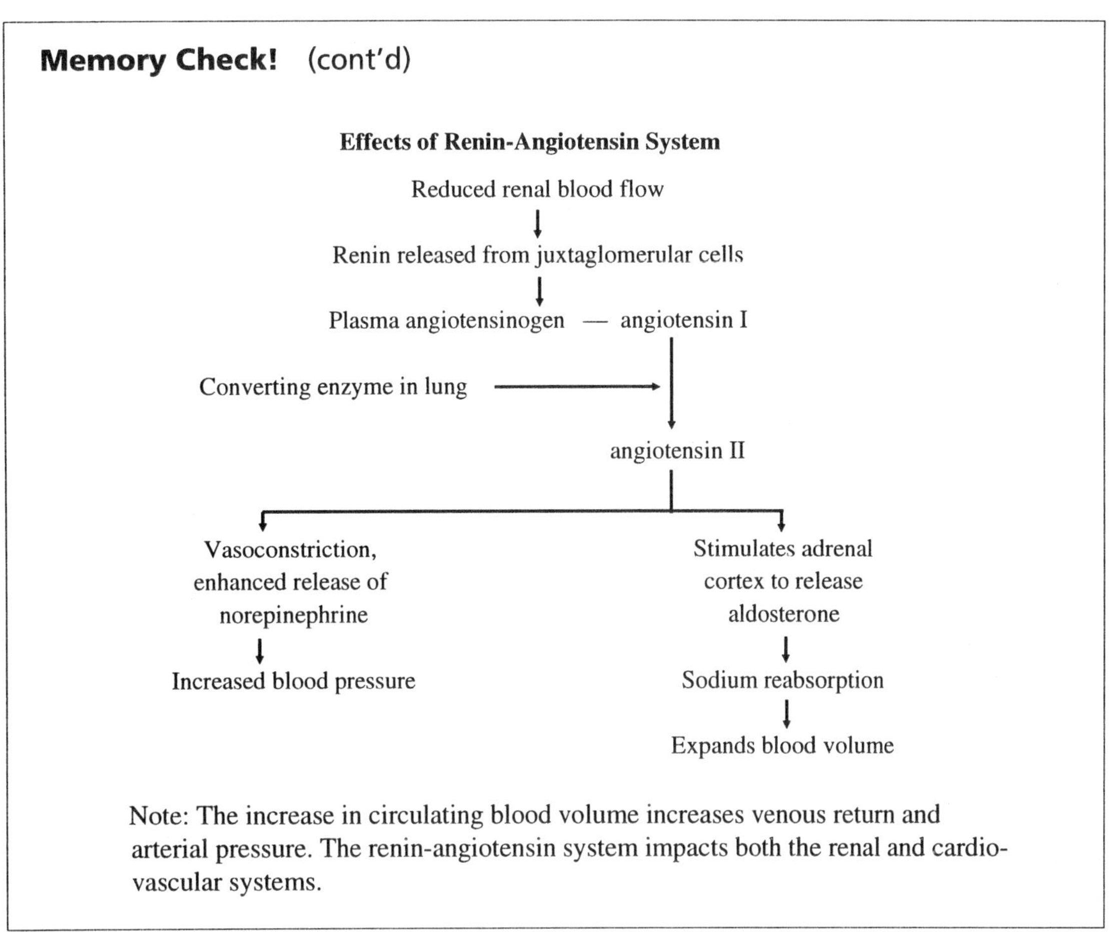

Note: The increase in circulating blood volume increases venous return and arterial pressure. The renin-angiotensin system impacts both the renal and cardiovascular systems.

c. Explain the basis of serum and urinalysis examinations to evaluate renal function. Review pages 803-804.

Memory Check!

Laboratory Tests for Kidney Function

- Blood urea nitrogen (BUN) measures the concentration of urea in the blood. Urea is formed from protein metabolism and is elevated in reduced glomerular filtration. Normal BUN is 10 to 20 mg/dl. The BUN rises in states of dehydration and acute and chronic renal failure as passage of fluid through the tubules is slowed.
- The serum creatinine level should have a stable value because creatinine is a byproduct of muscle metabolism and its levels of production are constant and are proportional to muscle mass. Normally, it is not reabsorbed. If normal serum levels of 0.7 to 1.2 mg/dl exist, it indicates normal renal function. When creatinine rises and accumulates in the plasma, it represents decreasing GFR. If doubled, renal function is probably half of normal. If three times, about 75 percent of renal function is lost.
- Creatinine clearance is the amount of blood theoretically "cleared" of creatinine by the kidney in one minute of filtration; 90 to 130 ml/min is normal. Creatinine clearance provides a good measure of renal blood flow and GFR as serum levels are related to a 24-hour urine volume. Inulin, a substance with a stable plasma concentration, can be used to assess clearance. The amount of inulin filtered is equal to the volume of plasma filtered multiplied by the plasma concentration of inulin.
- The urinalysis is an essential part of the examination of all patients who may have renal disease since materials in the urine can be diagnostic for many disorders. It is normal to have inorganic material such as Na^+, Cl^-, and K^+ and organic materials such as urea and creatinine in the urine. It is abnormal to find RBCs, more than a few WBCs, bacteria, protein, glucose, or ketones in the urine.

Objectives

After studying this chapter, the learner will be able to:

1. **Describe the pathophysiology of renal stones.**
Study pages 809-811; refer to Figures 28-1 and 28-2.

Calcium is a common constituent of renal stones; about 80 percent of stones or **renal calculi** are composed of calcium oxalate, calcium phosphate, or a combination of both. Another stone, the struvite stone, which is composed of magnesium ammonium phosphate, is caused by the action of some urea-splitting bacteria. These stones, unlike the others, are seen more often in women and account for 10 to 15 percent of all stones. Uric acid stones, about 7 percent of stones, may be seen with gout. Rarely, cystine stones are seen in individuals with a genetic defect in transporting cystine.

A colicky pain occurs as the rhythmic contractions of the ureter attempt to dislodge and advance the sharp-edged stone. The accumulation of urine behind the stone causes infection or damage to organs. This consequence to obstruction depends on the location of the obstruction. If high and complete, glomerular filtration may be affected. The pain may be in the flank or between the last rib and the lumbar vertebrae, or it may radiate into the groin, depending on the stone's location.

Treatment involves dilution of stone-forming substances by a high fluid intake, extraction of larger stones by instrumentation, fragmentation of stones by ultrasonic lithotripsy, and laser treatment. Some smaller stones may pass spontaneously.

2. **Characterize neurogenic bladder.**
Study pages 811-812; refer to Table 28-1.

Neurogenic bladder is a functional urinary tract obstruction caused by an interruption of the nerve supply to the bladder. The neurologic disruption can occur in the central nervous system or at the level of the spinal cord. Resulting bladder paralysis interferes with the normal flow of urine. Upper motor neuron lesions occur in the cortex or below the cortex but above the sacral level of the spinal cord and cause loss of voluntary control of voiding. Lower motor neuron lesions occur at the sacral level of the spinal cord and cause loss of both voluntary and involuntary control of urination.

Because of disordered sensation, symptoms are difficult to assess. Any infection may be treated with appropriate antibiotics.

3. **Describe renal and bladder tumors.**
Study pages 812-813; refer to Figure 28-3 and Tables 28-2 and 28-3.

Renal adenomas are uncommon, but they may become malignant and so are usually surgically removed. **Renal carcinoma** is the most common renal neoplasm and usually occurs in men between the ages of 50 and 60. An association between tobacco use and renal cell carcinoma exists. The tumors usually occur unilaterally and spread through the lymph nodes and blood vessels to the lungs, liver, and bones.

The manifestations are hematuria, flank pain, palpable flank mass, and weight loss. These signs and symptoms are infrequent; when they occur, they indicate an advanced stage of disease.

Treatment is usually surgical removal of the affected kidney combined with use of chemotherapy. Radiation therapy and biologic response modifiers may be useful.

Bladder tumors represent about 2 percent of all malignant tumors and are the fifth most common malignancy. The development of bladder cancer is most common in men older than 60 years of age.

The risk of primary bladder cancer is greater among individuals who smoke or work in the chemical, rubber, and textile industry and among women who take large amounts of phenacetin. Bladder cancer results from a genetic alteration in normal bladder epithelium. Metastasis is usually to lymph nodes, liver, bones, and lungs. Secondary bladder cancer develops by invasion of cancer from bordering organs such as cervical carcinoma in women and prostatic carcinoma in men.

Bladder tumors may be asymptomatic or accompanied by hematuria. Advanced cancers are associated with pelvic pain and frequent urination. Treatment depends on the type and size of the lesion and involves resection, chemotherapy, or radiotherapy.

4. Explain the development of urinary tract infections, the predisposing risk factors, and the most likely pathogens responsible for the infection.
Study page 813.

In these infections, predisposing factors are very important. Factors include fecal contamination of the urethra particularly in the female, sexual activity, catheterization or instrumentation of the urinary tract, urinary obstruction so the flushing effects of urination are reduced, and diaphragm spermatocidal usage.

The most common route in the development of acute urinary tract infection is by an ascending infection. Common pathogens in these infections are the gram-negative rods, namely *E. coli, Klebsiella, Proteus,* and *Pseudomonas.* Other possible infectious agents are gram-positive cocci, mycobacteria, and fungi.

5. Compare and contrast the signs, symptoms, and etiology of cystitis and pyelonephritis.
Study pages 813-815; refer to Figure 28-4 and Table 28-4.

(See box below.)

6. Describe the types of glomerulonephritis, its features, manifestations, and treatment.
Study pages 815-819; refer to Figure 28-5 and Tables 28-5 through 28-7.

Glomerular damage generally occurs from activation of biochemical mediators of inflammation, namely complement, leukocytes, and fibrin. Damage begins after antibody against glomerular basement membrane or antigen-antibody complexes have localized in the glomerular capillary wall. Complement is deposited with the antibodies. Complement activation attracts neutrophils and monocytes. The neutrophils and monocytes further the inflammatory reaction by releasing lysosomal enzymes which damage glomerular walls and increase glomerular capillary wall permeability. Membrane damage can lead to platelet aggregation and degranulation wherein platelets release vasoactive amines. Changes in membrane permeability permit the passage of protein molecules and red blood cells into the urine, causing proteinuria and hematuria.

The coagulation system also may be activated and lead to fibrin deposition in Bowman's space; this reduces renal blood flow and depresses glomerular filtration.

Mild proteinuria and hematuria occur during the early years of the disease. After 10 or 20 years, renal insufficiency will develop followed by nephrotic syndrome and an accelerated progression to end-stage renal failure.

The diagnosis of glomerular disease is confirmed by a urinalysis that shows proteinuria, red blood cells, white blood cells, and casts.

The basic principles for treating glomerulonephritis are related to treating the primary dis-

Cystitis and Pyelonephritis

	Cystitis (bladder) **Lower Tract Infection**	**Pyelonephritis (kidney tubules, pelvis, and interstitium)** **Upper Tract Infection**
Signs/Symptoms	Low abdominal pain, back pain, painful burning urination, frequent voiding/urgency, hematuria, cloudy urine	Fever, chills, backache, abdominal pain, nausea, vomiting, urinary urgency and frequency, costovertebral tenderness
Etiology	Urinary obstruction, prostatitis, ascending infection with gram-negative rods ("honeymoon cystitis"), irritable bladder from sphincter dysfunction, interstitial cytosis caused by an inflammatory autoimmune response	Inflammation or scarring of the interstitial tissue and tubules, causative organism is usually an ascending gram-negative rod but can be fungi or viruses; a risk factor is any urinary obstruction or condition that causes urine reflux or residual urine

ease, preventing or minimizing immune responses, and correcting accompanying problems such as edema, hypertension, and hyperlipidemia. Antibiotic therapy is essential for management of underlying infections. Dialysis or kidney transplantation ultimately may be necessary. (See box below.)

7. Identify and explain key features of nephrotic syndrome.
Study pages 819-820; refer to Table 28-8.

In **nephrotic syndrome**, there is increased glomerular permeability and protein leakage of 3.5 g or more in the urine per day.

The key features of nephrotic syndrome include proteinuria, edema, hypoalbuminemia, hyperlipidemia, and lipiduria. Proteinuria occurs with protein leakage from the serum into the urine; this process reduces blood oncotic pressure. Thus, water leaves the capillaries more easily and tissue edema follows. The edema is soft, pitting, and generalized. Hypoalbuminemia develops as albumin leaks through the capillaries and depletes its serum level. Hyperlipidemia occurs as the liver responds to the hypoalbuminemia by synthesizing replacement albumin. While synthesizing albumin, the liver also synthesizes lipoproteins in large amounts; therefore, hyperlipidemia develops. As tubular cells containing fat are sloughed into the urine, lipiduria can be seen. Also, free fat from the hyperlipidemia leaks across the glomerulus. Loss of protein immunoglobulins increases susceptibility to infection in nephrotic syndrome.

Treatment is with a normal protein, low-fat diet; salt restriction; diuretics; steroids; and occasionally, albumin replacement.

Common Types of Glomerulonephritis

Type and Cause	Pathophysiology
Poststreptococcal Group A beta-hemolytic streptococci	Diffuse, subepithelial deposits of immune and complement complexes, phagocytic infiltration, and occlusion of glomerular capillary blood flow decrease glomerular filtration
Rapidly progressive or crescentic Nonspecific response to glomerular injury	Diffuse accumulation of macrophages or epithelial cell proliferation into Bowman's space form crescents and occlude glomerular filtration, antiglomerular basement membrane antibodies lead to damaged tissue and renal failure
Membranoproliferative Usually idiopathic, associated with activation of complement pathways	Thickened basement membrane reduces glomerular capillary blood flow and decreases glomerular filtration
IgA nephropathy Usually idiopathic	Focal, some diffuse lesions, IgA deposits, and mediators decrease GFR
Minimal change disease or lipoid nephrosis Usually idiopathic	Diffuse fusion of epithelial processes, loss of negative charge in basement membrane, and increased permeability lead to proteinuria and nephrotic syndrome
Focal glomerulosclerosis Usually idiopathic	Similar pathology to minimal change disease
Membranous nephropathy Usually idiopathic, can be associated with systemic disease	Diffuse thickening of glomerular capillary wall increases permeability with proteinuria and nephrotic syndrome

8. Define and identify the common etiologies for prerenal, intrarenal, and postrenal disease.
Study pages 820-822; refer to Figure 28-6 and Tables 28-9 and 28-10.

Acute renal failure is the rapid deterioration of renal function with accompanying elevation of BUN and plasma creatinine; oliguria also develops. The etiology may be either prerenal because of renal hypoperfusion, intrarenal from renal functional impairment, or postrenal following obstruction of urinary flow.

The clinical progression has three phases: oliguria, diuresis, and recovery of renal function. BUN and plasma creatinine concentrations increase. The primary goal is to maintain life until renal function returns. (See first box below.)

9. Describe chronic renal failure; identify the systemic manifestation of uremia.
Study pages 822-825; refer to Tables 28-11 and 28-12.

Chronic renal failure symptoms and signs usually do not develop until GFR declines to 25 percent of normal. The chronic alteration is primarily because of loss of nephron mass. The clinical manifestations of chronic renal failure are described as **uremia**. The uremic state is characterized by a decline in renal function and the accumulation of toxins in the blood. If the lesions are tubular, electrolyte imbalances, volume depletions, and metabolic acidosis occur. In glomerular lesions, hematuria and nephrotic syndrome develop.

Uremia is a toxic condition associated with widespread effects on all body systems. (See second box below.)

Causes of Acute Renal Failure

Prerenal	Intrarenal	Postrenal
Hypovolemia Hemorrhage Hypotension Cardiac failure Interruption of renal artery flow	Prolonged renal ischemia Nephrotoxins Glomerulonephritis Intratubular obstructions or necrosis	Ureteral obstructions Edema, tumors, stones, clots Bladder outlet obstruction Prostatic hyperplasia, urethral strictures

Uremia

Skeletal	Cardiopulmonary	Neurologic	Hematologic
Bone demineralization	Hypertension Pericarditis Pulmonary edema	Fatigue Attention deficit Irritability Peripheral neuropathy Stupor Coma	Anemia Bleeding Infection Suppressed immunity
Metabolic	**Gastrointestinal**	**Integumentary**	**Reproductive**
Acidosis Hyperuricemia Hypocalcemia Hyperkalemia	Diarrhea Nausea Vomiting Anorexia Urinous breath	Pruritus Pigmentation	Infertility Decreased libido Impotence Amenorrhea

Note: If chronic renal failure cannot be managed with diet, diuretics, and fluid restriction, then dialysis or transplantation becomes necessary.

Practice Examination

1. Renal function tests include:

   a. the urinalysis.
   b. BUN and serum creatinine.
   c. SGOT/SGPT.
   d. Both a and b are correct.
   e. a, b, and c are correct.

2. Which substance is an abnormal constituent of urine?

   a. urea
   b. glucose
   c. sodium chloride
   d. creatinine

3. The presence of albumin in the urine would indicate probable damage to:

   a. glomeruli.
   b. renal columns.
   c. collecting tubules.
   d. pyramids.
   e. None of the above is correct.

4. Which statement is not true concerning urinary tract infections?

   a. Once cystitis develops, pyelonephritis will certainly occur.
   b. They are usually due to coliforms, especially *E. coli.*
   c. Organisms probably entered the bladder by way of the urethra.
   d. The patient may be asymptomatic.

5. Renal calculi may be composed of:

   a. calcium oxalate.
   b. uric acid.
   c. cholesterol.
   d. All of the above are correct.
   e. Both a and b are correct.

6. Which can be characteristic of ureteral stones?

   a. severe pain in back
   b. severe pain in abdomen
   c. nausea and vomiting
   d. All of the above are correct.
   e. Both a and c are correct.

7. Which are predisposing factors for acute urinary tract infections? (*More than one answer may be correct.*)

   a. congenital deformities of urinary tract
   b. the sex of the patient
   c. decreased urine flow
   d. increased urine flow
   e. increased fluid intake

8. A common cause of both pyelonephritis and cystitis is:

   a. urinary calculi.
   b. invading microorganisms, such as *E coli.*
   c. allergy reactions.
   d. heavy metals.

9. Uremia exhibits:

   a. polycythemia.
   b. retention of metabolic acids.
   c. low plasma calcium levels.
   d. increased erythropoiesis.
   e. Both a and d are correct.

10. Pyelonephritis (*more than one answer may be correct*):

    a. is an inflammation and infection of the urinary bladder.
    b. is characterized by fever, chills, and flank pain.
    c. is characterized by pyuria, bacteriuria, and hematuria.
    d. is more common in young women than in young men.

11. Which renal condition usually has a history of recent infection with beta-hemolytic streptococci?

    a. pyelonephritis
    b. chronic renal failure
    c. nephrosis
    d. glomerulonephritis
    e. calculi

12. Which statement is not true concerning glomerulonephritis?

    a. Significant damage to kidneys occurs during the body's response to an infection.
    b. Fever and flank pain occur.
    c. Complement activation attracts neutrophils.
    d. It is characterized by hematuria, proteinuria, and the presence of casts.
    e. Approximately 90% of individuals develop chronic disease.

13. Nephrotic syndrome is associated with ______ to plasma ______.

    a. increased glomerular permeability / urea
    b. decreased glomerular permeability / proteins
    c. decreased glomerular permeability / tubular filtrate
    d. increased glomerular permeability / proteins

14. Causes of acute renal failure include:

    a. cholecystitis.
    b. stones and strictures in kidneys or ureters.
    c. heart failure leading to poor renal perfusion.
    d. Both b and c are correct.
    e. a, b, and c are correct.

15. Which describe a patient in acute renal failure? (*More than one answer may be correct.*)

   a. elevated serum creatinine
   b. leukocytosis
   c. low BUN
   d. fever
   e. oliguria

16. Which is not a characteristic of chronic renal failure?

   a. hyperkalemia
   b. anuria
   c. anemia
   d. pruritus
   e. acidosis

17. Chronic renal failure:

   a. may result from hypertension.
   b. is usually the result of chronic inflammation of the kidney.
   c. may be treated with dialysis or transplants.
   d. All of the above are correct.
   e. Both a and c are correct.

18. An individual has an elevated blood level of urea and creatinine because of complete calculi blockage of one ureter. This is referred to as:

   a. prerenal disease.
   b. intrarenal disease.
   c. postrenal disease.
   d. preeclampsia.
   e. hypercalcemia.

19. Nephrotoxins such as the antibiotics may be responsible for:

   a. acute tubular necrosis.
   b. acute glomerulonephritis.
   c. pyelonephritis.
   d. cystitis.

20. Uremia, as seen in chronic renal failure, would include:

   a. metabolic acidosis.
   b. elevated BUN and creatinine.
   c. cardiovascular disturbances.
   d. All of the above are correct.

21. The earliest symptom of chronic renal failure is:

   a. pruritus.
   b. oliguria.
   c. polyuria.
   d. decreased BUN.

22. In chronic renal failure, tubulointerstitial disease leads to:

    a. sodium retention.
    b. sodium wasting.
    c. no significant changes in sodium levels.
    d. increased phosphate excretion.

Match the condition with the etiology.

23. ____ Goodpasture syndrome
24. ____ hypovolemia
25. ____ uremia

a. prerenal failure

b. postrenal failure

c. chronic glomerulonephritis

d. rapidly progressive glomerulonephritis

e. pruritus

Case Study

Mr. and Mrs. C. returned from a weekend of downhill skiing to find their nine-year-old-son, Eddie, with bloody urine. About six weeks earlier, they had spent a week skiing during which Eddie had a severe sore throat that was not treated because his teenage sitter did not take him to a physician.

Eddie was taken to his pediatrician where it was established that he had been lethargic and without appetite for the past ten days and had complained of back pain. His physical examination showed a temperature of 101° F and a blood pressure of 140/102. The remainder of the physical was noncontributory. Eddie's urinalysis showed blood, protein, and RBC casts with an elevated specific gravity. BUN and serum creatinine were elevated.

What do you think is the likely cause of Eddie's symptoms and signs? What do you think the pediatrician will do?

CHAPTER 29

Alterations of Renal and Urinary Tract Function in Children

Foundational Objective

a. Describe fluid balance in children; explain the implications of imbalances. Review page 804.

Memory Check!

- Infants and young children have a larger ratio of body water to body weight than adults. Children exchange half of their extracellular water each day. When children become ill, they tend to retain fluid because of lowered osmotic pressure. Children have limited ability to concentrate urine because of higher renal blood flow and shorter tubular length. Fluid and electrolyte balance is very sensitive to the slightest changes in any of these factors.

Objectives

After studying this chapter, the learner will be able to:

1. **Describe the common congenital anomalies that occur within the renal and urologic system.**
   Study pages 829-830; refer to Figures 29-1 through 29-3.

Structural defects range from minor, easily correctable anomalies to those incompatible with life. **Hypospadias**, with or without **chordee** and its band of fibrous tissue that deviates the penis ventrally, and **epispadias** are defects in the placement of the urethral meatus, the urethal opening is ventral and dorsal respectively. Hypospadias is the more common penile defect, with an incidence of 1 in 300 infant boys, and is usually easily corrected with surgery. Epispadias is a more complex problem, because it extends into the bladder; but it has a lower incidence rate, approximately 1 in 200,000 boys and 1 in 400,000 girls. This can also be surgically corrected but requires a more involved intervention.

Exstrophy of the bladder is a defect wherein the bladder and associated urinary tract structures are exposed to the surface of the body. This defect involves the abdominal wall and the pubic bone. Incidence is 1 in 40,000, of which three-fourths are boys. This defect allows urine to leak from the ureters onto the abdominal wall, leading to excoriation of the skin and the persistent odor of urine. The exposed bladder mucosa becomes edematous, bleeds easily, and is painful. Surgical repair requires several stages with the first during the first few days of life and the last at about age three. Neoplastic changes have been associated with exstrophy of the bladder.

Structural changes of the kidney may be categorized as those that affect renal function and those that do not; they may occur unilaterally or bilaterally. **Unilateral agenesis** occurs in approximately 1 in 1000 births and has little or no effect on function if one of the kidneys is normal. **Bilateral agenesis**, or Potter syndrome, occurs in approximately 1 in 3000 births and is usually associated with other anomalies; affected infants rarely live more than a few hours. **Hypoplastic kidney** may be small but functionally normal or underdeveloped and functionally abnormal. The bilateral form is a common cause of chronic renal failure. **Renal dysplasia** is associated with obstructions of the renal collecting system. **Ectopic kidney** is usually functionally normal but lies in the pelvic region rather than in the abdomen. **Horseshoe kidney**, or fused kidney, is associated with hydronephrosis, infection, and stone formation.

2. Note glomerular disorders in children; describe the pathophysiology and clinical manifestations of hemolytic uremic syndrome and its treatment.
Study pages 831-832.

Nephrotic syndrome and **glomerulonephritis** in children express pathophysiologic mechanisms similar to those observed in adults. **Hemolytic uremic syndrome** is associated with a viral or bacterial illness and is preceded one or two weeks by an upper respiratory or gastrointestinal infection. The antecedent infection causes endothelial injury to the glomerular arterioles. This event triggers the inflammatory cascade, resulting in platelet aggregation and fibrin clot formation that narrows the arterioles. Anemia results when erythrocytes and platelets that are damaged while passing through narrowed and inflamed glomerular arterioles are later removed by the spleen. This same thrombocyte and fibrin clot mechanism activates the fibrinolytic cascade that prompts the release of damaged platelets from the arterioles. These damaged platelets are also removed by the spleen. Thrombocytosis eventually results.

Classic symptoms of hemolytic uremic syndrome are pallor, bruising, and oliguria that may be accompanied by fever, vomiting, bloody diarrhea, abdominal pain, and jaundice. Central nervous system involvement, seizures, and lethargy may be features of severe disease.

Treatment is supportive and includes transfusions of red blood cells and platelets to treat the anemia and thrombocytopenia. Peritoneal dialysis may be required to regulate fluids and electrolytes until renal function returns to normal.

3. Identify the structural cause of vesicoureteral reflux and explain the potential effects on renal function.
Study page 833; refer to Figures 29-4 and 29-5.

Primary vesicoureteral reflux is caused by the congenital malpositioning of a ureter or ureters into the bladder that allows retrograde urine to flow up the ureters. If the urine contains microorganisms and can reach the renal parenchyma, chronic infection and scarring may result. The combination of reflux and infection can cause pyelonephritis. This condition is classified by a grading system, with grade I the most mild and grade V the most severe. **Secondary vesicoureteral reflux** occurs because an infection causes mucosal edema and interferes with the antireflux mechanisms of the urinary tract.

Symptoms associated with vesicoureteral reflux include fever, recurrent urinary tract infections, and poor feeding. Diagnosis is confirmed by a radiologic procedure that allows visualization of reflux during voiding. Treatment goals are to prevent infection and to protect and preserve renal function. Recurrent infection and grade V are indications for surgical repair.

4. Characterize Wilms tumor.
Study pages 834-835; refer to Table 29-1.

Wilms tumor, or nephroblastoma, is an embryonic tumor. The peak age of diagnosis is two to three years of age with an incidence of approximately 400 cases yearly in the United States. Wilms tumor may occur as a sporadic phenomenon or it may be inherited. The inherited form is an autosomal dominant disorder but is rare. The occurrence has been found to be caused by the deletion or inactivation of genes on the short arm of chromosome 11. This finding tends to support the theory of tumor-suppressor genes. Other congenital genitourinary anomalies have been associated with Wilms tumor in 18 percent of children.

These children may be asymptomatic or may present with vague abdominal pain, hematuria, fever, or hypertension. The tumor is smooth, firm, and usually encapsulated and separated from the renal parenchyma. Diagnosis is made by locating the tumor and assessing its site by radiologic procedures such as ultrasound, computerized tomography (CT scan), or magnetic resonance imaging (MRI). Treatment is surgical excision with a heminephrectomy or total nephrectomy. Depending on the stage of the tumor, chemotherapy or radiation therapy or both may be required.

5. Define primary and secondary enuresis; discuss their likely causes and common approaches to management.
Study pages 835-836; refer to Table 29-2.

Enuresis, or involuntary urination after voluntary bladder control should exist, can be classified in two categories: **primary enuresis** occurs when a child has never obtained continence and **secondary enuresis** occurs when a child has had and then loses bladder control. Secondary enuresis is also termed acquired enuresis. The origin may be neurologic, anatomical, or functional. Enuresis shows a familial tendency. Psychological problems have been related to enuresis in some cases and must be considered a legitimate cause in the absence of organic findings.

Management depends on cause and may include a combination of interventions such as medication, limited fluid intake, behavior modification, alarms, or periodic awakenings during sleep. Psychological counseling may also benefit the child and family.

Practice Examination

True/False

1. ____ Exstrophy of the bladder occurs because of birth trauma.

2. ____ Vesicoureteral reflux is caused by a congenitally malpositioned entry of the ureter or ureters into the bladder.

3. ____ Children are at no greater risk for fluid and electrolyte imbalances than adults.

4. ____ Grade V vesicoureteral reflux can be medically managed.

5. ____ Wilms tumor is an embryonic tumor of the kidney.

6. ____ Secondary enuresis occurs when the child has never been continent.

7. Nephrotic syndrome in children manifests as:

   a. proteinuria.
   b. hyperlipidemia.
   c. lipiduria.
   d. All of the above are correct.
   e. None of the above is correct.

8. Poststreptococcal glomerulonephritis in children:

   a. is a noninfectious renal disease.
   b. causes hypotension.
   c. causes dehydration.
   d. Both b and c are correct.

9. Infants cannot concentrate urine because of:

   a. shorter tubular length.
   b. increased tubular weight.
   c. increased blood flow to the kidneys.
   d. Both a and c are correct.
   e. a, b, and c are correct.

10. Vesicoureteral reflux causes urine to ______ up the ureters and places the young child at risk for ______.

    a. retrograde / glomerulonephritis
    b. regrade / nephrotic syndrome
    c. retrograde / pyelonephritis
    d. regrade / cystitis

11. Which manifestation may be associated with vesicoureteral reflux?

    a. recurrent urinary tract infections
    b. poor growth
    c. irritability
    d. Both a and b are correct.
    e. a, b, and c are correct.

12. Children are at risk for hemolytic uremic syndrome after:

    a. fever.
    b. vomiting and/or diarrhea.
    c. viral infections.
    d. All of the above are correct.

13. Organic causes of enuresis may include:

    a. congenital abnormalities of the urinary tract.
    b. a neurologic origin.
    c. diabetes insipidus.
    d. All of the above are correct.

14. Children with enuresis may be managed by:

    a. sleep interruption.
    b. psychotherapy.
    c. diet.
    d. All of the above are correct.

15. Which clinical manifestations suggest hemolytic uremic syndrome?

    a. oliguria
    b. pallor and bruising
    c. fever, vomiting, and diarrhea
    d. All of the above are correct.
    e. Both a and b are correct.

16. Identify the sequence of events in hemolytic uremic syndrome that cause anemia.

    1. The damaged cells are removed from the circulation by the spleen.
    2. The endothelial lining of the glomerular arterioles becomes swollen.
    3. Narrowed vessels damage erythrocytes.
    4. Fibrin split-products appear in the urine and serum.

    a. 1, 3, 4
    b. 2, 4, 1
    c. 3, 1, 2
    d. 2, 3, 1

17. Which factor influences the prognosis of a child with Wilms tumor?

    a. the child's height
    b. genetics
    c. stage
    d. congenital anomalies
    e. b, c, and d are correct.

18. What symptoms may a child with Wilms tumor develop?

    a. fever
    b. hypertension
    c. hematuria
    d. Both b and c are correct.
    e. a, b, and c are correct.

Match the description with the structural abnormality.

19. ____ small normally developed kidney
20. ____ usually normal kidneys remain in the pelvis
21. ____ urethral opening on the dorsal surface of the penis, a cleft along the ventral urethra in girls
22. ____ results from abnormal differentiation of renal tissue
23. ____ exposed bladder mucosa through a fissure in the abdominal wall
24. ____ urethral meatus opening on the ventral side of the penis
25. ____ absence of the kidneys

a. hypospadias
b. epispadias
c. bladder exstrophy
d. hypoplastic kidney
e. renal dysplasia
f. ectopic kidney
g. renal aplasia

Case Study

A three-year-old girl is brought to the emergency room of a local hospital because she has bloody stools. Her parents reveal a history of gastrointestinal illness two weeks ago after a weekend of camping. The girl has been well since the GI illness until yesterday when the bloody stools began. At that time, they noticed how pale she was and believe she has not voided at all today. Her assessment reveals pallor and bruising. A urine collection bag was placed on the child; however, she never voided while in the emergency room. A complete blood count revealed low Hgb, Hct, and platelets.

From the laboratory values, what diagnosis is likely? What treatment will she require?

CHAPTER 30

Structure and Function of the Reproductive Systems

Objectives

After review of this chapter, the learner will be able to:

1. **Describe the hormonal stimulation of the reproductive systems; note secondary sex characteristics.**
   Review pages 840-843; refer to Figures 30-1 through 30-3.

2. **Identify female external and internal genitalia and female sex hormones.**
   Review pages 843-849; refer to Figures 30-4 through 30-9 and Table 30-1.

3. **Describe the menstrual cycle, noting its differential hormonal effects, levels, and cellular events.**
   Review pages 849-852; refer to Figure 30-10 and Table 30-2.

4. **Identify male external and internal genitalia.**
   Review pages 852-857; refer to Figures 30-11 through 30-15.

5. **Describe spermatogenesis and male sex hormones.**
   Review pages 857-858; refer to Figures 30-16 and 30-17.

6. **Identify the structure of and cyclical hormones associated with female breast tissue; describe the lymphatic drainage.**
   Review pages 859-861; refer to Figures 30-18 and 30-19.

7. **Identify normal changes in the female and male reproductive systems that occur with advancing age.**
   Review page 861.

Practice Examination

1. GnRH reaches the anterior pituitary gland and causes the release of which of the following? (*More than one answer may be correct.*)

   a. growth hormone
   b. FSH
   c. ADH
   d. LH
   e. oxytocin

2. Which is not a structure of the female external genitalia?

   a. vagina
   b. clitoris
   c. vestibule
   d. labia minora
   e. labia majora

3. A new menstrual cycle has a rise in the levels of:

   a. LH.
   b. GH.
   c. estrogen.
   d. progesterone.
   e. FSH.

4. Progesterone:

   a. stimulates lactation.
   b. increases uterine tube motility.
   c. thins the endometrium.
   d. maintains the thickened endometrium.
   e. causes ovulation.

5. The ovaries produce:

   a. ova, estrogen, and oxytocin.
   b. ova only.
   c. ova and estrogen.
   d. testosterone and semen.
   e. None of the above is correct.

6. During which days of the menstrual cycle does the endometrium achieve maximum development?

   a. 2-6
   b. 7-12
   c. 14
   d. 20-24
   e. 26-28

7. Hormones necessary for the growth and development of female breasts are:

   a. estrogens and progesterone.
   b. oxytocin and ADH.
   c. androgens and steroids.
   d. gonadocorticoids.
   e. relaxin.

8. The structure that releases a mature ovum is the:

   a. corpus albicans.
   b. graafian follicle.
   c. primary follicle.
   d. corpus luteum.
   e. infundibulum.

9. A major duct of the female reproductive system is the:

   a. suspensory tube.
   b. uterosacral duct.
   c. broad duct.
   d. mesovarian duct.
   e. uterine tube.

10. Prostate is to the accessory gland as gonad is to the:

   a. ejaculatory duct.
   b. ovary.
   c. bulbourethral gland.
   d. accessory gland.
   e. urethra.

11. Cells that produce testosterone are called:

   a. interstitial endocrinocytes.
   b. testicular endocrine cells.
   c. sustentacular cells.
   d. spermatogonia.
   e. None of the above is correct.

12. The function of testosterone includes:

   a. development of male gonads.
   b. bone and muscle growth.
   c. influencing sexual behavior.
   d. growth of testes.
   e. All of the above are correct.

13. Immediately after the sperm cells leave the ductus epididymis, they enter the:

   a. ejaculatory duct.
   b. ductus deferens.
   c. urethra.
   d. exterior of the body.
   e. None of the above is correct.

14. A substance produced in the reproductive system mainly by the bulbourethral glands is:

   a. fructose.
   b. HCl.
   c. mucus.
   d. an alkaline, viscous fluid.

15. Which produce(s) a secretion that helps maintain the motility of spermatozoa?

   a. prostate
   b. penis
   c. greater vestibular glands
   d. interstitial tissues
   e. All of the above are correct.

16. Semen is:

    a. vaginal secretions needed to activate sperm.
    b. the product of the testes.
    c. the sperm and secretions of the seminal vesicles, prostate, and bulbourethral gland.
    d. responsible for engorgement of the erectile tissue in the penis.
    e. the secretion that causes ovulation in the female.

17. The vulva consists of the:

    a. labia majora and labia minora.
    b. clitoris.
    c. vaginal orifice.
    d. Both a and b are correct.
    e. a, b, and c are correct.

18. The major difference between female and male hormone production is:

    a. LH is without effect in the male.
    b. GnRH doesn't cause the release of FSH in the male.
    c. hormonal production is relatively constant in the male.
    d. Both a and b are correct.
    e. None of the above is correct.

19. The primary spermatocyte has:

    a. 46 chromosomes.
    b. the same number of chromosomes as a sperm.
    c. 23 chromosomes.
    d. a diploid number of chromosomes.
    e. Both a and d are correct.

20. During the follicular/proliferative phase of the menstrual cycle:

    a. vascularity of breast tissue increases.
    b. vascularity of breast tissue decreases.
    c. progesterone constricts the ducts.
    d. Both b and c are correct.

21. Most of the lymphatic drainage of the female breast occurs through the:

    a. axillary nodes.
    b. internal mammary nodes.
    c. subclavian nodes.
    d. brachial nodes.
    e. anterior pectoral nodes.

Match the aging reproductive changes with the term or response.

22. ____ primary follicles resist gonadotropin stimulation
23. ____ corpus luteum fails to develop
24. ____ less effective erection
25. ____ first menstruation

a. menarche

b. premenopause

c. menopause

d. vasomotor flush

e. vasocongestive response

f. luteal/secretory phase

g. follicular/proliferative phase

CHAPTER

31

Alterations of the Reproductive Systems Including Sexually Transmitted Diseases

Foundational Objectives

a. Identify the female and male reproductive structures. Review pages 843-848 and 852-857.

Memory Check!

- The female external genitalia collectively are called the vulva and comprise the structures visible externally: the mons pubis, the labia majora, the labia minora, the clitoris, and the vestibule. The urethral meatus, the vaginal opening, and two sets of glands—Skene glands and Bartholin glands—open onto the vestibule. The internal organs of the female reproductive system are two ovaries, two fallopian tubes or uterine tubes, the uterus, and the vagina. The ovaries are the primary female reproductive organs. They are located on both sides of the uterus and are suspended and supported by ligaments.
- The fallopian tubes extend from the ovaries to the uterus and open into the uterine cavity thus providing a direct communication from the peritoneal cavity to the uterine cavity. The uterus lies centrally in the pelvis and is divided structurally into the body, or corpus, and the cervix. The inner layer, the endometrium, consists of surface epithelium, glands, and connective tissue. The endometrium is shed during menstruation. At the lowest portion of the corpus is the internal os of the cervix. The external os is at the lower end of the cervix. The canal of the cervix provides a direct communication from the cavity of the uterine body through the internal os and the external os to the vagina.
- The vagina extends from the cervix of the uterus to the vaginal opening. Thus, there is continuous communication from outside the body to the peritoneal cavity through the reproductive system structures.
- The male reproductive structures are the penis; the testes in the scrotal sac; the duct system—which includes the epididymis, the vas deferens, the ejaculatory ducts, and the urethra; and the accessory glands which include the seminal vesicles, the prostate, and the bulbourethral glands.
- The testes are divided internally into lobules that contain the seminiferous tubules and Leydig cells. Sperm production takes place in the seminiferous tubules; Leydig cells secrete testosterone. On the posterior portion of each testis is a coiled duct, the epididymis. The head of the epididymis is connected with the seminiferous tubule of the testis and its tail is continuous with the vas deferens. The vas deferens is the excretory duct of the testis. It extends to the duct of the seminal vesicle and joins with it to form the ejaculatory duct. The ejaculatory duct joins the urethra, which is the common passageway to outside the body for both sperm and urine. The accessory glands communicate with the duct system. The prostate surrounds the neck of the bladder and the upper urethra. Its glandular ducts open into the urethra. The bulbourethral glands, or Cowper's glands, are located near the urethral meatus. The penis is composed of three elongated cylindrical masses of erectile tissue which comprise the shaft of the penis. The inner, ventral mass is the corpus spongiosum, which contains the urethra. The two outer, dorsal, parallel masses are the corpus cavernosa. The distal end of the penis or the glans is covered by the prepuce, or foreskin.

b. Describe the relationships of hormones to the normal menstrual cycle. Review pages 848-852; refer to Figure 30-10.

Memory Check!

- The three phases of the menstrual cycle are the follicular/proliferative phase, the luteal/secretory phase, and menstruation. During menstruation, the functional layer of the endometrium disintegrates and is discharged through the vagina. Menstruation is followed by the follicular/proliferative phase. During this phase, the anterior pituitary gland secretes FSH, which causes an ovarian follicle to develop. While the follicle is developing, it secretes estrogen, which causes cells of the endometrium to proliferate. By the time the ovarian follicle is mature, the endometrial lining is restored. At this point, ovulation occurs.
- Ovulation marks the beginning of the luteal/secretory phase of the menstrual cycle. The ovarian follicle begins its transformation into a corpus luteum. LH from the anterior pituitary stimulates the corpus luteum to secrete progesterone which initiates the secretory phase of endometrial development. If conception occurs, the nutrient-laden endometrium is ready for implantation. If conception and implantation do not occur, the corpus luteum degenerates and ceases its production of progesterone and estrogen. Without progesterone or estrogen to maintain it, the endometrium enters the ischemic phase and disintegrates. Then, menstruation occurs, marking the beginning of another cycle.

c. Characterize the structure and development of the female breast. Review pages 859-861; refer to Figure 30-18.

Memory Check!

- The female breast is composed of 15 to 20 pyramid-shaped lobes which are separated and supported by Cooper ligaments. Each lobe contains 20 to 40 lobules which subdivide into many functional units called acini. Each acinus is lined with a layer of epithelial cells capable of secreting milk and a layer of subepithelial cells capable of contracting to squeeze milk from the acinus. The acini empty into a network of lobular collecting ducts that reach the skin through openings in the nipple. The lobes and lobules are surrounded and separated by muscle strands and fatty connective tissue. An extensive capillary network surrounds the acini. Lymphatic drainage of the breast occurs largely through the axillary nodes.
- The nipple is a pigmented, cylindrical structure that has multiple openings. The areola is the pigmented, circular area around the nipple. A number of sebaceous glands are located within the areola and aid in lubrication of the nipple during lactation. The nipple's smooth muscle is innervated by the sympathetic nervous system.
- During childhood, breast growth is latent and growth of the nipple and areola keeps pace with body surface. At the onset of puberty in the female, estrogen secretion stimulates mammary growth. Full differentiation and development of breast tissue are mediated by a variety of hormones, including estrogen, progesterone, prolactin, growth hormone, thyroid hormone, insulin, and cortisol.
- During the reproductive years, the breast undergoes cyclic changes in response to changes in the levels of estrogen and progesterone associated with the menstrual cycle. Because the length of the menstrual cycle does not allow for complete regression of new cell growth, breast growth continues at a slow rate until approximately age 35. The number of acini increase with each cycle, so epithelial tissue proliferation is under the influence of hormones as long as secretion occurs.

Objectives

After studying this chapter, the learner will be able to:

1. **Distinguish between various menstrual disorders and their hormonal alterations or causes; identify manifestations of premenstrual syndrome.**
   Study pages 867-871; refer to Figure 31-1 and Tables 31-1 and 31-2.

Premenstrual syndrome (PMS) is the cyclic recurrence in the luteal phase of the menstrual cycle of physical, psychologic, or behavioral changes distressing enough to impair interpersonal relationships or usual activities. It has been estimated that 5 to 10 percent of menstruating women have severe to disabling premenstrual symptoms and 50 percent or more have moderately distressing symptoms. Currently, it is believed that PMS is the end result of abnormal tissue response of nervous, immunologic, vascular, and gastrointestinal systems to the normal changes of the menstrual cycle. This biological response may or may not be triggered by fluctuating estrogen and progesterone levels.

A predisposition to PMS runs in families and is likely due to genetics and/or environment. There is some evidence that supports a relationship between the severity and frequency of premenstrual symptoms and perfectionism, increased stress, poor nutrition, lack of exercise, low self-esteem, and history of sexual abuse or family conflict. Depression, anger, irritability, and fatigue have been reported as the most prominent and the most

Abnormal Menstrual Cycles

Disorder	Alteration
Primary dysmenorrhea	Excessive endometrial prostaglandin production
Painful menstruation	Increases myometrial contractions and constricts blood vessels
Amenorrhea	
Absence of menstruation	
Primary: menarche failure	Hypothalamus fails to synthesize GnRH so no ovulation occurs, no menstruation or secondary sex characteristics
Secondary: menstruation absence following menarche	Structural abnormalities, regulatory hormones inhibit ovulation
Dysfunctional uterine bleeding (DUB)	Progesterone deficiency or estrogen excess
Heavy or irregular bleeding caused by disturbance of menstrual cycle	Estrogen proliferates endometrium while progesterone limits it; large mass of tissue available for heavy, irregular bleeding
Polycystic ovarian syndrome (PCO) Anovulation causes enlarged, polycystic ovaries	Increased androgen secretion by ovaries, androgen is converted to estrogen peripherally, excessive endometrial tissue and dysfunctional bleeding
Premenstrual syndrome (PMS) Cyclic physical, psychologic, or behavioral changes impair relationships	Abnormal nervous, immunologic, vascular, and gastrointestinal tissue response to menstrual cycle; fluctuating estrogen and progesterone levels; genetic

distressing symptoms; physical symptoms seem less prevalent and problematic.

Treatment for PMS is symptomatic. After a trial of nonpharmacologic therapies, medications may be added to the treatment plan even if their efficacy in the treatment of PMS is questionable.

2. Describe pelvic inflammatory disease.
Study pages 871-873; refer to Figures 31-2 and 31-3.

Pelvic inflammatory disease (PID) is an acute inflammatory process caused by infection. PID involves organs of the upper genital tract, the uterus, fallopian tubes or uterine tubes, or ovaries. In its most severe form, the entire peritoneal cavity may be involved. Infection of the fallopian tubes is **salpingitis**; infection of the ovaries is **oophoritis**. Most cases of PID are caused by sexually transmitted microorganisms that ascend from the vagina to the uterus, fallopian tubes, and ovaries.

PID is considered a polymicrobial infection with the majority of cases being caused by nongonorrheal or nonchlamydial microbes. These organisms may induce a response that causes necrosis with repeated infections and may predispose a woman to PID. After one episode of pelvic infection, 15 to 25 percent of women develop long-term sequelae such as infertility, ectopic pregnancy, chronic pelvic pain, and pelvic adhesions. The incidence of complications increases markedly with repeated infections.

The clinical manifestations of PID are variable. Sixty-seven to 75 percent of women with salpingitis have subclinical infections. The first sign of the ascending infection may be the gradual onset of low bilateral abdominal pain often characterized as dull and steady. Symptoms are more likely to develop during or immediately after menstruation. The pain of PID may worsen with walking, jumping, or intercourse. Other manifestations of PID are difficult or painful urination and irregular bleeding. Other conditions causing pelvic pain must be excluded, such as ectopic pregnancy, threatened abortion, or appendicitis before treatment.

Treatment involves bed rest, avoidance of intercourse, and combined antibiotic therapy. Twenty-five to 40 percent of women require hospitalization for intravenous administration of antibiotics and treatment of peritonitis or tubo-ovarian abscess.

3. Define and cite causes of vaginitis, cervicitis, vulvitis, and bartholinitis.
Study pages 873-874; refer to Figure 31-4.

Vaginitis is an infection of the vagina mostly caused by sexually transmitted pathogens and *Candida albicans*. Since the acidic nature of vaginal secretions during the reproductive years provides protection against a variety of sexually transmitted pathogens, variables that alter the vaginal pH may predispose a woman to infection. The use of antibiotics may destroy *Lactobacillus acidophilus*, which helps maintain an acidic vaginal pH. Thus, there may be an overgrowth of *C. albicans* which could cause a yeast vaginitis.

Cervicitis is an inflammation of the cervix usually caused by one or more sexually transmitted pathogens. A mucopurulent exudate drains from the external os.

Vulvitis is an inflammation of the skin of the vulva and often of the perianal area. Vulvitis can be caused by contact with soaps, detergents, lotions, hygienic sprays, menstrual pads, perfumed toilet paper, or nonabsorbent or tight-fitting clothes.

Bartholinitis is an inflammation of one or both of the ducts that lead from the vaginal opening to the Bartholin glands. The causes of bartholinitis are microorganisms that infect the lower female reproductive tract; this disorder is usually preceded by cervicitis, vaginitis, or urethritis. Infection or trauma causes inflammatory changes that narrow the distal portion of the duct, leading to obstruction and stasis of glandular secretions and causing further inflammation.

4. Describe pelvic relaxation disorders.
Study page 874; refer to Figures 31-5 and 31-6 and Table 31-3.

The bladder, urethra, and rectum are supported by the endopelvic fascia and perineal muscles. This muscular and fascial tissue loses tone and strength with aging and may fail to maintain the pelvic organ in the proper position. Trauma such as childbirth or pelvic surgery damages or weakens the supporting structures.

Cystocele is descent of the bladder and the anterior vaginal wall into the vaginal canal. A cystocele may cause the woman to lose urine when she laughs, sneezes, coughs, or does anything that strains the abdominal muscles. Cystocele is usually accompanied by **urethrocele**, or sagging of the urethra. Urethrocele is usually caused by the shearing effect of the fetal head on the urethra during childbirth. A **rectocele** is the bulging of the rectum and posterior vaginal wall into the vaginal canal. An **enterocele** is herniation of the rectouterine pouch into the rectovaginal septum. **Uterine prolapse** is descent of the cervix or entire uterus into the vaginal canal.

Treatment includes isometric exercises to strengthen muscles, estrogens to improve tone and vascularity of fascial support, a pessary device to hold uterus in position, stool softeners, and surgery.

5. **Characterize the benign growth and proliferative conditions of the female reproductive system.**
   Study pages 876-879; refer to Figures 31-7 through 31-9.

   (See box below.)

6. **Characterize the malignant tumors of the female reproductive system.**
   Study pages 879-883; refer to Figures 31-10 and 31-11 and Tables 31-4 and 31-5.

   (See box on page 257 of *Workbook*.)

7. **Define terms used in female sexual dysfunction.**
   Study pages 883-886; refer to Table 31-6.

Sexual anorexia, or inhibited sexual desire, may be a biological manifestation of depression, alcohol or other substance abuse, prolactin-secretin pituitary tumors, or testosterone deficiency. Beta-adrenergic blockers used for heart disease may also inhibit sexual desire.

Vaginismus is an involuntary muscle spasm in response to attempted penetration. Common causes include prior sexual trauma, fear of sex, or organic disorders.

Anorgasmia is the inability of the woman to reach or achieve orgasm. Drugs such as narcotics, tranquilizers, antidepressants, and antihypertensive medications can inhibit orgasm.

Dyspareunia, or painful intercourse, is common. Inadequate lubrication may make penetration or intercourse unpleasant. Drugs with a drying effect, such as antihistamines, certain tranquilizers,

Benign Lesions of the Female Reproductive System

Lesion	Cause	Manifestations
Ovarian cyst		
Follicular cyst	Ovarian follicle doesn't release ovum, fluid isn't reabsorbed from degenerating follicle	Pelvic and abdominal pain, menstrual irregularities
Corpus luteum cyst	A persistent corpus luteum secretes progesterone	Pelvic pain, amenorrhea with subsequent heavy bleeding
Endometrial polyps	Estrogen stimulation	Premenstrual or intermenstrual bleeding
Leiomyomas (smooth muscle tumor)	Unknown, hormonal fluctuations alter size	Abnormal or increased uterine bleeding, pain, pressure
Adenomyosis (endometrial tissue in the myometrium)	Repeated pregnancies	Dysmenorrhea, uterine enlargement and tenderness
Endometriosis (ectopic endometrial tissue)	Depressed T_C cells tolerate ectopic tissue, genetics	Ectopic tissues respond to hormonal stimulation, bleeding causes pelvic adhesions and pain

Malignant Tumors of the Female Reproductive System

Tumor	Causes	Manifestations
Cervical cancer	STD, human papilloma virus, early sexual activity, multiple sex partners, smoking, diet, and vitamin deficiencies	Asymptomatic, vaginal bleeding or discharge, grade of epithelial thickness enables precursor lesion diagnosis
Vaginal cancer	Previous cervical cancer, nonsteroidal estrogens	Asymptomatic, vaginal bleeding or discharge
Endometrial cancer	Obesity, high-fat diet, no pregnancies, late menopause, hypertension	Vaginal bleeding
Ovarian cancer	Unknown, risk factors are similar to those for endometrial cancer	Systemic manifestations, pain and abdominal swelling, postmenopausal bleeding

and marijuana, and disorders such as diabetes, vaginal infections, and estrogen deficiency can decrease lubrication. Other causes of dyspareunia include infections and anatomical constraints around the introitus or the vulva.

Infertility is the inability to conceive after one year of unprotected intercourse and affects approximately 15 percent of all couples. Important causes of infertility in the female are malfunctions of the fallopian tubes, the ovaries, or the reproductive hormones. Endometriosis also may contribute to infertility.

8. By site, describe common disorders of the male reproductive system; distinguish between benign prostatic hypoplasia, prostatitis, and prostatic cancer.

Study pages 886-896; refer to Figures 31-12 through 31-24.

Urethritis is an inflammatory process usually caused by sexually transmitted microorganisms. Nonsexual origins of urethritis are inflammation or infection as a result of urologic procedures, insertion of foreign bodies into the urethra, anatomic abnormalities, or trauma.

Symptoms of urethritis include urethral tingling or itching or a burning sensation when urinating. Frequency, urgency, and purulent or clear mucous-like discharge from the urethra may occur. Treatment is appropriate antibiotic therapy for infectious urethritis and avoidance of mechanical irritation.

Urethral stricture is a narrowing of the urethra because of scarring. The scars may be congenital but are more likely to result from trauma or untreated or severe urethral infections.

Symptoms include urinary frequency and hesitancy, diminished force and size of the urinary stream, dribbling after voiding, and nocturia. Treatment is usually surgical and may involve urethral dilation, urethrotomy, or a variety of other surgical techniques.

Phimosis and **paraphimosis** are both disorders in which the penile foreskin, or prepuce, is "too tight" to be moved easily over the glans penis. In phimosis, the foreskin cannot be retracted back over the glans; in paraphimosis, the foreskin is retracted and cannot be moved forward to cover the glans. Phimosis can occur at any age and is most commonly caused by poor hygiene and chronic infection. Circumcision, if needed, is performed after infection has been eradicated. In paraphimosis, surgery must be performed to prevent necrosis of the glans caused by constricted blood vessels.

Peyronie disease is a fibrotic condition that causes lateral curvature of the penis during erection. The problem usually affects middle-aged men and is associated with painful erection, painful intercourse for both partners, and poor erection distal to the involved area. There is no definitive treatment for Peyronie disease. Spontaneous remissions occur about 50 percent of the time. Pharmacologic therapies that increase oxygenation may hasten resolution. Surgical resection of the fibrous plaque followed by grafting has been successful.

Balanitis is an inflammation of the glans penis and usually occurs in conjunction with an inflammation of the prepuce. It is associated with poor hygiene and phimosis. The accumulation under the foreskin of glandular secretions, sloughed epithelial cells, and *Mycobacterium smegmatis* can irritate the glans directly or lead to infection. Balanitis is most commonly seen in men with poorly controlled diabetes mellitus and candidiasis. Antimicrobials are used to treat infection, and circumcision can prevent recurrences.

Penile cancer is rare in the United States. Although the exact etiology is unknown, cancer of the penis is likely a result of chronic irritation caused by smegma beneath a phimotic foreskin.

Varicocele, hydrocele, and spermatocele are common intrascrotal disorders. **Varicocele** is an abnormal dilation of a vein within the spermatic cord, and most occur on the left side. They may be painful or tender. They occur in 10 to 15 percent of males, frequently after puberty. The cause of varicocele is incompetent or congenitally absent valves in the spermatic veins that normally prevent backflow of blood. Thus, blood pools in the veins rather than flowing into the venous system. Decreased blood flow through the testis interferes with spermatogenesis and can cause infertility.

A **hydrocele** is a collection of fluid within the tunica vaginalis and is the most common cause of scrotal swelling. Hydroceles in infants are congenital malformations that frequently resolve spontaneously by one year of age. Hydroceles in adults may be caused by an imbalance between the secreting and absorptive capacities of scrotal tissues.

The **spermatocele** is a cyst located between the head of the epididymis and the testis that usually is asymptomatic or produces mild discomfort that is relieved by scrotal support. Neither hydroceles nor spermatoceles are associated with infertility.

Cryptorchidism is a condition in which one or both testes fail to descend into the scrotum. It is the most common congenital condition involving the testes. In approximately 75 to 90 percent of infants with cryptorchidism, the testes descend into the scrotum by one year of age. The cause of cryptorchidism is not clear, but it may result from a developmental delay, a defect of the testis, deficient maternal gonadotropin stimulation, or some mechanical factor that prevents descent through the inguinal canal.

Untreated cryptorchidism is associated with lowered sperm count and impaired fertility. Undescended testes are susceptible to neoplastic processes. Treatment often begins with administration of human chorionic gonadotropin. If hormonal therapy is not successful, the testis is located and moved into the scrotum surgically.

Torsion of the testis is a condition wherein the testis rotates on its vascular pedicle; this interrupts its blood supply. Onset may be spontaneous or follow physical exertion or trauma. If the torsion cannot be reduced manually, surgery must be performed within six hours after the onset of symptoms to preserve normal testicular function.

Orchitis is an acute inflammation of the testes and is uncommon except as a complication of systemic infection or as an extension of an associated epididymitis. Mumps is the most common infectious cause of orchitis and usually affects postpubertal males. The onset is sudden and occurs three to four days after the onset of parotitis. Irreversible damage to spermatogenesis results in about 30 percent of affected testes.

Treatment is supportive and includes bed rest, scrotal support, elevation of the scrotum, hot or cold compresses, and analgesic agents for relief of pain. Appropriate antimicrobial drugs should be used for bacterial orchitis. Corticosteroids are indicated in proved cases of nonspecific granulomatous orchitis.

Testicular cancers are rare, accounting for approximately 1 percent of all male cancers; yet they are the most common solid tumor of young adult men. The cure rate is greater than 95 percent.

The etiology of testicular neoplasms is unknown. Because young men are affected most frequently, it is believed that high levels of androgens may contribute to carcinogenesis. A genetic predisposition exists. Cryptorchidism also is statistically associated with the development of testicular cancer. Apparently, the undescended testis has a developmental defect or undergoes gradual involution and degeneration over time which may contribute to neoplastic changes.

Painless testicular enlargement usually is the first sign of testicular cancer. Enlargement is gradual and may be accompanied by a sensation of testicular heaviness or dull ache in the lower abdomen. Occasionally, acute pain occurs because of rapid growth; then, there may be hemorrhage and necrosis. Besides surgery, treatment involves radiation and chemotherapy singly or in combination. Orchiectomy does not affect sexual function.

Epididymitis, inflammation of the epididymis, generally occurs in sexually active young males. In young men, the usual cause is a sexually transmitted microorganism. In men over 35 years of age, intestinal bacteria and *Pseudomonas aeruginosa* found in urinary tract infections and prostatitis may also cause epididymitis. The pathogenic microorganism reaches the epididymis by ascending the vas deferens from an infected urethra or bladder.

Acute and severe scrotal or inguinal pain is caused by inflammation of the epididymis and surrounding tissues. The individual may have pyuria and bacteriuria and a history of urinary symptoms including urethral discharge. Complications of epididymitis include abscess formation, infarction of the testis, recurrent infection, scarring of epididymal endothelium, and infertility. Treatment includes antibiotic therapy for the infection and various measures to provide symptomatic relief. The individual's sexual partner should be treated with antibiotics if the causative microorganism is a sexually transmitted pathogen.

Benign prostatic hyperplasia (BPH) is also called benign prostatic hypertrophy and causes problems as enlarged prostatic tissue compresses the prostatic urethra. More than half of all men between 60 and 69 years of age have prostatic enlargement. During the third decade of life, the prostate reaches adult size. Between 40 and 45 years of age, benign hyperplasia begins and continues slowly until death. Current etiologic theories of BPH implicate estrogen/androgen synergism or undefined prostatic growth factors with possible additional hormonal involvement.

BPH begins in the periurethral glands, which are the inner glands or layers of the prostate. As nodular hyperplasia and cellular hypertrophy progress, the compressed prostatic urethra usually, but not always, causes bladder outflow obstruction. The urge to urinate frequently, some delay in starting urination, and decreased force of the urinary stream develop. Over a period of several years, the bladder is unable to empty all of the urine, and urine retention becomes chronic.

Progressive bladder distention causes sacculations or diverticular outpouchings of the bladder wall. The ureters may be obstructed as they pass through the hypertrophied detrusor muscle. Bladder or kidney infection then develops. Hyperplastic tissue may be removed surgically.

Prostatitis is an inflammation of the prostate usually limited to a few of the gland's excretory ducts. Prostatitis is categorized as acute bacterial prostatitis, chronic bacterial prostatitis, or nonbacterial prostatitis.

Acute bacterial prostatitis is an ascending infection of the urinary tract that tends to occur in men between the ages of 30 and 50 but also is associated with BPH in older men. Coliform bacteria are common causes of acute bacterial prostatitis.

Symptoms include dysuria and urinary frequency and lower abdominal and suprapubic discomfort. The individual may also have a slow, small urinary stream, inability to empty the bladder, and the need to urinate frequently during the night. Systemic signs of infection include sudden onset of a high fever, fatigue, joint pain, and muscle pain. Long-term, broad-spectrum antibiotics may be required to resolve the infection and control its spread. Pain relievers, antipyretics, bed rest, and adequate hydration are also used therapeutically.

Chronic bacterial prostatitis is characterized by recurrent urinary tract infections and the persistence of pathogenic bacteria. This prostatitis is the most common recurrent urinary tract infection in men.

Symptoms are variable and may be similar to those of acute bacterial prostatitis. The prostate may be only slightly enlarged, but fibrosis causes it to be firm and irregular in shape. Treatment of chronic bacterial prostatitis is difficult mainly because fibrosis blocks passage of antibiotics into prostatic tissues. Therefore, therapeutic levels are hard to achieve. The usual treatment is a 12-week course of antibiotics. If chronic bacterial prostatitis is not cured medically, a radical transurethral prostatectomy may be required.

Nonbacterial prostatitis is the most common prostatitis syndrome and consists of prostatic inflammation without evidence of bacterial infection. Its etiology is unclear.

Men with nonbacterial prostatitis may complain of continuous or spasmodic pain in the suprapubic, infrapubic, scrotal, penile, or inguinal area. The prostate gland generally feels normal upon palpation. Nonbacterial prostatitis is diagnosed by exclusion. There is no generally accepted treatment for nonbacterial prostatitis. A course of antibiotics for both affected individuals and sexual partners may minimize symptoms.

Prostatic cancer accounts for more than 13 percent of all cancer deaths and more than 28 percent of all cancers in men in the United States; only lung cancer accounts for more male deaths. Prostatic cancer rarely occurs in men under the age of 50. Incidence increases with advancing age; over 80 percent of all prostate cancers are diagnosed in men over age 65. More than 95 percent of prostatic neoplasms are adenocarcinomas and most occur in the periphery of the prostate. Local extension is usually posterior, although late in the disease the tumor may invade the rectum or encroach on the prostatic urethra and cause bladder outlet obstruction. Sites of distant metastasis occur via lymph and blood vessels and include the lymph nodes, bones, lungs, liver, and adrenals. The pelvis, lumbar spine, femur, thoracic spine, and ribs are the most common sites of bone metastasis.

Prostatic cancer often causes no symptoms until it is far advanced. The first manifestations of disease are slow urinary stream, hesitancy, incomplete emptying, frequency, nocturia, and dysuria. Unlike the symptoms of obstruction caused by BPH, the symptoms of obstruction caused by prostatic cancer are progressive and do not temporarily remit. Symptoms of late disease include bone pain at sites of bone metastasis, edema of the lower extremities, enlarged lymph nodes, liver enlargement, pathologic bone fractures, and mental confusion associated with brain metastases.

Transrectal ultrasound (TRUS), prostatic-specific antigen (PSA) blood tests, and digital examination can validate the symptoms of prostatic cancer. Treatment options include hormonal therapy, chemotherapy, radiation therapy, surgery, or any combination of these. Symptomatic relief of urinary obstruction, bladder outlet obstruction, colon obstruction, and spinal cord compression may be required.

9. Describe sexual dysfunction in the male.
Study page 896.

Male **sexual dysfunction** is the impairment of erection, emission, and ejaculation. In men over 40 years of age, organic factors are involved in more than 50 percent of dysfunctional cases. Neurologic disorders can interfere with the important sympathetic, parasympathetic, and central nervous system mechanisms of erection, emission, and ejaculation. Men who are taking antihypertensives, antidepressants, antihistamines, antispasmodics, sedatives or tranquilizers, barbiturates, diuretics, sex hormone preparations, narcotics, or psychoactive drugs or who consume ethyl alcohol experience sexual dysfunction.

10. Differentiate between benign and malignant female breast disease.
Study pages 896-906; refer to Figures 31-25 through 31-28 and Tables 31-8 through 31-13.

Many terms have been used to describe benign breast lesions of epithelial origin. **Fibrocystic disease** or physiologic nodularity is one description, and it is manifested by palpable lumps in the breast. These lumps fluctuate with the menstrual cycle and may become progressively worse until menopause. This terminology is not altogether accurate since physiologic nodularity is present in approximately 50 percent of menstruating women. Also, some of the lesions called fibrocystic disease are associated with an increased risk of breast cancer.

Breast cancer is the most common cancer in American women and the second biggest killer after lung cancer. Lifetime risk for breast cancer is approximately one in every eight women. The risk of breast cancer increases as age advances and is the greatest in women aged 45 to 64. The risk factor and possible etiologies of breast cancer can be classified as reproductive, hormonal, environmental, and familial. (See box on page 261 of *Workbook*.)

11. Describe gynecomastia.
Study page 906.

Gynecomastia is the overdevelopment of breast tissue in a male. Gynecomastia accounts for approximately 85 percent of all masses that develop in the male breast and affects approximately 35 percent of the male population. Incidence is greatest among adolescents and men older than age 50.

Gynecomastia usually involves an imbalance of the estrogen-testosterone ratio. The ratio can be altered by tumor- and drug-induced hyperestrogenism that elevates the estrogen levels while testosterone levels remain normal. Testosterone levels may be extremely low with normal estrogen levels in hypergonadism. Gynecomastia also can be caused by increased breast tissue responsiveness to estrogen or decreased responsiveness to androgen. Estrogen-testosterone imbalances are associated with hypogonadism, Klinefelter syndrome, testicular neoplasms, cirrhosis of the liver, infectious hepatitis, chronic renal failure, chronic obstructive lung disease, hyperthyroidism, tuberculosis, and chronic malnutrition.

Hyperplasia results in a firm, palpable mass at least 2 cm in diameter located beneath the areola. Identification and treatment of the cause are likely to resolve the gynecomastia.

Benign/Malignant Female Breast Disorders

Disorder	Risks	Pathophysiology	Manifestations	Treatment
Fibrocystic disease Microcysts Macrocysts Adenosis Apocrine change Fibrosis Fibroadenomas Ductal hyperplasia	Puberty to lifetime, nonproliferative lesions demonstrate no added risk for cancer, proliferative lesions without atypia have slightly increased risk, proliferation with atypia have a high risk for cancer development	Increased estrogen levels, alterations in estrogen-to-progesterone ratio	Fluctuating pain, pain increases as menstruation approaches, fluctuating lesion size, multiple lesions	Cyst drainage, surgical excision, pain relief by synthetic androgen
Breast cancer	Increasing age: Lifetime, 1 in 8 at age 30, 1 in 2500 at age 40, 1 in 200 at age 50, 1 in 50 at age 60, 1 in 25 at age 70, 1 in 15 at age 80, 1 in 10 No term pregnancies, long reproductive life, ionizing radiation, high-fat diet, alcohol ingestion, first-degree relatives	Estrogens have a proliferative effect on mammary gland epithelium, estrogens may increase susceptibility to environmental carcinogens, transforming growth factor (TgF), autosomal dominant inheritance on chromosome 17	Painless lumps, skin retraction over lesion, nipple puckering and discharge After metastasis: palpable axillary lymph nodes, bone pain, site-specific signs and symptoms	Surgery to remove lesion, radiation to prevent metastasis, chemotherapy, hormones for hormone-dependent tumors

12. State the current status of sexually transmitted diseases (STDs).
Study page 907; refer to Table 31-14.

The study and categorization of **STDs** has broadened to include bacterial, viral, and other agents as causes of STDs. The viral-induced STDs are generally considered incurable. It is estimated that more than 12 million cases of STDs are contracted by Americans a year. The incidence and increase in STDs is due to increased premarital sex, an increase in the divorce rate, nonmonogamy among married people, and bisexuality. These factors contribute to the increase in numbers of sexual partners and an increased exposure to STDs. The number of individuals who fail to take protective measures when engaging in sexual activities also contributes to the problem.

13. Characterize the bacterial, bacterial-like STDs, focusing on infectious agents and manifestations.
Refer to Table 31-16.

(See first box on page 262 of *Workbook.*)

14. Characterize the viral STDs, focusing on infectious agents and manifestations.
Refer to Table 31-16.

(See second box on page 262 of *Workbook.*)

Bacterial, Bacterial-like STDs

Disease/Infectious Agent	Manifestations
Gonorrhea *Neisseria gonorrhoeae*	Possibly asymptomatic, urethritis, cervicitis, mucopurulent discharge, anorectal infection, pharyngitis, conjunctivitis, ophthalmia
Syphilis *Treponema pallidum*	Primary: nonpainful chancre at site of invasion Secondary: systemic involvement with skin rash and lymphadenopathy Tertiary: gummas
Chancroid *Haemophilus ducreyi*	Papule erodes into painful ulcer, superficial exudate, painful lymphadenopathy
Bacterial vaginosis *Gardnerella vaginitis*	Thin and scant malodorous vaginal discharge
Urogenital infections Lymphogranuloma venereum *Chlamydia trachomatis*	Commonly associated with other STDs, purulent discharge, cervicitis, urethritis, proctitis, newborn conjunctivitis and pneumonia, tender lymph nodes and inguinal buboes

Note: Treatment of bacterial, bacterial-like STDs is with appropriate antibiotics.

Viral STDs

Disease/Infectious Agent	Manifestations
Genital herpes Herpes simplex virus (HSV-1 or HSV-2) (latent virus)	Painful blisterlike lesions on external genitalia and genital tract
Condylomata acuminata (warts) Human papillomavirus (HPV)	Soft, skin-colored single or clustered growths

Note: Treatment for HSV is not curative, but oral and topical antiviral agents (acyclovir) are used to lower recurrence; HPV lesions are treated with topical agents and surgery.

15. Characterize the parasitic STDs by infectious agents and manifestations.
Refer to Table 31-16.

Parasitic STDs

Disease/Infectious Agent	Manifestations
Trichomoniasis *Trichomonas vaginalis*	Pain during intercourse, dysuria, spotting
Scabies *Sarcoptes scabiei*	Intense pruritus
Pediculosis pubis (crabs) *Phthirus pubis*	Pruritus

Note: Treatment is by antitrichosomal agents, scabicides, and prescription creams.

Practice Examination

1. Secondary amenorrhea is:

   a. failure to begin menstruation by age 20.
   b. menarche failure.
   c. increased myometrial vasculature constriction.
   d. the absence of menstruation following menarche.

2. What is the likely pathophysiology of PMS?

   a. Elevated prolactin levels cause salt and water retention.
   b. Elevated aldosterone levels cause salt and water retention.
   c. An abnormal nervous, immunologic, vascular, and gastrointestinal response to the menstrual cycle likely occurs.
   d. Both a and b are correct.

3. Acute pelvic inflammatory disease (PID) (*more than one answer may be correct*):

   a. primarily affects males.
   b. is usually caused by viruses.
   c. never causes peritonitis.
   d. involves the epididymis.
   e. may cause infertility or tubular pregnancy.

4. Anovulatory cycles having prolonged estrogen levels and absent progesterone production are found in:

   a. cervical cancer.
   b. corpus luteum cysts.
   c. adenomyosis.
   d. endometrial hyperplasia.
   e. Both b and c are correct.

5. Depressed T cell function is associated with:

   a. follicular cysts.
   b. endometrial polyps.
   c. leiomyomas.
   d. adenomyosis.
   e. endometriosis.

6. A 42-year-old retired prostitute who became sexually active at age 14 is at risk to develop:

   a. endometriosis.
   b. cervical carcinoma.
   c. breast cancer.
   d. uterine carcinoma.

7. Painful intercourse is:

   a. inability to achieve orgasm.
   b. inhibited sexual desire.
   c. muscle spasm in response to attempted penetration.
   d. dyspareunia.

8. Elevated serum gonadotropins suggest:

   a. testicular disease.
   b. genital organ inflammation.
   c. prostatic carcinoma.
   d. gynecomastia.

9. Phimosis is:

   a. thickening of the fascia in the erectile tissue of the corpora cavernosa.
   b. the condition of a retracted foreskin that cannot be moved forward.
   c. a condition in which the foreskin cannot be retracted.
   d. caused by poor hygiene and chronic infection.
   e. Both c and d are correct.

10. A varicocele is an intrascrotal disorder:

    a. that results in a collection of fluid within the tunica vaginalis.
    b. occurring because of independent or congenitally absent valves in the spermatic veins.
    c. located between the head of the epididymis and the testis.
    d. that does not interfere with spermatogenesis.

11. Cryptorchidism is:

    a. underdevelopment of the testes.
    b. the absence of scrotal tissue.
    c. relieved by scrotal support.
    d. failure of testes to descend into the scrotum.
    e. an imbalance between secreting and absorptive capacities of scrotal tissues.

12. The infectious cause of orchitis is:

    a. streptococci.
    b. gonococci.
    c. chlamydial organisms.
    d. mumps virus.

13. Which organisms can cause epididymitis?

    a. Enterobacteriaceae
    b. *Neisseria gonorrhoeae*
    c. *Chlamydia trachomatis*
    d. All of the above are correct.
    e. None of the above is correct.

14. In benign prostatic hyperplasia, enlargement of periurethral tissue of the prostate causes:

    a. obstruction of the urethra.
    b. inflammation of the testis.
    c. decreased urinary outflow from the bladder.
    d. abnormal dilation of a vein within the spermatic cord.
    e. tension of the spermatic cord and testis.

15. A major cause of recurrent urinary tract infections in the male is:

    a. orchitis.
    b. balanitis.
    c. epididymitis.
    d. chronic bacterial prostatitis.
    e. nonbacterial prostatitis.

16. A symptom or sign of late-stage, metastatic prostatic cancer is:

    a. a slow urinary stream.
    b. frequency of urination.
    c. incomplete emptying.
    d. mental confusion.
    e. a, b, and c are correct.

17. Male sexual dysfunction may be caused by:

    a. infection around the introitus.
    b. diabetes mellitus.
    c. infected hymenal remnants.
    d. None of the above is correct.

Match the characteristic with the benign or malignant female breast disorder.

18. ____ fluctuating lesion size	a. fibrocystic disease
19. ____ palpable axillary lymph nodes	b. breast cancer
20. ____ gene on chromosome 17	

Match the STD with its causative agent.

21. ____ gonorrhea
22. ____ syphilis
23. ____ condylomata acuminata
24. ____ pediculosis pubis
25. ____ lymphogranuloma

a. *Haemophilus ducreyi*
b. *Mycoplasma hominis*
c. *Neisseria gonorrhoeae*
d. *Gardnerella vaginalis*
e. *Treponema pallidum*
f. human papillomavirus
g. *Sarcoptes scabiei*
h. *Phthirus pubis*
i. *Chlamydia trachomatis*
j. *Trichomonas vaginalis*

Case Study

Mrs. B. is a 46-year-old female who consults her physician about the nature of a lump in her left breast. About three months ago, her spouse noticed a small lump in her left breast; however, she was unconcerned since she experienced small lumps in her breast around the times of her menses. Yet, this lump seemed to be growing and did not seem to fluctuate in size as in the past. Three small lumps that fluctuated in size were noticed by Mrs. B in her right breast. She states she is in excellent health, exercises daily, and neither smokes nor drinks alcohol.

Mrs. B. is the mother of two preteen children. After the birth of her last child, she took birth control pills for eight years and then selected an alternative method of birth control. Her onset of menses occurred at age 10. Her family history reveals that her mother and one of three aunts died of breast cancer; otherwise, the history is noncontributing.

On examination, a 2- to 3-cm mass was palpated in the upper quadrant of her left breast. This mass was firm, fixed to the chest wall, and slightly tender to touch. The skin and nipple appeared normal. Under the left axilla, a node about the size of a pea was palpable. Three 1- to 2-cm soft, movable masses were palpated in Mrs. B.'s right breast.

Mammography confirmed the presence of a 3-cm mass in the left breast and four 1.5-cm masses in the right breast. All other diagnostic procedures were negative.

What do you think about Mrs. B.'s examination and her risk factors?

CHAPTER 32

Structure and Function of the Digestive System

Objectives

After review of this chapter, the learner will be able to:

1. **List sequentially the parts of the alimentary canal from mouth to anus.**
   Refer to Figure 32-1.

2. **Describe the structural layers of the gastrointestinal tract.**
   Review page 918; refer to Figure 32-2.

3. **Describe the mouth and esophagus, noting specific structure and function.**
   Review pages 918-920; refer to Figure 32-3.

4. **Describe the stomach, noting specific structure, function, and secretions.**
   Review pages 921-924; refer to Figures 32-5 through 32-8 and Table 32-1.

5. **Describe the small intestine, noting specific structure, function, and secretions.**
   Review pages 924-928; refer to Figures 32-9 through 32-11 and Table 32-1.

6. **Describe the structure and function of the large intestine and identify normal intestinal flora and their activities.**
   Review pages 929-931; refer to Figure 32-12.

7. **Describe the structure, function, and secretions of the liver and describe the gallbladder.**
   Review pages 931-936; refer to Figures 32-13 through 32-18.

8. **Explain the relationship between cell types and function of the pancreas.**
   Review pages 936-939; refer to Figure 32-18.

9. **Describe the alterations in the digestive system associated with normal aging.**
   Review page 940.

Practice Examination

1. The muscularis of the gastrointestinal tract is:

   a. skeletal muscle throughout the tract, particularly in the esophagus and large intestine.
   b. the layer that contains the blood capillaries for the entire wall of the tract.
   c. composed principally of keratinized epithelium.
   d. composed of circular fibers and longitudinal fibers.

2. The digestive functions performed by the saliva and salivary amylase respectively are:

   a. moistening and protein digestion.
   b. deglutition and fat digestion.
   c. peristalsis and polysaccharide digestion.
   d. lubrication and carbohydrate digestion.

3. The nervous pathway involved in salivary secretion requires stimulation of:

   a. receptors in the taste buds and somatic motor impulses to salivary glands.
   b. receptors in the mouth, sensory impulses, and parasympathetic impulses to salivary glands.
   c. taste receptors, sensory impulses, and somatic motor impulses to salivary glands.
   d. pressoreceptors in blood vessels and autonomic impulses to salivary glands.

4. Food would pass rapidly from the stomach into the duodenum if it were not for the:

   a. fundus.
   b. epiglottis.
   c. rugae.
   d. cardiac sphincter.
   e. pyloric sphincter.

5. The secretion of gastric juice:

   a. occurs only when swallowed food comes in contact with the stomach.
   b. is entirely under the control of the hormone gastrin.
   c. is entirely under the control of the hormone enterogastrone.
   d. is stimulated by the presence of saliva in the stomach.
   e. occurs in three phases: cephalic, gastric, and intestinal.

6. During nervous control of gastric secretion, the gastric glands secrete before food enters the stomach. This stimulus to the glands comes from:

   a. gastrin.
   b. impulses over somatic nerves from the hypothalamus.
   c. motor impulses from the cerebral cortex and cerebellum.
   d. parasympathetic impulses over the vagus nerve.

7. Pepsinogen:

   a. must be activated by HC1.
   b. is secreted by the chief cells.
   c. is a precursor to pepsin.
   d. All of the above are correct.

8. Beginning at the lumen of the tube, the sequence of layers of the gastrointestinal tract is:

   a. mucosa, submucosa, muscularis, serosa.
   b. submucosa, mucosa, serosa, muscularis.
   c. submucosa, mucosa, muscularis, skeletal muscle.
   d. serosa, muscularis, mucosa, submucosa.

9. Normally, when chyme leaves the stomach:

   a. the nutrients are ready for absorption into the blood.
   b. the amount of inorganic salts have been increased by the action of hydrochloric acid.
   c. its pH is neutral.
   d. the proteins have been partly digested into polypeptides.
   e. All of the above are correct.

10. Which layer of the small intestine includes microvilli?

    a. submucosa
    b. mucosa
    c. muscularis
    d. serosa

11. Which is not an example of mechanical digestion?

    a. chewing
    b. churning and mixing of food in the stomach
    c. peristalsis and mastication
    d. conversion of protein molecules into amino acids

12. Pancreatic juice is to trypsin as gastric juice is to:

    a. salivary amylase.
    b. pepsin.
    c. mucin.
    d. intrinsic factor.

13. Which part of the small intestine is most distal from the pylorus?

    a. jejunum
    b. pyloric sphincter
    c. duodenum
    d. cardiac sphincter
    e. common bile duct

14. The pancreas:

    a. lies mostly on the left side of the abdominal cavity, anterior to the stomach and the spleen.
    b. secretes all of its products directly into the bloodstream.
    c. is a gland with its duct ultimately opening into the duodenum.
    d. contains cells with endocrine function for the determination of secondary sex characteristics.
    e. is classified as a digestive exocrine gland, not having endocrine functions.

15. The chief role played by the pancreas in digestion is to:

    a. secrete insulin and glucagon.
    b. churn the food and bring it into contact with digestive enzymes.
    c. secrete enzymes which digest food in the small intestine.
    d. assist in absorbing the digested foods.

16. Among the structural features of the small intestine are villi, microvilli, and circular folds. Their function is to:

    a. liberate hormones.
    b. promote peristalsis.
    c. liberate digestive enzymes.
    d. increase the surface area for absorption.

17. The fate of carbohydrates in the small intestine is:

    a. digestion to monosaccharides.
    b. conversion to simple sugars by the activity of trypsin.
    c. hydrolysis to amino acids.
    d. conversion to glycerol and fatty acids.

18. The absorptive fate of the end products of digestion may be summarized as:

    a. most fatty acids are absorbed into the blood; glucose and amino acids are absorbed into the lymphatic system.
    b. amino acids and monosaccharides are absorbed into blood capillaries; most fatty acids are absorbed into lymph.
    c. amino acids and fatty acids are absorbed into the lymph capillaries; glycerol and glucose are absorbed into the blood capillaries.
    d. fatty acids are absorbed into blood capillaries; glycerol, glucose, and amino acids are absorbed into lymph.

19. A lobule of the liver contains a centrally located:

    a. vein with radiating hepatocytes and sinusoids.
    b. arteriole with radiating capillaries and Kupffer cells.
    c. hepatic sinus with radiating sinusoids.
    d. hepatic duct with radiating Kupffer cells and cords of hepatic cells.

20. An obstruction of the common bile duct would cause blockage of bile coming from:

    a. the gallbladder.
    b. the liver but not from the gallbladder.
    c. both the liver and the gallbladder.
    d. the pancreatic duct but not from the gallbladder.

21. The human adult liver does not:

    a. store glycogen.
    b. produce erythrocytes.
    c. convert ammonia to urea.
    d. produce blood coagulation proteins.

22. The chyme that enters the large intestine is converted to feces by activity of:

    a. specific mucosal enzymes.
    b. gastric and duodenal hormones.
    c. bacteria and water reabsorption.
    d. the microvilli, villi, and circular muscles.

Match the substance with its function.

23. ____ mucus
24. ____ intrinsic factor
25. ____ cholecystokinin

a. stimulates gallbladder to eject bile
b. activates pepsinogen
c. required for vitamin B_{12} absorption
d. increases gastrointestinal mobility
e. protects gastric mucosa from digestion
f. stimulates liver to secrete bile

CHAPTER

33

Alterations of Digestive Function

Foundational Objective

a. Describe the structure and function of the gastrointestinal tract and accessory organs of digestion. Review pages 940-942; refer to Figure 32-1.

Memory Check!

- The gastrointestinal system includes the oral structures (mouth, salivary glands, pharynx), the alimentary tract (esophagus, stomach, small intestine, large intestine, appendix, anus), and the accessory organs of digestion (liver, gallbladder, bile ducts, pancreas). The function of the alimentary tract is to digest masticated food, to absorb digestive products, and to excrete the digestive residue and certain waste products excreted by the liver through the bile duct.
- The esophagus is a straight tube that carries food from the pharynx to the stomach. The stomach is a distensible organ. The stomach's mucosal cells secrete hydrochloric acid and proteolytic enzymes which aid in digestion. The mucosa of the lower part of the stomach is lined by mucous cells. The distal end of the stomach is called the pylorus. The small intestine is divided into the duodenum, jejunum, and ileum. The large intestine or colon consists of the cecum, ascending colon, transverse colon, descending colon, sigmoid colon, and rectum. The vermiform appendix is a nonfunctional vestigial structure attached to the cecum. The colon is a storage reservoir for undigested food and a site for water absorption.
- The alimentary tract has four layers: mucosa, submucosa, muscularis, and serosa. The mucosal layer consists of epithelial cells lining the lumen's surface, supporting connective tissue called the lamina propria, and a unique thin, muscular layer called the muscularis mucosae. The structure of the inner mucosal layer varies to provide specialized function at each part of the tract. The esophagus is lined by stratified squamous epithelium which enables rapid gliding of masticated food from the mouth to the stomach. The stomach has a thick glandular mucosa which provides mucus, acid, and proteolytic enzymes to help digest food. The small intestinal mucosa has a villous structure to provide a large surface of cells for active absorption. The large intestinal mucosa is lined by abundant mucus-secreting cells which facilitate storage and evacuation of the residue. Beneath the mucosa is the submucosa which gives structural support to the tract because of its abundant collagenous tissue. The muscle layer contracts rhythmically to move materials through the alimentary tract. The serosal layer is a thin, smooth membrane present on the outer surface of the alimentary tract. It keeps the tortuous loops of bowel from becoming tangled and is continuous with the mesentery. The mesentery is a connective tissue attachment of the bowel to the abdominal wall; it contains blood vessels, lymphatics, and nerves.

(Continued)

Memory Check! (cont'd)

- A wave of muscle contraction carries a bolus of swallowed food down the esophagus where a sphincter at the lower end of the esophagus prevents regurgitation. Contractions in the stomach mix the food and push the partially digested contents into the duodenum. The muscle of the pylorus only partially closes the outlet to the stomach, so intestinal contents can regurgitate into the stomach if the small intestine is not emptying properly. Normally, movement of lumenal contents in the small intestine is more rapid in the upper small intestine and slows as chyme moves distally. Contents pass from the ileum into the colon where reverse proximal movement is partially prevented by the ileocecal valve. Water is absorbed in the colon and the contents become solid; the solid residue is moved to the left side of the colon and rectum. When the rectum becomes distended, an urge for defecation develops.
- The liver and the pancreas are glandular organs with excretory ducts emptying into the duodenum at a site called the ampulla of Vater. The excretory ducts of the liver are called bile ducts. The gallbladder is a storage reservoir connected to the bile ducts by the cystic duct.
- Most of the blood from the abdominal organs is carried to the liver via the portal vein. Therefore, blood is filtered by the glandular cells of the liver before it returns to the heart via the hepatic vein and vena cava. Because portal blood has little oxygen left after passing through the abdominal organs, the liver has the hepatic artery to provide oxygenated blood. The bulk of the liver is composed of hepatocytes which are aligned in cords with sinusoids between the cords to diffuse the blood from the portal areas to the central vein. Between adjacent hepatocytes are tiny canaliculi that carry bile produced by the hepatocytes to the portal area where they empty into epithelial-lined bile ducts. In the sinusoids, waste products and nutrients are removed and metabolized by the hepatocytes. The metabolites may be returned to the blood, stored in the hepatocytes, or excreted into bile canaliculi. The liver also contains many mononuclear cells or Kupffer cells that line the sinusoids. They phagocytize particulate material from the blood. Metabolically, the liver (1) produces bile salts, (2) excretes bilirubin, (3) metabolizes nitrogenous substances, (4) produces serum proteins, and (5) detoxifies drugs and poisons.
- The gallbladder is a distension of the common bile duct that becomes a storage reservoir for bile. The gallbladder empties its contents into the duodenum after meals when bile salts are needed for fat absorption. This reservoir function is not essential, as the gallbladder can be removed without loss of digestive function.
- The pancreas is a long, narrow glandular organ lying horizontally and retroperitoneally in the midabdomen region. The pancreatic duct runs the length of the pancreas and empties into the duodenum after joining the bile duct. The bulk of the pancreas is made up of glands that secrete digestive enzymes into the pancreatic duct. When activated by intestinal juices, these enzymes digest carbohydrate, fat, and protein. Pancreatic enzymes are essential for life. Scattered among the pancreatic glands are clusters of endocrine cells known as the islets of Langerhans, which produce insulin and other hormones.
- The digestive process begins in the mouth, where a carbohydrate-splitting enzyme or amylase from the salivary glands mixes with food during mastication. In the stomach, proteolytic pepsin and hydrochloric acid are added to speed the digestive process. The greatest volume of digestive enzymes originates from the pancreas and is added to the digesting mixture of food in the duodenum. In addition, bile salts secreted by the liver and stored in the gallbladder are added to emulsify lipids into small water-soluble micelles. The final phase of the digestive process occurs at the surface of small intestinal epithelial cells. Complex endocrine and nervous mechanisms coordinate the timing of the secretion of digestive enzymes, hydrochloric acid, and bile salts. The sight of food may cause salivation and gastric secretions because of nervous stimulation. Distention of the stomach causes release of gastrin which stimulates acid production and gastric emptying. Movement of food into the duodenum causes the pancreas to secrete more fluid and enzymes and the gallbladder to release bile. The products of both enter the duodenum.

Objectives

After studying this chapter, the learner will be able to:

1. **Describe the common terms used in identifying the manifestations of gastrointestinal dysfunction.**
Study pages 945-947; refer to Figure 33-1 and Table 33-1.

Anorexia is the absence of a desire to eat despite physiologic stimuli that would normally produce hunger. Anorexia is a nonspecific symptom often associated with nausea, abdominal pain, and diarrhea. Disorders of other systems besides the digestive system are accompanied by anorexia. These include cancer, heart disease, and renal disease.

Vomiting is the forceful emptying of stomach and intestinal contents or chyme through the mouth. The vomiting reflex is stimulated by presence of ipecac or copper salts in the duodenum, severe pain, or distention of the stomach or duodenum. Torsion or trauma affecting the ovaries, testes, uterus, bladder, or kidney also elicit vomiting.

Nausea and retching usually precede vomiting. **Nausea** is a subjective experience associated with many different conditions. **Retching** is a strong involuntary effort to vomit. In retching, the lower esophageal sphincter and body of the stomach relax but the duodenum and antrum of the stomach go into spasm. The reverse peristalsis forces chyme from the stomach and duodenum up into the esophagus. Since the upper esophageal sphincter is closed, chyme does not enter the mouth. As the abdominal muscles relax, the contents of the esophagus drop back into the stomach. This process may be repeated several time before vomiting occurs.

Vomiting occurs when the stomach is full of gastric contents and the diaphragm is forced high into the thoracic cavity by strong abdominal muscle contractions. The higher intrathoracic pressure forces the upper esophageal sphincter to open and chyme is discharged from the mouth. Spontaneous vomiting not preceded by nausea or retching is called **projectile vomiting**. This vomiting is caused by direct stimulation of the vomiting center because of neurologic lesions involving the brain stem. The metabolic consequences of vomiting are fluid, electrolyte, and acid-base disturbances.

Constipation is difficult or infrequent defecation involving decreased numbers of bowel movements per week, hard stools, and difficult evacuation. Constipation is frequently caused by unhealthy dietary and bowel habits combined with inadequate exercise. It also can occur as a result of intestinal immobility or obstruction disorders.

Constipation resulting from lifestyle or bowel habits usually has a long duration. Dysfunctional constipation is more likely to be sudden and can accompany the development of organic lesions.

Diarrhea is increased frequency of defecation accompanied by changes in fecal fluidity and volume. In **osmotic diarrhea**, the presence of nonabsorbable substances in the intestine causes water to be drawn into the lumen by osmosis. The excess water and the nonabsorbable substances increase stool weight and volume. This causes large-volume diarrhea. **Secretory diarrhea** is a form of large-volume diarrhea caused by excessive mucosal secretion of fluid and electrolytes. Excessive intestinal secretion is caused mostly by bacterial enterotoxins released by cholera or strains of *Escherichia coli.* A lesion that impairs autonomic control of motility such as diabetic neuropathy can cause large-volume diarrhea. Excessive motility decreases transit time, mucosal surface contact, and opportunities for fluid absorption. **Motility diarrhea** can be caused by resection of the small intestine, surgical bypass of an area of the intestine, or fistula formation between loops of the intestine.

Small-volume diarrhea is usually caused by inflammatory disorders of the intestine or by fecal impaction from severe constipation. In the latter case, the diarrhea consists of mucus and fluid produced by the colon to lubricate the impacted feces and move it toward the anal canal.

Abdominal pain is observed in a number of gastrointestinal diseases. Abdominal organs are sensitive to stretching and distention, which can activate nerve endings in both hollow and solid structures. Histamine, bradykinin, and serotonin, when released during inflammation, stimulate organic nerve endings and produce abdominal pain. The edema and vascular congestion that accompany inflammation also cause painful stretching. Any obstruction of blood flow because of distention of bowel obstruction or mesenteric vessel thrombosis produces ischemic pain. **Parietal pain** arises from the parietal peritoneum and is more localized and intense than **visceral pain**, which arises from the organs themselves. **Referred pain** is visceral pain felt at some distance from a diseased or affected organ. Referred pain is usually well localized and is felt in the skin or deeper tissues which share a central, common afferent pathway with the affected organ.

Numerous disorders cause gastrointestinal tract bleeding. Acute **gastrointestinal bleeding** is usually characterized by **hematemesis**, or the presence of blood in the vomitus; **hematochezia**, or frank bleeding from the rectum; or **melena**, which is dark, tarry stools. **Occult bleeding** is slow, chronic blood loss that results in iron-deficiency anemia as iron stores in the bone marrow are slowly depleted.

2. Compare and contrast the various disorders of digestive motility.
Study pages 947-952; refer to Figures 33-2 and 33-3 and Tables 33-2 and 33-3.

(See box below.)

3. Describe the pathogenesis of acute and chronic gastritis.
Study pages 952-954.

Gastritis is an inflammatory disorder of the gastric mucosa that may be acute or chronic and that affects the fundus or antrum or both. Antiinflammatory drugs are known to cause **acute gastritis** which erodes the epithelium, probably because

Motility Disorders

Disorder	Causes	Manifestations
Dysphagia (swallowing difficulty)	Esophageal obstruction Tumors, strictures, or diverticula Impaired esophageal motility Neural dysfunction, muscular disease, CVA Achalasia (decreased ganglion cells in myenteric plexus, muscle cell atrophy)	Distention and spasm of esophagus after swallowing, regurgitation of undigested food
Gastroesophageal reflux (chyme reflux into esophagus)	Increased abdominal pressure, ulcers, pyloric edema and strictures, hiatal hernia	Regurgitation of chyme within one hour of eating
Hiatal hernia (protrusion of upper stomach through diaphragm into thorax)	Congenitally short esophagus, trauma, weak diaphragmatic muscles at gastroesophageal junction, increased abdominal pressure	Gastroesophageal reflux, dysphagia, epigastric pain
Pyloric obstruction (narrow pylorus)	Peptic ulcer or carcinoma near pylorus	Epigastric fullness, nausea and pain, vomitus without bile
Intestinal obstruction (impaired chyme flow through intestinal lumen)	Hernia, telescoping of one part of intestine into another, twisting, inflamed diverticula, tumor growth, loss of peristaltic activity	Colicky pain to severe and constant pain, vomiting, diarrhea, constipation, dehydration and hypovolemia and acidosis with their complications

they inhibit prostaglandins that normally stimulate the secretion of protective mucus. Alcohol, histamine, digitalis, and metabolic disorders such as uremia are contributing factors for gastritis.

The clinical manifestations of acute gastritis can include vague abdominal discomfort, epigastric tenderness, and bleeding. Healing usually occurs spontaneously within a few days. Discontinuing injurious drugs, using antacids, or decreasing acid secretion with drugs facilitates healing.

Chronic gastritis is a progressive disease that tends to occur in elderly individuals. This gastritis causes thinning and degeneration of the stomach wall.

Chronic fundal gastritis is the most severe type, as the gastric mucosa degenerates extensively. The loss of chief cells and parietal cells diminishes secretion of pepsinogen, hydrochloric acid, and intrinsic factor. Pernicious anemia develops because intrinsic factor is unavailable to facilitate vitamin B_{12} absorption. Chronic fundal gastritis becomes a risk factor for gastric carcinoma, particularly in individuals who develop pernicious anemia. A significant number of individuals with chronic fundal gastritis have antibodies to parietal cells, intrinsic factor, and gastric cells in their sera, thus suggesting an autoimmune mechanism in the pathogenesis of the disease.

Chronic antral gastritis is more frequent than fundal gastritis. It is not associated with decreased hydrochloric acid secretion, pernicious anemia, or the presence of parietal cell antibodies. *Helicobacter pylori* is a major etiologic factor associated with the inflammation seen in chronic gastritis. The longstanding inflammatory process and gastric atrophy may develop without a history of abdominal distress. Individuals may report vague symptoms including anorexia, fullness, nausea, vomiting, and epigastric pain. Gastric bleeding may be the only clinical manifestation of gastritis.

4. Compare duodenal, gastric, and stress ulcers; identify the complications of surgical management of ulcers.
Study pages 954-959; refer to Figures 33-4 through 33-6 and Tables 33-4 and 33-5.

A **peptic ulcer** is a break or ulceration in the protective mucosal lining of the lower esophagus, stomach, or duodenum. Such breaks expose submucosal areas to gastric secretions and autodigestion.

Risk factors for peptic ulcer disease are smoking and habitual use of NSAIDs or alcohol. Some chronic diseases such as emphysema, rheumatoid arthritis, and cirrhosis are associated with the development of peptic ulcers. Infection of the gastric and duodenal mucosa with *H. pylori* may cause peptic ulcers. Studies of life stress and ulcer disease are inconclusive regarding causation of peptic ulcers.

Postgastrectomy syndromes are a group of signs and symptoms that occur after gastric resection. They are caused by alterations in motor and control functions of the stomach and upper small intestine. **Dumping syndrome** is the rapid emptying of hypertonic chyme from the surgically reduced and smaller stomach into the small intestine 10 to 20 minutes after eating.

Alkaline reflux gastritis is stomach inflammation caused by reflux of bile and alkaline pancreas secretions that contain proteolytic enzymes which disrupt the mucosal barrier. Clinical manifestations include nausea, vomiting in which the vomitus contains bile, and sustained epigastric pain that worsens after eating and is not relieved by antacids.

Afferent loop obstruction is a problem caused by volvulus, hernia, adhesion, or stenosis in the duodenal stump on the proximal side of the surgery. The symptoms of afferent loop obstruction include intermittent severe pain and epigastric fullness after eating.

Diarrhea is frequent elimination of a large volume of stool. Postgastrectomy diarrhea appears to be related to rapid gastric emptying of large amounts of high carbohydrate liquids. **Weight loss** frequently follows gastric resection because the stomach is less able to mix, churn, and break down food.

Anemia after gastrectomy results from iron, vitamin B_{12}, or folate deficiency.

(See box on page 277 of *Workbook.*)

5. Define malabsorption syndrome and maldigestion; characterize pancreatic insufficiency and lactase and bile salt deficiency.
Study pages 959-960.

Malabsorption syndromes interfere with nutrient absorption in the small intestine; the intestinal mucosa fails to absorb or transport the digested nutrients into the blood. **Malabsorption** is the result of mucosal disruption caused by gastric or intestinal resection, vascular disorders, or intestinal

Features of Ulcers

Feature	Duodenal	Gastric	Stress
Age incidence	25-50 years	50-70 years	Related to severe stress, trauma, sepsis, head injuries
Sex prevalence	Men	No sex difference	
Stress factors	Average	Increased	Increased
Acid production	Increased	Normal to low	Increased
Ulcerogenic drugs	Increased use of alcohol and tobacco	Moderate use of alcohol and tobacco	
Associated gastritis	Seldom	Common	
Helicobacter pylori	Often present	May be present	
Pain	Pain-food-relief, common nocturnal pain, remission and exacerbations	Pain-food-relief, uncommon nocturnal pain, chronic, no remission and exacerbations	Asymptomatic until hemorrhage or perforation
Hemorrhage	Common	Less common	Very common (most frequent complication)
Malignancy	Almost never	Possible	

Note: Medical treatment is directed toward inhibiting or buffering acid secretions to relieve symptoms and promote healing. Antacids, dietary management, anticholinergic histamine blockers, and physical and emotional rest are used to accomplish relief and promote healing. *H. pylori* is treated with a combination of antibiotics and bismuth.

disease. **Maldigestion** is failed or faulty digestion because of deficiencies of chemical enzymes.

Pancreatic insufficiency occurs because of deficient production of lipase, amylase, trypsin, or chymotrypsin by the pancreas. Causes of pancreatic insufficiency include chronic pancreatitis, pancreatic carcinoma, pancreatic resection, and cystic fibrosis. Fat maldigestion is the chief problem. A large amount of fat in the stool is the most common sign of pancreatic insufficiency.

Lactase deficiency inhibits the breakdown of lactose or milk sugar into monosaccharides and therefore prevents lactose digestion and absorption across the intestinal wall. Lactase deficiency is most common in blacks. The undigested lactose remains in the intestine where bacterial fermentation causes gases to form. The osmotic gradient in the intestine also increases, which causes irritation and osmotic diarrhea.

Conjugated bile acids or bile salts are necessary for the digestion and absorption of fats. When bile from the liver enters the duodenum, the bile salts aggregate with fatty acids and monoglycerides to form micelles. Micelle formation solubilizes fat molecules and allows them to pass through the unstirred layer at the brush border. Advanced liver disease, which causes **bile salt deficiency**, obstruction of the common bile duct, intestinal immotility, and diseases of the ileum, leads to poor intestinal absorption of fat and fat-soluble vitamins A, D, E, and K. Increased fat in the stool leads to diarrhea and decreased plasma proteins. The loss of fat-soluble vitamins causes night blindness, bone demineralization, and bleeding abnormalities.

6. Compare ulcerative colitis and Crohn disease.
Study pages 960-961; refer to Table 33-6.

(See box below.)

7. Distinguish between diverticular disease and appendicitis.
Study pages 962-963; refer to Figure 33-7.

Diverticula are herniations or saclike outpouchings of mucosa through the muscle layers of the colon wall. **Diverticulosis** is asymptomatic diverticular disease. **Diverticulitis** represents symptomatic inflammation. The most frequent site of diverticula is the sigmoid colon at weak points in the colon wall where arteries penetrate the muscularis. Habitual consumption of a low-residue diet reduces fecal bulk and reduces the diameter of the colon. According to the law of Laplace, wall pressure increases as the diameter of the lumen decreases. Pressure within the narrow lumen can increase enough to rupture the diverticula and cause abscess formation or peritonitis. An increase of dietary fiber intake frequently relieves symptoms. Surgical resection may be required if there are severe complications.

Appendicitis is an inflammation of the vermiform appendix. Obstruction of the lumen with feces, tumors, or foreign bodies followed by bacterial infection is the most likely cause of appendicitis. The obstructed lumen does not allow drainage of the appendix, and as mucosal secretion continues, intraluminal pressure increases. The increased pressure decreases mucosal blood flow and the appendix becomes hypoxic. The mucosa ulcerates, which promotes bacterial inflammation and edema. Gangrene develops from thrombosis of the luminal blood vessels followed by perforation.

Epigastric or periumbilical pain is the typical symptom of an inflamed appendix. Right lower quadrant pain that exhibits rebound tenderness is

Ulcerative Colitis and Crohn Disease

Feature	Ulcerative colitis	Crohn disease
Family history	Less common	More common
Location of lesions	Large intestine, no "skip" lesions, mucosal layer involved	Large or small intestine, "skip" lesions common, entire intestinal wall involved
Granulomas	Rare	Common
Anal and perianal fistulas and abscesses	Rare	Common
Narrowed lumen and possible obstruction	Rare	Common
Abdominal pain	Common, mild to severe	Common, mild to severe
Diarrhea	Common	Common
Bloody stools	Common	Less common
Abdominal mass	Rare	Common
Small intestinal malabsorption	Rare	Common
Steatorrhea	Rare	Common
Cancer risk	Increased	Not increased

associated with extension of the inflammation to the surrounding tissues. Nausea, vomiting, and anorexia follow the onset of pain. Leukocytosis and a low-grade fever are common. Perforation, peritonitis, and abscess formation are the most serious complications of appendicitis.

Appendectomy is the treatment for simple or perforated appendicitis.

8. Characterize the disorders of overnutrition and undernutrition.
Study pages 963-965.

Overnutrition, or excessive caloric intake, leads to **obesity**, or excessive body fat, which is associated with three leading causes of death: cardiovascular disease, cancer, and diabetes mellitus. Obesity also is a risk factor for breast, cervical, endometrial, and liver cancer in women. Obese men are at greater risk for prostatic, colon, and rectal cancer than nonobese men.

Obesity is classified by cause as either exogenous, resulting from an excess of ingested calories, or endogenous, resulting from inherent metabolic problems. Physiologically, obesity can be (1) hyperplastic, that is, caused by a greater-than-normal number of fat cells; or (2) hypertrophic, that is, caused by a greater-than-normal size of fat cells. In children, the adipose tissue is dispersed over the entire body and is both hyperplastic and hypertrophic with few metabolic abnormalities. Adult-onset obesity is hypertrophic, with the adipose tissue centrally located, and metabolic abnormalities are more common. Genotype is an important predisposing factor.

A number of theories have been postulated to explain the physiology of obesity. In the lipoprotein-lipase (LPL) theory, lipase hydrolyzes fats into their components which then reenter the fat cells and are converted back into fats; LPL promotes fat storage and hypertrophic cells.

The lipostatic theory states that obese individuals have a higher set-point, which makes it difficult to maintain weight loss.

Another theory of obesity is based on the thermogenesis of brown fat cells that are responsible for heat production. Subcutaneous brown fat cells release excess energy through heat production instead of converting the energy to fat stores; obese people are believed to have very few brown fat cells.

The sodium-potassium-adenosine triphosphatase (ATPase) pump transports sodium out of the cell and potassium into the cell and splits adenosine triphosphate, thus releasing energy. Obese people have fewer ATPase pumps, which could lead to less energy release and obesity.

One psychologic theory proposes that obese people are directed more by the sight, smell, and taste of food than by hunger and satiety. Another psychologic theory is that eating creates the desire to eat more.

Diabetes mellitus is often associated with obesity. The excess serum glucose is stored as glycogen in the liver or as triglycerides in adipose cells, thus enhancing hypertrophy and hyperplasia of fat cells.

Treatment for obesity caused by excessive nutrient intake is a regimen of reduced nutrient intake and increased energy expenditure. Individuals with adult-onset obesity can reduce the size of the adipose cells and achieve a standard weight. Those with child-onset obesity may never achieve standard weight. Additional treatments such as psychotherapy, behavioral modification, medications, and surgery may be needed.

Many young adults and adolescents in the United States are affected by two complex and related eating disorders, anorexia nervosa and bulimia. **Anorexia nervosa** is characterized by refusal to eat because of distorted body image perceptions that one is too fat. As the disease progresses, fat and muscle depletion give the individual a skeletonlike appearance. The loss of 25 to 30 percent of ideal body weight can eventually lead to death caused by starvation-induced cardiac failure. Treatment objectives for anorexia nervosa include reversing the compromised physical state, promoting insights and knowledge about the disorder, and modifying food habits.

Bulimia is characterized by binging or the consumption of normal to large amounts of food followed by self-induced vomiting or purging of the intestines with laxatives. Although individuals with bulimia are afraid of gaining weight, their weight usually remains within normal range. Because of negative connotations associated with vomiting and purging, individuals who have bulimia often binge and purge secretly. Bulimics may binge and purge as often as 20 times a day. Continual vomiting of acidic chyme can cause pitted teeth, pharyngeal and esophageal inflammation, and tracheoesophageal fistulas. Overuse of laxatives can cause rectal bleeding.

Starvation can be either short-term or long-term. Therapeutic short-term starvation is part of many weight-reduction programs, while therapeutic long-term starvation is used in medically controlled environments to facilitate rapid weight loss in morbidly obese individuals. Pathologic long-term starvation can be caused by poverty or chronic diseases such as cardiovascular, pulmonary, hepatic, and digestive disorders, malabsorption syndromes, and cancer.

Short-term starvation consists of several days of total dietary abstinence or deprivation. Glucose is the preferred energy source for cells. Once all available energy has been absorbed from the intestine, glycogen in the liver is converted to glucose through **glycogenolysis**, or the splitting of glycogen into glucose. This process peaks within four to eight hours after glycogenolysis, and **gluconeogenesis** in the liver begins by the formation of glucose from noncarbohydrate molecules. Both of these processes deplete stored nutrients and thus cannot meet the body's energy needs indefinitely. Proteins continue to be catabolized in gluconeogenesis to a minimal degree to provide carbon for the synthesis of glucose.

The main characteristics of **long-term starvation** are decreased dependence on gluconeogenesis and increased use of products of lipid and pyruvate metabolism for cellular energy sources. Once the supply of adipose tissue is depleted, proteolysis begins. The breakdown of muscle protein is the last process to supply energy for life. Death results from severe alteration in electrolyte balance and loss of renal, pulmonary, and cardiac function.

Adequate ingestion of appropriate nutrients is the obvious treatment for starvation. Starvation caused by chronic disease, long-term illness, or malabsorption is treated by enteral or parenteral nutrition.

9. Describe the complications of liver dysfunction.
Study pages 965-970; refer to Figures 33-8 through 33-10 and Table 33-7.

The complications of liver disease include portal hypertension, ascites, hepatic encephalopathy, jaundice, and hepatorenal syndrome. (See box on page 281 of *Workbook*.)

10. Compare the viral hepatitis types.
Study pages 970-972; refer to Table 33-8.

The clinical manifestations of the different types of hepatitis are very similar and usually consist of three phases: the prodromal, icteric, and recovery phases. The **prodromal phase** of hepatitis begins about two weeks after exposure and ends with appearance of jaundice. Fatigue, anorexia, malaise, nausea, vomiting, headache, hyperalgia, cough, and low-grade fever precede the onset of jaundice. The infection is highly transmissible during this phase.

The **icteric phase** begins about one to two weeks after the prodromal phase and lasts two to six weeks. The icteric phase is the actual phase of illness. The liver is enlarged, smooth, and tender, and percussion over the liver causes pain.

The posticteric or **recovery phase** begins with resolution of jaundice at about six to eight weeks after exposure. In most cases, liver function returns to normal within 2 to 12 weeks after the onset of jaundice.

Fulminant hepatitis is a clinical syndrome resulting in severe impairment or necrosis of liver cells and potential liver failure. It may occur as a complication of hepatitis C or hepatitis B and is compounded by infection with the delta virus. The hepatic necrosis is irreversible. Treatment of fulminant hepatitis is supportive. Liver transplantation may be lifesaving. Survivors usually do not develop cirrhosis or chronic liver disease.

(See first box on page 282 of *Workbook.*)

11. Describe cirrhosis and contrast various types.
Study pages 972-974; refer to Figure 33-11 and Table 33-9.

Cirrhosis is an irreversible inflammatory disease that disrupts liver structure and function. Structural changes result from fibrosis, which is a consequence of inflammation. (See second box on page 282 of *Workbook.*)

12. Compare cholelithiasis to cholecystitis.
Study pages 974-976; refer to Figure 33-12.

Obstruction and inflammation are the most common disorders of the gallbladder. Obstruction is caused by gallstones, which are aggregates of substances in the bile. The gallstones may remain in the gallbladder or enter the cystic duct. If gallstones become lodged in the cystic duct, they obstruct the flow of bile into and out of the gallbladder and cause inflammation. Gallstone formation is termed **cholelithiasis**, while inflammation of the gallbladder or cystic duct is known as **cholecystitis**.

Liver Disease Complications

Complication	Causes	Manifestations
Portal hypertension	Obstruction or impeded blood flow in portal venous system or vena cava, cirrhosis, viral hepatitis, parasitic infection, hepatic vein thrombosis, right heart failure	Esophageal and stomach varices with vomiting of blood, splenomegaly, ascites
Ascites	Portal hypertension and reduced serum albumin levels increase capillary hydrostatic pressure which pushes water into the peritoneal cavity, cirrhosis, heart failure, constrictive pericarditis, abdominal malignancies, nephrotic syndrome, malnutrition	Abdominal distension, displaced diaphragm and dyspnea, peritonitis
Hepatic encephalopathy	Blood that contains toxins such as ammonia is shunted from gastrointestinal tract to systemic circulation, toxins reach brain	Subtle changes in cerebral function, confusion, tremor of hands, stupor, convulsions, coma
Jaundice Hemolytic (unconjugated bilirubin)	Excessive hemolysis of red blood cells because of immune reactions, infections, toxic substances, or transfusions of incompatible blood	Dark urine, light-colored stools, anorexia, malaise, fatigue, pruritus
Obstructive (conjugated bilirubin)	Obstruction of bile flow by gall-stones or tumor prevents flow into duodenum, drugs	
Hepatocellular (conjugated and un-conjugated bilirubin)	Intrahepatic disease, obstruction by bile calculi, genetic enzyme defects, infections	
Hepatorenal syndrome	Decrease in blood volume, intrarenal vasoconstriction because the liver may fail to remove excessive vaso-active substances from the blood	Oliguria, sodium and water retention, hypotension, BUN and creatinine increases

Characteristics of Viral Hepatitis

Characteristic	Hepatitis A	Hepatitis B	Hepatitis D	Hepatitis C	Hepatitis E
Transmission route	Fecal-oral, parenteral, sexual	Parenteral, sexual	Parenteral, fecal-oral, sexual	Parenteral	Fecal-oral
Incubation period	30 days	60-180 days	30-180 days	35-60 days	15-60 days
Carrier state	No	Yes	Yes	Yes	No
Severity	Mild	Severe, may be prolonged	Severe	Unknown	Severe in pregnant women
Chronic hepatitis	No	Yes	Yes	Yes	No
Prophylaxis	Hygiene, immune serum globulin	Hygiene, HBV vaccine	Hygiene, HBV vaccine	Hygiene, screening blood	Hygiene, safe water

Note: Treatment is supportive, physical activity is restricted, low-fat and high-carbohydrate diet is recommended, and interferon is useful in chronic B and C types.

Cirrhosis of the Liver

Type	Cause	Manifestations
Alcoholic cirrhosis	Toxic effects of chronic and excessive alcohol intake, alcohol is oxidized by the liver to acetaldehyde which damages hepatocytes	Typical, decreased sexual function
Primary biliary cirrhosis	Unknown, possibly an autoimmune mechanism that scars ducts	Typical, circulating IgG
Secondary biliary cirrhosis	Obstruction by neoplasms, strictures, or gallstones scars the ducts proximally	Typical
Post-necrotic cirrhosis	Viral hepatitis due to HAV or hepatitis C, drugs or other toxins, autoimmune destruction	Typical

Note: Typical manifestations include hepatomegaly, splenomegaly, ascites, and jaundice. Serologic studies reveal elevated enzymes and bilirubin, decreased albumin, and prolonged prothrombin time.

Gallstones are of two types: cholesterol and pigmented. Cholesterol stones are the most common. Cholesterol gallstones form in bile that is supersaturated with cholesterol produced by the liver. Usually within the gallbladder, supersaturation sets the stage for cholesterol crystal formation and aggregation into "macrostones." If the stones become lodged in the cystic or common duct, they cause pain and cholecystitis. Pigmented stones occur later in life and are associated with cirrhosis. Pigmented stones are created by unconjugated bilirubin binding with calcium. Risk factors for cholelithiasis include obesity, middle age, female gender, American Indian ancestry, and gallbladder, pancreatic, or ileal disease.

Abdominal pain and jaundice are the cardinal manifestations of cholelithiasis. Vague symptoms include heartburn, flatulence, epigastric discomfort, and fatty food intolerances. Biliary colic pain is caused by the lodging of one or more gallstones in the cystic or common duct. The pain can be intermittent or steady and located in the right upper quadrant with radiation to the mid-upper back. Jaundice indicates that the stone is located in the common bile duct.

Laparoscopic cholecystectomy is the preferred treatment for gallstones that cause obstruction or inflammation. Alternative treatments are the administration of drugs that dissolve the stones and ultrasonic lithotripsy.

Cholecystitis can be acute or chronic and is almost always caused by the lodging of a gallstone in the cystic duct. Obstruction causes the gallbladder to become distended and inflamed, followed by decreased blood flow, ischemia, necrosis, and possible perforation. Fever, leukocytosis, rebound tenderness, and abdominal muscle guarding are common findings. Serum bilirubin and alkaline phosphatase levels may be elevated.

13. Describe the pathogenesis of pancreatitis.
Study page 976.

Pancreatitis, or inflammation of the pancreas, is a relatively rare but potentially serious disorder. It is believed that **acute pancreatitis** develops because of an injury or disruption of the pancreatic ducts or acini that permits leakage of pancreatic enzymes into pancreatic tissue. The leaked enzymes initiate autodigestion and acute pancreatitis. Bile reflux into the pancreas occurs if gallstones obstruct the common bile duct; the refluxed bile also injures pancreatic tissue. Toxic enzymes also are released into the bloodstream and cause injury to vessels and other organs such as the lungs and kidneys. **Chronic pancreatitis** is caused mostly by alcohol abuse.

Mild to severe epigastric or midabdominal pain is the cardinal symptom of acute pancreatitis. The pain is caused by distended pancreatic ducts and capsule, chemical irritation and inflammation of the peritoneum, and irritation or obstruction of the biliary tract. Fever and leukocytosis accompany the inflammatory response. Nausea and vomiting are caused by hypermotility or paralytic ileus secondary to the pancreatitis or peritonitis. Elevated serum amylase is a characteristic diagnostic feature. Hypotension and shock frequently occur because plasma volume is lost as enzymes and kinins released into the circulation increase vascular permeability and dilate vessels. The results are hypovolemia, hypotension, and myocardial insufficiency.

The goal of treatment for acute pancreatitis is to stop the process of autodigestion and prevent systemic complications. Parenteral fluids are given to restore blood volume and prevent hypotension and shock. Severe, unremitting pancreatitis may require peritoneal lavage to remove toxic exudates or surgical drainage of the pancreas.

14. Characterize the various cancers of the digestive system.
Study pages 977-983; refer to Figures 33-13 through 33-15 and Tables 33-10 and 33-11.

Cancers of the Digestive System

Type	Risks	Manifestations
Esophagus Squamous cell carcinoma Adenocarcinoma	Malnutrition, alcohol, tobacco, chronic reflux	Chest pain, dysphagia
Stomach Adenocarcinoma Squamous cell carcinoma	Dietary salty foods, nitrates, nitrosamines, gastric atrophy	Anorexia, malaise, weight loss, upper abdominal pain, vomiting, occult blood, symptoms of organ involved in metastasis from stomach
Colorectal Adenocarcinoma (left colon grows in ring; right colon grows in mass)	Chromosomal deletions, polyps, diverticulitis, ulcerative colitis, high refined CHO, low-fiber/ high-fat diet	Pain, anemia, bloody stool, mass—right colon, obstruction—left colon, distention, elevated CEA
Liver Hepatocarcinoma Cholangiocarcinoma	HBV, HCV, HDV, cirrhosis, intestinal parasites, aflatoxin	Pain, anorexia, bloating, weight loss, portal hypertension, ascites, +/- jaundice, elevated serum proteins and enzymes
Gallbladder Secondary metastases Adenocarcinoma Squamous cell carcinoma	Cholelithiasis	Steady pain, diarrhea, anorexia, vomiting, +/- jaundice
Pancreas Adenocarcinoma	Chronic pancreatitis, cigarette smoking, alcohol, diabetic women	Weight loss, weakness, nausea, vomiting, abdominal pain, depression, +/- jaundice, possible hypoglycemia if an insulin-secreting tumor

Note: Treatment for esophageal, stomach, gallbladder, and pancreatic cancer is essentially surgical. Liver neoplasms are treated by surgery and chemotherapy. Colorectal cancer therapy uses surgery, radiation, and chemotherapy.

Practice Examination

1. During vomiting, there is:

   a. forceful diaphragm and abdominal muscle contractions, airway closure, esophageal sphincter relaxation, and deep inspiration.
   b. deep inspiration, airway closure, forceful diaphragm and abdominal muscle contractions, and esophageal sphincter relaxation.
   c. airway closure, forceful diaphragm and abdominal muscle contractions, deep inspiration, and esophageal sphincter relaxation.
   d. esophageal sphincter relaxation, forceful diaphragm and abdominal muscle contractions, deep inspiration, and airway closure.

2. Which does not cause constipation?

   a. opiates
   b. megacolon
   c. sedentary lifestyle
   d. hyperthyroidism
   e. emotional depression

3. Osmotic diarrhea is caused by:

   a. lactase deficiency.
   b. bacterial enterotoxins.
   c. ulcerative colitis.
   d. Crohn disease.
   e. Both c and d are correct.

4. Melena is:

   a. bloody vomitus.
   b. gaseous bowel distension.
   c. blood in the stool.
   d. loss of appetite.
   e. black, tarry stools.

5. A common manifestation of hiatal hernia is:

   a. gastroesophageal reflux.
   b. diarrhea.
   c. belching.
   d. postprandial substernal pain.
   e. Both a and d are correct.

6. Gastroesophageal reflux is:

   a. caused by rapid gastic emptying.
   b. excessive lower esophageal sphincter functioning.
   c. associated with abdominal surgery.
   d. caused by spontaneously relaxing lower esophageal sphincter.

7. Intestinal obstruction causes:

   a. decreased intraluminal tension.
   b. hyperkalemia.
   c. decreased nutrient absorption.
   d. Both a and b are correct.
   e. a, b, and c are correct.

8. Peptic ulcers may be located in the:

   a. stomach.
   b. esophagus.
   c. duodenum.
   d. colon.
   e. a, b, and c are correct.

9. Gastric ulcers:

   a. may lead to malignancy.
   b. occur at a younger age than duodenal ulcers.
   c. always have increased acid production.
   d. exhibit nocturnal pain.
   e. Both a and c are correct.

10. Duodenal ulcers:

    a. occur four times more frequently in females than in males.
    b. may be complicated by hemorrhage.
    c. are associated with sepsis.
    d. may cause inflammation and scar tissue formation around the sphincter of Oddi.

11. In malabsorption syndrome, flatulence and abdominal distension are likely caused by:

    a. protein deficiency and electrolyte imbalance.
    b. undigested lactose fermentation by bacteria.
    c. fat irritating the bowel.
    d. impaired absorption of amino acids and accompanying edema.

12. The characteristic lesion of Crohn disease is:

    a. found in the ileum.
    b. precancerous.
    c. granulomatous.
    d. malignant.
    e. Both a and c are correct.

13. Low-residue diets play a role in the pathogenesis of:

    a. appendicitis.
    b. diverticulitis.
    c. ulcerative colitis.
    d. Crohn disease.
    e. cholecystitis.

14. A 14-year-old male has been admitted to the emergency room suffering with acute-onset abdominal pain in the lower right quadrant. Abdominal rebound tenderness is intense, and he has a fever and leukocytosis. This individual most likely is suffering:

    a. acute appendicitis.
    b. diverticulitis.
    c. ulcerative colitis.
    d. cholelithiasis.
    e. cholecystitis.

15. Adult-onset obesity is:

    a. both hyperplastic and hypertrophic.
    b. dispersed over the entire body.
    c. hypertrophic.
    d. unrelated to genotype.
    e. None of the above is correct.

16. Short-term starvation involves:

    a. glycogenolysis.
    b. gluconeogenesis.
    c. proteolysis.
    d. Both a and b are correct.
    e. a, b, and c are correct.

17. The most common manifestation of portal hypertension is:

    a. rectal bleeding.
    b. cirrhosis.
    c. intestinal bleeding.
    d. duodenal bleeding.
    e. vomiting of blood from esophageal bleeding.

18. Hepatic encephalopathy is manifested by:

    a. ascites.
    b. splenomegaly.
    c. dark urine.
    d. oliguria.
    e. cerebral dysfunction.

19. Which would be consistent with a diagnosis of viral hepatitis? (*More than one answer may be correct.*)

    a. elevated AST serum enzymes
    b. decreased serum albumin levels
    c. prolonged coagulation times
    d. increased serum bilirubin levels
    e. decreased ALT serum enzymes

20. Which viral hepatitis is not associated with a chronic state or a carrier state?

    a. hepatitis A
    b. hepatitis B
    c. hepatitis C
    d. serum hepatitis
    e. hepatitis D

21. Which type of jaundice is due to increased destruction of erythrocytes?

    a. obstructive
    b. hemolytic
    c. hepatocellular
    d. Both b and c are correct.

22. Which most often causes biliary cirrhosis?

    a. malnutrition
    b. alcoholism
    c. hepatitis A or C
    d. autoimmunity
    e. biliary obstruction

23. Symptoms of cholelithiasis include all of the following except:

    a. nausea and vomiting.
    b. right upper quadrant tenderness.
    c. jaundice.
    d. decreased serum bilirubin levels.
    e. abdominal distress.

24. In pancreatitis:

    a. the tissue damage likely results from release of pancreatic enzymes.
    b. high cholesterol intake is causative.
    c. diabetes is uncommon in chronic pancreatitis.
    d. bacterial infection is the etiological cause.

25. Predisposing factors in the development of colon cancer include all of the following except:

    a. familial polyposis.
    b. ulcerative colitis.
    c. low-fiber/high-fat diet.
    d. high-fiber diet.
    e. high refined CHO diet.

Case Study

Dr. R. is a 55-year-old male professor whose department chair is an unrelenting harasser. Dr. R.'s family investments have failed and his early planned retirement is no longer possible. Persistent upper abdominal pain for the last two months has convinced him that he needs a diagnostic work-up.

At the physician's office, Dr. R. revealed a history of smoking one pack of cigarettes a day for 25 years. His eating habits are irregular. However, he indicated a pain-antacid-relief pattern. The pain was more intense right after eating. He frequently takes aspirin for headaches and to relieve rheumatoid stiffness while golfing. His family and remaining history were unremarkable except that he had lost 10 pounds during the last six weeks.

Which type of peptic ulcer do you suspect? How could your suspicion be confirmed?

CHAPTER

34

Alterations of Digestive Function in Children

Foundational Objective

a. Describe the structure and function of the gastrointestinal tract and accessory organs of digestion. Review *Workbook* pages 272-273; refer to Figure 32-1.

Memory Check!

- See *Workbook*'s narrative for Foundational Objective **a** in Chapter 33.

Objectives

After studying this chapter, the learner will be able to:

1. **Describe the pathophysiology and treatment associated with cleft lip and palate.** Study page 992; refer to Figure 34-1.

Cleft lip is caused by incomplete fusion of the nasomedial or intermaxillary process during the second month of fetal development and occurs in approximately 1 in 1000 births. The defect in cleft lip usually is beneath one or both nostrils and may involve the external nose, nasal cartilages, nasal septum, and alveolar processes. It also may be associated with a flattening and broadening of the facial features probably due to the absence of constraining structures which are omitted by the cleft.

Cleft palate occurs in approximately 1 in 1250 births and is frequently associated with cleft lip but can occur alone. The defect may affect only the uvula and soft palate but may extend forward toward the nostrils through the hard palate. If it extends through the hard palate, open communication between the structures of the nasopharynx and the oral cavity leads to sinusitis and otitis media.

In most cases, cleft lip and cleft palate are caused by genetic and nongenetic factors; a multifactorial inheritance exists. A major difficulty seen with cleft lip or palate is poor feeding. The infant with isolated cleft lip but an intact palate may feed without great difficulty. On the other hand, cleft palate may significantly interfere with feeding. Bottle feeding may require a large, soft nipple with an oversized opening. Breast feeding may be impossible for some cleft palate infants without a prosthesis for the roof of the mouth.

Treatment is surgical correction that is usually accomplished in stages. Supportive therapy may include prosthodontics and orthodontics and speech therapy.

2. **Describe the structural defects of esophageal atresia and tracheoesophageal fistula.** Study pages 992-993; refer to Figure 34-2.

Congenital malformations of the esophagus occur in approximately 1 in 3000 to 4500 births. **Esophageal atresia** is a condition wherein the esophagus ends in a blind pouch and may be accompanied by a connection between the esophagus and the trachea called a **tracheoesophageal fistula** (TEF). These conditions develop from aberrant differentiation of the trachea at four to six weeks of embryonic development. The blind esophageal pouch in atresia fills rapidly with secretions or food and overflows; regurgitated food and fluid may enter the lungs. Thirty percent of children with this anomaly have other associated congenital defects, particularly cardiovascular defects.

Diagnosis may not be made until recurrent aspiration and pneumonias become problematic. Diagnosis is confirmed by the inability to pass a catheter into the stomach as the x-ray shows the catheter coiled at the level of the defect. Treatment is surgical correction.

3. Describe the structural defect and pathophysiology associated with pyloric stenosis.
Study pages 993-995.

Pyloric stenosis is an obstruction of the pylorus because of hypertrophy of the pyloric sphincter. Obstruction becomes evident between one to two weeks and three to four months of age. Boys are affected five times more frequently than girls, and whites are more frequently affected than Orientals or blacks. Pyloric stenosis is seen more frequently in term than in premature infants. Increased gastrin secretion in the mother tends to increase the probability of pyloric stenosis and may be linked to maternal stress. Hereditary factors also may be involved.

Generally, stenosis is manifested in a previously healthy infant who begins to have marked forceful vomiting at three to four weeks of age that does not resolve. Weight loss and fluid and electrolyte imbalances follow and may end in death if intervention is not provided. A small, movable mass at the site of the hypertrophic pylorus may be palpable in the left upper quadrant of the abdomen.

Stenosis is usually suspected on clinical manifestations and confirmed by ultrasonography or an upper gastrointestinal series that demonstrates the lesion. Treatment is surgical release of the hypertrophic fibers or pyloromyotomy after stabilization of the infant's fluid and electrolyte balance.

4. Describe congenital aganglionic megacolon, or Hirschprung disease.
Study pages 996-997; refer to Figure 34-3.

Congenital aganglionic megacolon, or **Hirschprung disease**, is a condition generally associated with failure of the parasympathetic nervous system to produce intramural ganglion cells in the enteric nerve plexuses. This failed innervation causes a section of the colon to be immotile and creates a functional intestinal obstruction in the affected area. This section becomes distended with feces, thus the name "megacolon." Eighty percent of these disorders are limited to the rectal end of the sigmoid colon. Hirschprung disease accounts for one-third of all intestinal obstructions in infants and occurs in 1 in 5000 births, with a greater incidence in males.

Clinical manifestations are mild to severe chronic constipation, although diarrhea may be the first sign because only liquid may pass the aganglionic section. Severe edema of the colon begins to obstruct blood and lymphatic flow, causing **enterocolitis** and tissue destruction. Bacteria can infiltrate the bowel wall from the lumen and may case gram-negative sepsis. Severe fluid and electrolyte imbalance caused by diarrhea may become life-threatening.

Diagnosis is confirmed by rectal biopsy that demonstrates the aganglionic bowel. Definitive treatment consists of resection of the aganglionic segment and constant attention to bowel hygiene thereafter.

5. Describe intussusception.
Study page 998; refer to Figure 34-5.

Intussusception is the telescoping or invagination of one portion of the intestine into another that causes an intestinal obstruction. The most commonly affected area is the ileum, which invaginates into the cecum through the ileocecal valve. Collapse is in the direction of peristaltic flow. Eighty to 90 percent of intestinal obstructions in infants and children are caused by intussusception, and boys are more commonly affected. Intussusception generally occurs between 3 and 35 months of age; 75 percent occur before one year of age.

The pathophysiology of intussusception is like that of megacolon because the telescoping bowel obstructs blood and lymphatic flow, which causes rapid edema and tissue necrosis. Gangrene may follow.

The obstruction is usually accompanied by passage of dark and gelatinous or "currant jelly" stools. Diagnosis is made on clinical manifestations and confirmed by ultrasonography. Reduction of the intussusception must be done immediately and is frequently performed using hydrostatic pressure of the contrast media used for x-ray or an enema to push the invaginated bowel segment from its intussusception. This is successful 60 to 70 percent of the time, although some children require surgery to correct the intussusception or related complications. This condition is fatal if untreated.

6. **Describe the pathophysiology and potential complications related to gastroesophageal reflux.**
   Study pages 998-999.

Gastroesophageal reflux (GER) is the return of gastric contents into the esophagus because of poor function of the lower esophageal sphincter. GER is more common in premature than in term newborn infants and usually resolves by 6 to 12 months of age without significant effect on the infant. GER has been implicated as a possible factor in sudden infant death syndrome (SIDS). The cause of GER is unknown, although delayed maturation of the sphincter or impaired hormonal response mechanisms are suspected. Other factors include location of the gastroesophageal junction and the angle of the junction and mucosal gathering.

Clinical manifestations include forceful vomiting with a 75 percent occurrence within the first week of life, aspiration pneumonia in one-third of those affected, and poor weight gain. **Esophagitis** may result from exposure of the esophagus to acidic gastric contents that may cause either strictures or anemia from prolonged occult blood loss.

Diagnosis may be made from clinical manifestations or confirmed by barium swallow or esophageal pH probe studies that demonstrate an abrupt drop in esophageal pH during the reflux episodes. Mild GER resolves without treatment, although some children require elevated prone positioning after feedings to help reduce reflux. Pharmacologic therapies include medication to increase lower gastrointestinal motility and gastric emptying time in an effort to decrease the opportunity for reflux; medications that decrease gastric acidity can be used. Surgical correction or fundoplication is rarely required but may be performed if medical management is ineffective.

7. **Describe the gastrointestinal and digestive abnormalities associated with cystic fibrosis.**
   Study page 999; refer to Table 34-1.

Cystic fibrosis (CF) is a multisystem disease that is primarily manifested in the pancreas. The classic triad of pathophysiology of cystic fibrosis is pancreatic enzyme deficiency leading to maldigestion, overproduction of mucus in the respiratory tract leading to chronic obstructive pulmonary disease, and elevated levels of sodium and chloride in sweat. Very viscous exocrine secretions tend to obstruct glandular ducts. Approximately 85 percent of children with CF have pancreatic insufficiency. The lack of pancreatic enzymes results in maldigestion of proteins, carbohydrates, and fats, leading to chronic malnutrition. Pancreatic ducts also may be blocked with viscous secretions that eventually may damage pancreatic cells and lead to diabetes mellitus. Maldigestion of fats causes steatorrhea or fatty stools. Other complications include anemia, biliary cirrhosis, vitamin K deficiency, and rectal prolapse because of the passage of large, bulky stools.

Pancreatic enzyme function may be estimated by 72-hour fecal fat measurement; fecal content of trypsin and chymotrypsin also may be measured. Pancreatic enzyme replacement may be administered with meals, and a high-calorie/high-protein diet is usually prescribed.

8. **Describe gluten-sensitive enteropathy.**
   Study pages 999-1002; refer to Figure 34-6.

Gluten-sensitive enteropathy, formerly called celiac sprue or celiac disease, is the loss of mature villous epithelium caused by ingestion of gluten, the protein component of cereal grains. The gluten is toxic to the intestinal epithelial cells. Pathogenesis appears to involve dietary, genetic, and immunologic factors. The disease occurs mostly in whites.

Diarrhea is an early sign in most infants. The stools are pale, bulky, greasy, and foul-smelling; they may contain oil droplets. Vomiting and abdominal pain are prominent in infants but unusual in older children. Anorexia is prevalent and growth is usually diminished. Consequences of malabsorption such as rickets, tetany, frank bleeding, or anemia may be obvious. The child may bleed easily.

An intestinal biopsy is required to detect the classic mucosal changes caused by gluten-sensitive enteropathy. Serum gluten antibodies also may be measured.

Treatment requires immediate and permanent institution of a diet free of wheat, rye, barley, oats, and malt. Lactose (milk sugar) is also excluded since lactose intolerance is presumed. Infants are given vitamin D, iron, and folic acid supplements to treat deficiencies.

9. Compare kwashiorkor and marasmus.
Study page 1002.

Kwashiorkor and **marasmus** are common types of malnutrition in children. They are collectively known as **protein energy malnutrition** (PEM). Both are states of long-term starvation. Kwashiorkor is a severe protein deficiency, and marasmus is a severe deficiency of all nutrients. Both are problems in impoverished populations.

In kwashiorkor, protein synthesis is reduced in all tissues. Physical and mental growth are stunted. The lack of sufficient plasma proteins results in generalized edema. The liver swells with stored fat because no hepatic proteins are synthesized to form and release lipoproteins. Kwashiorkor also causes malabsorption, reduced bone density, and impaired renal function.

In marasmus, metabolic processes including liver function are preserved, but growth is severely retarded. Caloric intake is too low to support protein synthesis for growth or the storage of fat. Muscle and fat wasting occur. Anemia is common and may be severe. The presence of subcutaneous fat, hepatomegaly, and fatty liver distinguishes kwashiorkor from marasmus.

Practice Examination

True/False

1. ____ Pyloric stenosis is caused by the prolapse of gastric tissue into the pylorus and results in edema and obstruction.

2. ____ Tracheoesophageal fistula is often associated with esophageal atresia.

3. ____ Poor weight gain associated with gastroesophageal reflux may be ignored because it is a self-limiting disorder.

4. ____ Intussusception involves a blind pouch in the esophagus.

5. ____ "Currant jelly" stools are a common finding in cystic fibrosis.

6. ____ Increased gastrin secretion in pregnant women may contribute to pyloric stenosis in their infants.

7. ____ Diabetes mellitus may be a complication of cystic fibrosis.

8. ____ The pharmacologic approach to gastroesophageal reflux includes pancreatic enzyme replacement.

9. ____ Congenital aganglionic megacolon is the result of faulty innervation of the colon.

10. ____ The pharmacologic approach to cystic fibrosis includes the administration of medications that increase lower gastrointestinal motility in an effort to aid passage of large, bulky stools.

11. ____ Rectal manometry is useful in the diagnosis of aganglionic megacolon.

Fill-in-the-Blank

12. __________ has been implicated as a possible factor in sudden infant death syndrome.

13. Congenital aganglionic megacolon is diagnosed by rectal manometry and rectal __________.

14. A pH probe will demonstrate a __________ in esophageal pH during a period of reflux.

15. Cleft palate is frequently complicated by communication between the __________ and __________ cavities.

16. __________ may be a complication of cystic fibrosis secondary to passing large stools.

Match the description with the alteration.

17. ____ involves the rectal segment of the sigmoid colon
18. ____ acute onset of abdominal pain and distention
19. ____ cardiovascular defects accompany
20. ____ may initially present with diarrhea
21. ____ food regurgitation
22. ____ may contribute to aspiration pneumonia
23. ____ incompetent lower esophageal sphincter
24. ____ "currant jelly" stools
25. ____ enema may be treatment

a. congenital aganglionic megacolon
b. tracheoesophageal fistula
c. intussusception
d. gastroesophageal reflux
e. esophageal atresia

Case Study

Baby B. is a term infant male born vaginally to a 21-year-old white woman; he is her first child. Three weeks after birth, he began to vomit without apparent reason. At the pediatrician's office, it was determined that the infant had fed well and gained weight until now. The vomiting occurs immediately after eating and the vomitus consists of the bulk of the feeding.

What is Baby B.'s likely problem, and what can be done?

CHAPTER 35

Structure and Function of the Musculoskeletal System

Objectives

After review of this chapter, the learner will be able to:

1. **Identify the structural elements and function of bone.**
   Review pages 1013-1015; refer to Table 35-1.

2. **Describe the features of compact and spongy bone; classify bones.**
   Review pages 1015-1016; refer to Figures 35-1 and 35-3.

3. **Describe the process of bone remodeling and healing.**
   Review pages 1017-1018; refer to Figure 35-4.

4. **Structurally and functionally, classify joints.**
   Review pages 1018-1023; refer to Figures 35-5 through 35-8.

5. **Describe the arrangements of muscle fiber in a skeletal muscle; explain the structure and function of a motor unit.**
   Review pages 1023-1029; refer to Figures 35-9 through 35-12 and Tables 35-3 and 35-4.

6. **Describe skeletal muscle contraction at the molecular level.**
   Review pages 1029-1030; refer to Figure 35-13.

7. **Identify the energy sources for muscular contraction.**
   Review pages 1030-1031; refer to Table 35-5.

8. **Indicate the types of skeletal muscle contractions and the interaction between groups of muscles.**
   Review pages 1031-1032.

9. **Describe the changes in the musculoskeletal system that accompany normal aging.**
   Review page 1032.

Practice Examination

1. The skeletal system (*more than one answer may be correct*):

   a. supports tissues.
   b. binds organs together.
   c. protects CNS structures.
   d. participates in blood cell formation.
   e. lines body cavities.

2. Sialoprotein:

   a. promotes resorption.
   b. binds calcium.
   c. stabilizes the basement membrane of bones.
   d. promotes calcification.

Match the microscopic feature of bone with its description.

3. ____ Volkmann's canals	a. small canals that connect bone cells
4. ____ trabeculae	b. concentric rings
5. ____ lamellae	c. cavities where bone cells are housed
	d. contains blood vessels
	e. irregular meshwork

6. The diaphysis is the:

   a. rounded end of long bones.
   b. shaft of long bones.
   c. lattice framework of spongy bones.
   d. surface of a synovial cavity.

7. A function of the epiphyseal plate that is not a function of the articular cartilage is to:

   a. enable articulation of bones.
   b. enable bone to increase in length.
   c. repair damaged bone tissue.
   d. provide sensory nerves to bone.

8. The remodeling of bone is done by basic multicellular units that consist of bone precursor cells. Precursor cells:

   a. differentiate into osteoclasts and osteoblasts.
   b. are located on free surfaces of bone and along vascular channels.
   c. Neither a nor b is correct.
   d. Both a and b are correct.

9. Identify the sequence of bone healing in fractures and surgical injuries.

1. procallus formation	a. 2, 1, 3, 4, 5
2. callus formation	b. 3, 1, 2, 4, 5
3. hematoma formation	c. 3, 2, 1, 4, 5
4. callus replacement with lamellar or trabecular bone	d. 1, 2, 3, 4, 5
5. periosteum and endosteum remodeling	e. 1, 2, 3, 5, 4

10. Joints are classified functionally and structurally. Which is a proper function and structural relationship?

a. amphiarthrosis/fibrous
b. diarthrosis/synovial
c. synarthrosis/synchondrosis
d. diarthrosis/fibrous
e. synarthrosis/cartilaginous

11. In older individuals, the bone remodeling cycle:

a. is faster because osteoclastic activity is enhanced.
b. is enhanced because mineralization increases.
c. has more precursor cells.
d. has fewer bone cells because the bone marrow becomes infiltrated with fat.
e. Both a and b are correct.

12. Which is not included in a motor unit?

a. muscle fibers
b. motor nerve axons
c. anterior horn cell
d. upper motor neuron

13. The perimysium is to a fasciculus as the:

a. periosteum is to a bone.
b. muscle is to epimysium.
c. myofibril is to a muscle fiber.
d. epimysium is to the endomysium.
e. muscle cell is to the endomysium.

Match the microscopic feature of muscle fibers with its description.

14. ____ sarcomere
15. ____ sarcolemma
16. ____ sarcoplasmic reticulum

a. membrane covering the muscle cell
b. flattened, tubelike network
c. unit of contraction
d. calcium transport
e. tubules that run perpendicular to muscle myofibrils

17. Which is not a characteristic of type I muscle fibers?

    a. sparse capillary supply
    b. slow contraction speed
    c. high resistance to fatigue
    d. profuse capillary supply
    e. oxidative metabolism

18. Which protein is found in the thick myofilaments?

    a. actin
    b. myosin
    c. troponin
    d. tropomyosin
    e. a, c, and d are correct.

19. An important function of the transverse tubules is to:

    a. provide organic nutrients to muscle fibers.
    b. initiate fiber contraction.
    c. enable regeneration of muscle fibers.
    d. allow for intracellular calcium uptake.

20. The ion necessary for coupling is:

    a. sodium.
    b. calcium.
    c. potassium.
    d. magnesium.
    e. phosphate.

21. Aerobic respiration:

    a. permits the body brief periods during which it does not require oxygen.
    b. causes an increase in the amount of lactic acid.
    c. yields more molecules of ATP than anaerobic respiration.
    d. uses more glycogen to produce ATP than anaerobic respiration.
    e. leads to oxygen debt.

22. Repayment of oxygen debt:

    a. converts lactic acid to glycogen.
    b. replenishes ATP stores.
    c. replenishes phosphocreatine stores.
    d. Both b and c are correct.
    e. a, b, and c are correct.

23. The strength of muscle contraction depends on the:

    a. extent of the load.
    b. initial length of muscle fibers.
    c. recruitment of additional motor units.
    d. nerve innervation ratios.
    e. All of the above are correct.

24. Attempting to push an object too heavy to move is an example of a/an ______ contraction.

   a. isotonic
   b. concentric
   c. flaccid
   d. tetanic
   e. isometric

25. Which does not happen with muscle as individuals grow older?

   a. Type II fibers may decrease.
   b. Mitochondrial volume decreases.
   c. The amount of RNA increases to compensate for decreased size of motor units.
   d. All of the above occur with advancing age.

CHAPTER 36

Alterations of Musculoskeletal Function

Foundational Objectives

a. Describe the processes that maintain bone integrity. Review pages 1017-1018; refer to Figure 35-4.

> **Memory Check!**
>
> - In the first phase of the remodeling cycle, a stimulus such as hormone, drug, vitamin, or physical stressor activates the osteoclasts. In phase two, the osteoclasts resorb bone and leave in its place an elongated cavity termed a resorption cavity. The resorption cavity in compact bone follows the longitudinal axis of the haversian system; in spongy bone the resorption cavity parallels the surface of the trabeculae. In phase three, new bone or secondary bone is laid down by osteoblasts lining the walls of the resorption cavity. In compact bone, successive layers are laid down until the resorption cavity is reduced to a narrow haversian canal around a blood vessel. This process destroys old haversian systems and forms new haversian systems. New trabeculae are formed in spongy bone.
> - The remodeling process is capable of repairing microscopic bone injuries, but gross injuries such as fractures and surgical wounds heal by a different process. In bone wound healing, the stages are as follows:
>
>   1. Hematoma formation
>   2. Procallus formation
>   3. Callus formation
>   4. Osteoblasts continue to replace the callus with either lamellar bone or trabecular bone.
>   5. The periosteal and endosteal surfaces are remodeled to the size and shape of the bone before injury.

b. Describe the types of joints. Review pages 1018-1023; refer to Figures 35-5 through 35-8.

> **Memory Check!**
>
> - Joints are classified by the degree of movement they permit or by the connecting tissues that hold them together. Based on movement, a joint is classified as (1) a synarthrosis or an immovable joint, (2) an amphiarthrosis or a slightly movable joint, or (3) a diarthrosis or a freely movable joint. On the basis of connective structures, joints are classified as fibrous, cartilaginous, or synovial.
>
> (*Continued*)

Memory Check! (cont'd)

- A joint united directly to bone by fibrous connective tissues is called a fibrous joint. Generally, fibrous joints are synarthroses, or immovable, but many fibrous joints allow some movement. The degree of movement depends on the distance between the bones and the flexibility of the fibrous connective tissue.
- There are two types of cartilaginous joints or amphiarthroses. A symphysis is a cartilaginous joint in which bones are united by a pad or disk of fibrocartilage. The articulating surfaces are usually covered by a thin layer of hyaline cartilage and a thick pad of fibrocartilage which acts as a shock absorber and stabilizer. Examples of symphyses are the symphysis pubis and the intervertebral discs. A synchondrosis is a joint in which hyaline cartilage connects the two bones. The joints between the ribs and the sternum are synchondroses. Slight movement at the synchondroses between the ribs and the sternum allows the chest to move outward and upward during breathing.
- Synovial joints or diarthroses are the most movable and complex joints in the body. A synovial joint consists of a fibrous joint capsule or articular capsule, a synovial membrane, a joint cavity or synovial cavity, synovial fluid, and an articular cartilage. The joint capsule consists of parallel, interlacing bundles of dense, white fibrous tissue. It has a rich supply of nerves, blood vessels, and lymphatic vessels. The nerves are sensitive to the rate and direction of motion, compression, tension, vibration, and pain.
- The synovial membrane is the smooth, delicate inner lining of the joint capsule. It lines the nonarticular portion of the synovial joint and any ligaments or tendons that traverse the joint cavity. The synovial membrane is capable of rapid repair and regeneration.
- The joint cavity or synovial cavity is an enclosed, fluid-filled space between the articulating surfaces of the two bones that enables the two bones to move "against" one another. Synovial fluid within the cavity lubricates the joint surfaces, nourishes the pad of the articular cartilage, and contains free-floating synovial cells and various leukocytes that phagocytose joint debris and microorganisms.
- Articular cartilage is a layer of hyaline cartilage that covers the end of each bone. The function of articular cartilage is to reduce friction and to distribute the weight-bearing forces.

c. Define terms associated with muscle fibers. Review pages 1023-1029; refer to Figures 35-9 through 35-12 and Table 35-3.

Memory Check!

- Each anterior horn cell, its axon, and the innervated muscle fibers is called a motor unit. The motor unit behaves as a single entity and contracts as a whole when it receives an adequate electrical impulse. A muscle fiber is a single muscle cell. This long cell is cylindrical in structure and surrounded by a membrane capable of excitation and impulse propagation. The muscle fiber contains bundles of myofibrils in a parallel arrangement along the longitudinal axis of the muscle. The myofibrils contain sarcomeres that are the actual contracting units. The sarcomeres consist of actin and myosin, which are the contractile proteins.
- Besides the myofibrils, the major components of the muscle fiber include the muscle membrane, sarcotubular system, sarcoplasm, and mitochondria. The muscle membrane is a two-part membrane. It includes the sarcolemma, which contains the plasma membrane of the muscle cell, and the cell's basement membrane. At the motor nerve endplate, where the nerve impulse is transmitted, the sarcolemma forms the highly convoluted synaptic cleft. The protein systems of the sarcolemma transport nutrients and synthesize proteins. They also provide the sodium-potassium pump and include the cell's cholinergic receptor. The basement membrane serves as the cell's microskeleton and maintains the shape of the muscle cell.

(Continued)

Memory Check! (cont'd)

- The sarcoplasm is the cytoplasm of the muscle cell and contains numerous enzymes and proteins that are responsible for the cell's energy production, protein synthesis, and oxygen storage. Unique to the muscle is the sarcotubular system, which includes the transverse tubules and the sarcoplasmic reticulum. The sarcoplasmic reticulum is involved in calcium transport that initiates muscle contraction at the sarcomere. The sarcoplasmic reticulum is composed of tubules that run parallel to the myofibrils and are termed sarcotubules. The transverse tubules are closely associated with the sarcotubules and run across the sarcoplasm and communicate with the extracellular space. Both tubules allow for intracellular calcium uptake, regulation, release during muscle contraction, and storage of calcium during muscle relaxation.

d. Identify the major events of muscle contraction and relaxation. Review pages 1029-1030; refer to Figure 35-13.

Memory Check!

Major Events of Muscle Contraction and Relaxation

Excitation and Contraction

A nerve impulse reaches the end of a motor neuron and releases acetylcholine

↓

Acetylcholine diffuses across the neuromuscular junction and binds to acetylcholine receptors on the muscle fiber

↓

Stimulation of acetylcholine receptors initiates an impulse that travels along the sarcolemma, through the transverse tubules, and to the sarcoplasmic reticulum

↓

Calcium is released from the sarcoplasmic reticulum into the sarcoplasm; calcium binds to troponin molecules on the thin myofilaments

↓

Tropomyosin molecules shift to expose actin's active engagement sites

↓

Energized myosin cross-bridges of the thick myofilaments bind to actin and use their ATP energy to pull the thin myofilaments toward the center of each sarcomere

↓

As the thin myofilaments slide past the thick myofilaments, the entire muscle fiber shortens

Relaxation

After the impulse passes, the sarcoplasmic reticulum begins actively pumping calcium back into the sarcoplasm

↓

As calcium leaves the troponin molecules of the thin myofilaments, tropomyosin returns to its position and blocks actin's active engagement sites

↓

Myosin cross-bridges cannot bind to actin and can no longer sustain the contraction

↓

The thick and thin myofilaments are no longer connected, so the muscle fiber returns to its longer, resting length

Objectives

After studying this chapter, the learner will be able to:

1. **Compare the types of fractures; describe the causes, manifestations, and treatment of fractures.**
   Study pages 1037-1040; refer to Figure 36-1 and Table 36-1.

Fractures are classified as complete or incomplete and open or closed. In a **complete** fracture, the bone is broken all the way through; in an **incomplete** fracture, the bone is damaged but remains in one piece. Complete or incomplete fractures also are considered **open** if the skin is broken or **closed** if it is not. A fracture wherein the bone breaks into two or more fragments is termed a **comminuted** fracture. Fractures also are classified according to the direction of the fracture line.

The signs and symptoms of a fracture include unnatural alignment, swelling, muscle spasm, tenderness, pain, and impaired sensation. The immediate pain of a fracture is severe and usually due to the traumatic injury. Subsequent pain often is produced by muscle spasm. Numbness is caused by the pinching of a nerve by the trauma or by bone fragments. Pathologic fractures are not usually associated with trauma or trauma-related pain. Stress fractures are painful because of accelerated remodeling and are usually relieved by rest. Range of motion in the joint is limited, and movement may evoke audible clicking sounds or crepitus.

Fracture treatment involves realigning the bone fragments to their normal or anatomic position and holding the fragments in place so that bone union can occur. Several methods are available to reduce or align a fracture, including closed manipulation, traction, and open surgical reduction. Splints and plaster casts are used to immobilize and hold a reduction in place. Improper reduction or immobilization of a fractured bone may result in nonunion, delayed union, or malunion.

(See box on page 304 of *Workbook.*)

2. **Define terms associated with skeletal system stress.**
   Study pages 1040-1045; refer to Figures 36-4 and 36-5 and Table 36-2.

Dislocation is the temporary displacement of two bones in which the two bone surfaces lose contact entirely. If the contact between the surfaces is only partially lost, the injury is called **subluxation**. Dislocations and subluxations are often accompanied by fracture. As the bone separates from the joint, it may bruise or tear adjacent nerves, blood vessels, ligaments, supporting structures, and soft tissue.

A tear in a tendon is a **strain**. Major trauma or excessive stress can tear a tendon at any site in the body. The tendons of the hands, feet, knee, upper arm, thigh, ankle, and heel are frequently injured sites. Ligament tears are known as **sprains**. Ligament tears and ruptures can occur at any joint but are most common in the wrist, ankle, elbow, and knee joints. A complete separation of a tendon or ligament from its attachment is an **avulsion**. An avulsion is the result of abnormal stress on the ligament or tendon and is commonly seen in young athletes, especially sprinters, hurdlers, and runners.

Trauma can also cause painful inflammation of tendons, or **tendinitis**, and bursae, or **bursitis**. Besides trauma, causes of tendinitis include crystal deposits, postural misalignment, and hypermobility in a joint. **Epicondylitis** is inflammation of a tendon where it attaches to a bone. Examples of epicondylitis include tennis elbow, which is an inflammation of the lateral epicondyle of the humerus, and medial epicondylitis, which is referred to as golfer's elbow. Acute **bursitis** occurs primarily in the middle years and is caused by repeated trauma. Septic bursitis is caused by wound infection or bacterial infection of the skin overlying the bursae. The shoulder is the most common site of bursitis.

Muscle strain is often the result of sudden, forced motion causing the muscle to become stretched beyond its normal capacity. Muscles are injured more often than tendons in young people; the opposite is true in older populations. Regardless of the cause of trauma, muscle cells usually are able to regenerate, although regeneration may take up to six weeks.

Myositis ossificans is thought to be caused by scar tissue calcification and subsequent ossification. An example is seen in football players after injury to thigh muscles.

Types of Fractures

Type	Characteristic	Cause
	Common Complete Fractures	
Open fracture	Communicating wound between bone and skin	Moderate to severe energy that exceeds tissue tolerance
Oblique fracture	Fracture line at 45° angle to long axis of bone	Angulation and compressive energy
Spiral fracture	Fracture line encircling bone	Twisting energy with distal part unable to move
Transverse fracture	Fracture line perpendicular to long axis of bone	Energy directly toward bone
Impacted fracture	Fracture fragments are pushed into each other	Compressive energy directly to distal fragment
Pathologic fracture	Fracture occurs at any point in the bone	Minor energy to already weakened bone
	Common Incomplete Fractures	
Greenstick fracture	Break on one cortex of bone with spongy bone splintering	Minor direct or indirect energy in children or elderly
Stress fracture	Microfracture	Bone is subjected to repeated stress beyond its strength, muscles are stronger than bone

Myoglobinuria can be a life-threatening complication of severe muscle trauma manifested by excess myoglobin, an intracellular muscle protein, in the urine. Muscle damage releases the myoglobin. The most severe form is often called crush syndrome. Less severe and more localized forms are called compartment syndromes, which can lead to Volkmann ischemic contracture in the forearm or leg. Crush syndrome first gained notoriety in injuries seen following the London air raids in World War II. More recently, it has been reported in individuals found unresponsive because of drug overdoses and those who are immobile for long periods of time. Myoglobinuria can also be seen following viral infections, administration of certain anesthetic agents, strychnine poisoning, tetanus, excessive muscular activity, heatstroke, electrolyte disturbances, fractures, status epilepticus, electroconvulsive therapy, and high-voltage electrical shock.

3. **Differentiate between osteoporosis, osteomalacia, Paget disease, and osteomyelitis.**
   Study pages 1045-1049; refer to Figure 36-6.

   (See box on page 305 of *Workbook*.)

4. **Compare osteoarthritis to rheumatoid arthritis; characterize other inflammatory joint diseases.**
   Study pages 1049-1060; refer to Figures 36-7 through 36-12.

Ankylosing spondylitis is a chronic, inflammatory joint disease characterized by stiffening and fusion or ankylosis of the spine and sacroiliac joints. Like rheumatoid arthritis, ankylosing spondylitis is a systemic, immune inflammatory disease. The disease is strongly associated with the presence of histocompatibility antigen HLA-B27 on the chromosomes of affected individuals; this

Common Disorders of Bone

Disorder	Causes	Pathophysiology	Manifestations
Osteoporosis	Decreased levels of estrogen and testosterone, reduced physical activity, excessive doses of heparin, insufficient calcium, excess cortisol	Reduced bone mass or density, imbalance in bone resorption and formation	Pain and bone deformity, fracture, increased radiolucency
Osteomalacia (adults) Rickets (children)	Deficiency of vitamin D lowers absorption of calcium from intestines	Inadequate and delayed mineralization, osteoid tissue is not mineralized	Pain, bone fractures, vertebral collapse, radiolucent bands perpendicular to bone surface pseudofracture
Paget disease	Unknown	Excessive resorption of spongy bone followed by accelerated formation of softened bone	Thickening of bones, radiographic findings of irregular bone trabeculae with thickened and disorganized patterns
Osteomyelitis	Most often a staphylococcal infection, contaminated open wound	Acute inflammation of marrow and bone, necrosis	Acute and chronic inflammation, fever, pain, lymphadenopathy, necrotic bone by radionuclide bone scanning

suggests a genetic predisposition to the disease. In ankylosing spondylitis, the primary pathologic site is at the point where ligaments, tendons, and the joint capsule are inserted into bone rather than in the synovial membrane as in rheumatoid arthritis. The end result of ankylosing spondylitis is fibrosis, ossification, and fusion of the joint.

Ankylosing spondylitis begins with inflammation of fibrocartilage in cartilaginous joints, particularly in the vertebrae. As inflammatory cells infiltrate and erode fibrocartilage in joint structures, repair begins to occur. Repair begins with the proliferation of fibroblasts. The collagen synthesized by fibroblasts becomes organized into fibrous scar tissue. Eventually, the scar tissue calcifies and ossifies. With time, all the cartilaginous structures of the joint are replaced by ossified scar tissue and the joints fuse or lose flexibility.

The most common symptoms of early ankylosing spondylitis are low back pain and stiffness. The pain initially is insidious but progressively becomes persistent. Forward flexion, rotation, and lateral flexion of the spine are restricted and painful. As the disease progresses, the individual becomes increasingly stooped. The thoracic spine becomes rounded, the head and neck are held forward on the shoulders, and the hips are flexed. Along with low back pain, many individuals may have peripheral joint involvement, uveitis or inflammation of eye structures, fibrotic changes in the lungs, cardiomegaly, aortic incompetence, amyloidosis, and Achilles tendinitis.

Treatment of individuals with ankylosing spondylitis consists of physical therapy to maintain skeletal mobility and prevent the natural progression of contractures. Antiinflammatory and analgesic medications are prescribed to suppress some of the pain and stiffness and to facilitate exercise. Surgical procedures and radiotherapy are sometimes used to provide relief for individuals with end-stage disease or intolerable deformity.

Gout is a metabolic disorder that disrupts the body's control of uric acid production or excretion. High levels of uric acid accumulate in the blood and in other body fluids, including synovial fluid. When the uric acid reaches a certain concentration in

Noninflammatory and Inflammatory Joint Disease

Feature	Osteoarthritis	Rheumatoid arthritis
Pathologic feature	Noninflammatory, loss of proteoglycans from articular cartilage in synovial joints, bone sclerosis, bone spurs	Inflammatory, damage or destruction of synovial membrane extends to articular cartilage joint capsule and surround ing ligaments and tendons, pannus
Onset age	> 40, increases with age, equal sex distinction	Middle age, prevalence in females
Risk factors	Primary: autosomal recessive Secondary: joint stress, congenital abnormalities, joint instability, drugs	Genetics, environmental
Joints affected	Peripheral and central, weight bearing	Phalangeal, wrists, knee
Cause	Proteoglycan destruction	Microbial invasion, autoimmunity
Manifestations	Pain, stiffness, enlargement, tenderness, limited motion, muscle wasting, dislocation, deformity	Same as OA with systemic involvement, subcutaneous nodules, deviation of joints, rheumatoid factor and circulating immune complexes

fluids, it crystallizes. The crystals are deposited in connective tissues throughout the body.

When crystallization occurs in synovial fluid, painful inflammation of the joint develops. This condition is known as **gouty arthritis**. With time, crystal deposition in subcutaneous tissues causes the formation of small, white nodules or **tophi** and their inflammatory sequelae. Crystal aggregates deposited in the kidneys can form urate renal stones and lead to renal failure. In classic gouty arthritis, inflammation of the joint is caused by the formation of monosodium urate crystals. In **pseudogout**, the crystals are of calcium pyrophosphate-dihydrate. Either crystal causes the onset of acute inflammatory response.

Approximately 95 percent of affected individuals, almost always men, have **primary gout** wherein the hyperuricemia is due to an overproduction of uric acid. The defect in primary gout is unknown but is likely an inherited enzyme defect. In **secondary gout**, the hyperuricemia is the result of an acquired chronic disease or a drug that interferes with balance between production and excretion of uric acid. Hyperuricemia from overproduction of uric acid can be due to increased metabolic processes such as leukemia, increased cellular breakdown like hemolytic anemia, neoplastic processes, and genetic metabolic disorders in which hyperuricemia is just one of many clinical manifestations. Diuretics are thought to cause secondary gout as they decrease the renal tubular excretion of urate. Chronic renal disease, hypertension, and starvation also decrease uric acid excretion.

The pathophysiology of gout is closely linked to purine metabolism, cellular metabolism of purines, and kidney function. Uric acid is a breakdown product of purine nucleotides. Some individuals with gout have an accelerated rate of purine synthesis and other individuals break down purine nucleotides at an accelerated rate. Both conditions result in an overproduction of uric acid. Kidney function is involved in the pathophysiology of gout because most uric acid is eliminated from the body through the kidneys. Urate undergoes both reabsorption and excretion within the renal tubules. Sluggish urate excretion by the kidney may be caused by decreased glomerular filtration of urate or an acceleration in urate reabsorption.

The presence of urate crystals anywhere triggers the acute inflammatory response as the neutrophils are attracted to phagocytose the crystals. Tissue damage occurs when the phagocytizing neutrophils release the contents of their digestive lysosomes. Lysosomal contents are released from neutrophils as they die following their life span of about two days, by leakage after injury by biochemical reactions with ingested urate crystals or through rupture of neutrophils during attempts to ingest exceptionally large urate crystals.

Attacks of gouty arthritis occur abruptly, usually in a peripheral joint. The primary symptom is severe pain. Approximately 50 percent of the initial attacks occur in the metatarsophalangeal joint of the great toe. Other involved joints are the heel, ankle, instep of the foot, knee, wrist, or elbow.

Tophaceous gout, the chronic stage of disease, can begin as early as three years or as late as 40 years after the initial attack of gouty arthritis. Progressive inability to excrete uric acid expands the urate pool until tophi appear in cartilage, synovial membranes, tendons, and soft tissue. The helix of the ear is the most common site of tophi, which are the diagnostic lesions of chronic gout. Each tophus consists of a deposit of urate crystals surrounded by a granuloma made of mononuclear phagocytes that have developed into epithelial giant cells. Tophaceous deposits appear in other areas and produce irregular swellings of the fingers, hands, knees, and feet. Though the tophi themselves are painless, they often cause progressive stiffness and persistent aching of the affected joint.

Acute gouty arthritis is treated with antiinflammatory drugs. The individual should have a low purine diet and high fluid intake to increase urinary output. Antihyperuricemic drugs can be given to reduce serum urate concentrations.

5. Describe examples of secondary muscular dysfunction.
Study pages 1060-1061.

Muscular symptoms arise from causes unrelated to the muscle itself. These secondary muscular phenomena include contracture, stress-related muscle tension, and immobility.

Several conditions cause the muscle fibers to shorten without contracting; this is called a **contracture**. A physiologic muscle contracture occurs without muscle action potential in the sarcolemma and is explained as failure of the calcium pump even in the presence of plentiful adenosine triphosphate (ATP). A physiologic contracture is seen in McArdle disease, which is an enzyme deficiency, and malignant hyperthermia. The contracture is usually temporary if the underlying pathology can be corrected.

A pathologic contracture is considered a permanent muscle shortening due to muscle spasm or weakness. It is associated with plentiful ATP and will occur in spite of a normal action potential. The most common form of contracture is seen in muscular dystrophy and central nervous system (CNS) injury. Contractures may also develop secondary to scar tissue contraction in the flexor tissues of a joint.

Stress-induced muscle tension has been associated with chronic anxiety as well as a variety of stress-related muscular symptoms, including neck stiffness, back pain, and headache. The underlying pathophysiology presumably is caused by increased activity of the reticular-activating system and increased firing of the efferent loop of the gamma fibers which produce further muscle contraction and increased muscle tension.

Progressive relaxation training and biofeedback are possible ways to treat muscle tension. The hope is to enhance the individual's ability to relax specific muscle groups in order to relieve tension. This could reduce CNS and ANS arousal.

The term **disuse atrophy** describes the pathologic reduction in normal size of muscle fibers following inactivity due to bed rest, trauma, casting, or local nerve damage. Atrophy may be prevented by frequent forceful isometric muscle contractions and passive lengthening exercises.

6. Distinguish between muscle membrane abnormalities.
Study page 1061.

The hyperexcitable membrane seen in myotonic disorders and the intermittently unresponsive membrane seen in the periodic paralyses are defects in the plasma membrane of the muscle fiber. **Myotonia** is a delayed relaxation after voluntary muscle contraction such as gripes, eye closure, or muscle percussion. It is due to the prolonged depolarization of the muscle membrane. Myotonia is seen mostly in inherited disorders. Its symptoms are mild except in myotonic muscular dystrophy. Myotonia is treated by drugs that reduce muscle fiber excitability.

In **periodic paralysis**, the muscle membrane is unresponsive to neural stimuli. Periodic paralysis is triggered by exercise and any process or medication that alters serum potassium. The disorder is often inherited in an autosomal dominant pattern. Oral and intravenous potassium can relieve acute attacks. A low-salt diet and drugs are useful for long-term therapy.

7. Compare the metabolic, inflammatory, and toxic myopathies.
Study pages 1061-1063.

Myopathies

Myopathy	Causes	Manifestations
	Metabolic Myopathy	
	Altered thyroid hormone levels change muscle protein synthesis and electrolyte balance	
	Thyrotoxicosis	Proximal weakness, paresis of extraocular muscles
	Hypothyroidism	Flabby and weak muscles, sluggish movements
McArdle disease	Absence of muscle phosphorylase, unable to catabolize glycogen or produce lactic acid	Exercise intolerance, fatigue, painful muscle cramps, muscle weakness and wasting
Acid maltase deficiency	Autosomal recessive, absence of acid maltase, accumulation of glycogen in lysosomes of muscle and other cells	Adult: similar to muscular dystrophy or polymyositis, severe respiratory muscle weakness
Pompe disease (infantile form of acid maltase deficiency)		Infant: hypotonia, areflexia, enlarged heart and tongue and liver, early death
Myoadenylate deaminase deficiency	Absence of myoadenylate deaminase, cannot form phosphocreatine and ATP during exercise	Exercise intolerance
Carnitine palmitoyl transferase (CPT) and carnitine deficiency	Absence of CPT and carnitine, fatty acid byproducts and energy are not transported to the myofibrils	CPT: mild muscular symptoms, episodes of renal failure because of myoglobinuria Carnitine: progressive muscle weakness
	Inflammatory Myopathy	
	Infectious	
	Tuberculosis and sarcoidosis	Granulomas in muscle and other tissues

(Continued)

Myopathies (cont'd)

Myopathy	Causes	Manifestations
	Trichinosis	Larvae from infected pork migrate to host lymphatics: pain, rash, and muscle stiffness
	Viral infections	Muscle pain and tenderness similar to symptoms of influenza
Polymyositis (generalized muscle inflammation) Dermatomyositis (polymyositis with skin lesions)	Cell-mediated, immune system abnormalities	Necrosis of muscle fibers, malaise, fever, muscle swelling pain and tenderness, lethargy, symmetric proximal muscle weakness; both diseases show dysphagia, vasculitis, Raynaud phenomenon, cardiomyopathy, fibrosis, coexisting pulmonary collagen disorders; dermatomyositis exhibits skin rash, calcinosis, and eyelid edema
	Toxic Myopathy	
	Alcohol abuse, direct toxic effect and nutritional deficiency causes necrosis of muscle fibers	Benign cramps and pain, severe weakness, myoglobinuria and renal failure
	Antimalarial and amebicidal agents impair lysosomal processes	Generalized muscle weakness
	Sedatives and narcotics	Myoglobinuria
	Repeated therapeutic drug injection	Local muscle fiber necrosis, fibrotic bands

8. Classify bone tumors by tissue of origin, whether benign or malignant, and their pattern of bone destruction.

Study pages 1063-1066; refer to Figure 36-13 and Table 36-3.

Bone tumors may originate from bone cells, cartilage, fibrous tissue, marrow, or vascular tissue. On the basis of mesodermal tissue of origin, bone tumors are classified as osteogenic, chondrogenic, collagenic, or myelogenic. The mesoderm contributes to primitive fibroblasts and reticulum cells. The fibroblast is the progenitor of the osteoblast, the chondroblast, and the fibrous connective tissue cell.

Benign bone tumors destroy small areas of bone, tend to be limited to the anatomic confines of the host bone, and have a well-demarcated border. Benign bone tumors push against neighboring tissue, have a symmetrical, controlled growth pattern, and tend to compress and displace neighboring normal bone tissue which weakens the bone's structure until it leads to pathologic fracture.

The geographic pattern, the moth-eaten pattern, and the permeative pattern are patterns of bone destruction in bone tumors. Tumors exhibiting the geographic pattern have well-defined margins that can be easily separated from the surrounding normal bone. There is a uniform and well-defined lytic area in the bone of these benign lesions.

In the moth-eaten pattern, the cancerous lesion has a less-defined or demarcated margin that cannot be easily separated from normal bone. Areas of partially destroyed bone adjacent to completely lytic areas are found. This pattern of bone destruction is characteristic of rapidly growing, **malignant bone tumors**. An aggressive, malignant tumor causes the permeative pattern of bone destruction. The margins of the tumor are poorly demarcated, and abnormal bone merges with surrounding normal bone tissue. Malignant bone tumors tend to be large and aggressive in their bone destruction, to invade surrounding tissue, and to metastasize.

Origin of Benign and Malignant Bone Tumors

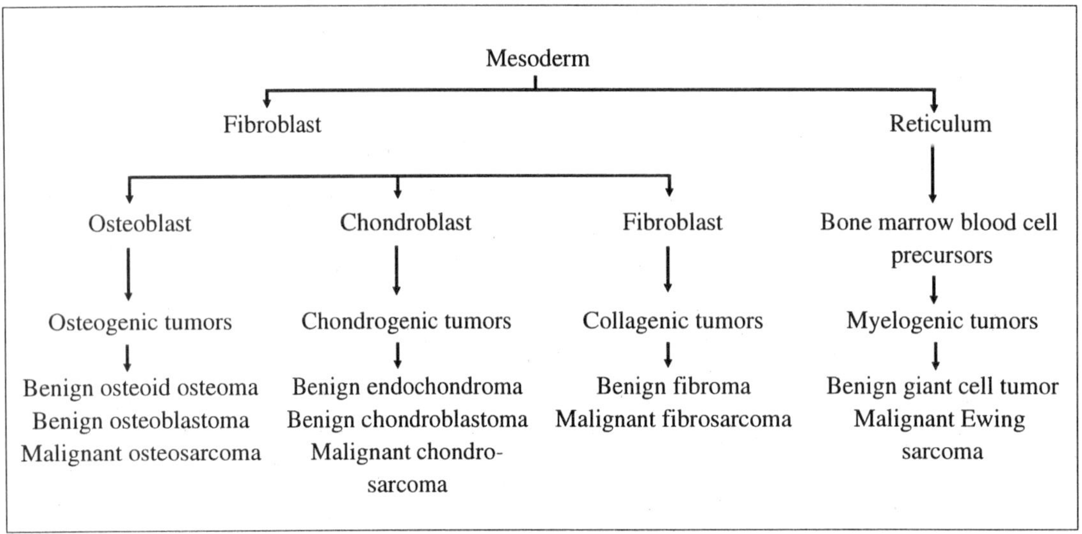

Note: Diagnosis depends on serum metabolite and enzyme levels, radiologic studies, CT scans, MRI, blood counts, and biopsy.

9. Characterize the common types of bone tumors.
Study pages 1065-1066.

Osteosarcoma is a malignant bone-forming tumor that is large and destructive and most often found in bone marrow; it has a moth-eaten pattern of bone destruction. Osteosarcomas always contain osteoid and callus and also may contain chondroid and fibrinoid tissue. The osteoid is deposited between the trabeculae of the callus. The "streamers" of osteoid infiltrate the normal compact bone, destroy it, and replace it with dense callus and masses of osteoid. The bone tissue never matures to compact bone. Ninety percent of osteosarcomas are located in the metaphyses of long bones. Fifty percent of osteosarcomas occur around the knee area. The tumor breaks through the cortex, lifts the periosteum, and forms a soft tissue mass that is not covered by new bone.

Common initial symptoms are pain and swelling; pain is usually worse at night. Systemic symptoms are uncommon. Preoperative chemotherapy has improved the treatment for localized osteosarcoma. Chemotherapy can be given both preoperatively and postoperatively. Combination treatment includes radiation therapy and surgery.

Chondrosarcoma, a chondrogenic tumor, is a large, ill-defined malignant tumor that infiltrates trabeculae in spongy bone. It occurs most often in the metaphysis or diaphysis of long bones. The tumor contains large lobules of hyaline cartilage that are separated by bands of fibrous tissue and anaplastic cells. It expands and enlarges the contour of the bone, causes extensive erosion of the cortex, and expands into the soft tissues.

Symptoms associated with the chondrosarcoma have an insidious onset. Local swelling and pain are usual symptoms. At first, the pain is intermittent; then, it gradually intensifies and becomes constant. Surgical excision is generally regarded as the treatment of choice; however, individuals demonstrate recurrences and so amputation is considered.

Fibrosarcoma, a malignant collagenic tumor, is a solitary tumor that most frequently affects the metaphyseal region of the femur or tibia. The tumor is composed of a firm, fibrous mass of tissue containing collagen, malignant fibroblasts, and occasional osteoclast-like giant cells.

Pain and swelling are the usual symptoms and indicate that the tumor has broken through the cortex. Local tenderness, a palpable mass, limitation of motion, or a pathologic fracture are other symptoms and signs. Radical surgery and amputation are the treatments of choice for fibrosarcoma.

Giant cell tumors are common primary bone tumors. The giant cell tumor is a solitary, circumscribed tumor that causes extensive bone resorption because of its osteoclastic origin. The tumor is rich in osteoclast-like giant cells and anaplastic stromal cells and is found in the center of the epiphysis in the femur, tibia, radius, or humerus. The tumor has a slow, relentless growth rate and is usually contained within the original contour of the affected bone. It may extend into the articular cartilage. It has recurrence rate as high as 80 percent.

The most common symptoms associated with the giant cell tumor are pain, local swelling, and limitation of movement. Cryosurgery and resection of the tumor decrease recurrence and are more successful treatments than curettage and radiation; amputation may be necessary.

Myeloma is a malignant neoplastic proliferation of plasma cells. Myelomas cause cortical and medullary bone lysis and infiltrate the bone marrow.

The most common symptom of myeloma is pain that is initially aching, intermittent, and aggravated by weight bearing. As the disease progresses, the pain becomes severe and prolonged. Myeloma has a poor prognosis and the treatment is generally palliative. Radiotherapy and chemotherapy have very limited success.

10. Identify the incidence, manifestations, treatment, and prognosis of rhabdomyosarcoma.
Study page 1067.

The malignant tumor of striated muscle is a **rhabdomyosarcoma**. The incidence of rhabdomyosarcoma is extremely rare, but it is highly malignant because of its rapid metastasis. These tumors are located in the muscle tissue of the head, neck, and genitourinary tract 75 percent of the time. The remainder are in the trunk and extremities.

The diagnosis of rhabdomyosarcoma is made by incisional biopsy and histological examination of the specimen. Pleomorphic, embryonal, and alveolar types can be differentiated. The pleomorphic type is a highly malignant tumor of the extremities of adults.

Treatment consists of a combination of surgical excision, radiation therapy, and systemic chemotherapy. Cure in cases with distant metastasis is unlikely.

Practice Examination

1. In a complete fracture:

   a. the fracture crosses or involves the entire width or thickness of the bone.
   b. more than two bone fragments are present.
   c. separation of ligaments exists.
   d. post-traumatic infection is always present.
   e. the surface opposite the break is intact.

2. In an oblique fracture, the energy or force is:

   a. twisting with the distal part unable to move.
   b. compressive and at an angle.
   c. directly to an already weakened bone.
   d. directly to the distal fragment.

3. Which is a definite sign of a fracture?

   a. abrasion
   b. shock
   c. muscle spasm
   d. unnatural alignment
   e. All of the above are correct.

Match the term with its characteristic.

4. ____ subluxation
5. ____ sprain

a. articular cartilages lose contact entirely
b. articular cartilages are partially separated
c. complete separation of a tendon or a ligament
d. a ligament tear

6. Compartment syndromes:

a. involve large compartments of hemorrhage.
b. bleed into joints.
c. lead to muscle ischemia.
d. may result from myoglobinuria.
e. Both b and c are correct.

7. The most common cause of osteomyelitis is:

a. hematogenous spread of infection.
b. rheumatoid disease.
c. direct contamination of an open wound.
d. deficiency of calcium.
e. deficiency of vitamin D.

8. Osteoporosis is:

a. inadequate mineralization.
b. impaired synthesis of bone organic matrix.
c. reduced bone mass or density.
d. formation of sclerotic bone.
e. None of the above is correct.

9. Osteomalacia causes:

a. loss of bone matrix.
b. inadequate mineralization.
c. radiolucency.
d. All of the above are correct.
e. Both b and c are correct.

10. Bone tumors may originate from all of the following except:

a. epithelial tissue.
b. cartilage.
c. fibrous tissue.
d. vascular tissue.
e. mesoderm.

11. In benign bone tumors, there is:

    a. a uniform and well-defined lytic area.
    b. a moth-eaten pattern of bone destruction.
    c. abnormal bone merging with surrounding normal bone tissue.
    d. an area of partially destroyed bone adjacent to completely lytic areas.

12. An osteosarcoma is a/an:

    a. collagenic, malignant bone tumor.
    b. myelogenic, benign tumor.
    c. myelogenic, malignant tumor.
    d. osteogenic, benign bone tumor.
    e. osteogenic, malignant tumor.

13. The major symptom of bone cancer is a:

    a. flattering gait.
    b. persistent pain that worsens at night.
    c. lack of sensation.
    d. general swelling over a bone.
    e. coolness over a bone.

14. Giant cell tumors:

    a. are collagenic tumors.
    b. are located in the diaphysis of a long bone.
    c. have extensive osteoblastic activity.
    d. have high recurrence rates.
    e. are multifocal.

15. Myeloma:

    a. is a malignant proliferation of plasma cells.
    b. has a poor prognosis.
    c. infiltrates the bone marrow.
    d. Both a and c are correct.
    e. a, b, and c are correct.

16. Rheumatoid arthritis begins with:

    a. destruction of the synovial membrane and subsynovial tissue.
    b. inflammation of ligaments.
    c. destruction of the articular cartilage.
    d. softening of the articular cartilage.
    e. destruction of the joint capsule.

17. The causes of osteoarthritis include which of the following? (*More than one answer may be correct.*)

    a. collagenases
    b. proteoglycan destruction
    c. rheumatoid factor
    d. circulating immune complexes
    e. infections

18. Ankylosing spondylitis (*more than one answer may be correct*):

    a. is a systemic immune inflammatory disease.
    b. is characterized by stiffening or fusion of the spine.
    c. causes instability of synovial joints.
    d. begins with inflammation of fibrocartilage.
    e. in manifested early by low back pain and stiffness.

19. In gout:

    a. the pathogenesis is formation of monosodium urate crystals in joints and tissues.
    b. purine metabolism is altered.
    c. affected individuals likely have an inherited enzyme defect.
    d. the hyperuricemia can be the result of acquired chronic disease or a drug.
    e. All of the above are correct.

20. A muscle contracture is:

    a. likely caused by increased activity in the reticular activating system and the gamma loop in the muscle fiber.
    b. muscle shortening possible because of CNS injury.
    c. often helped by relaxation training and biofeedback.
    d. a consequence of reduced muscle protein synthesis.
    e. All of the above are correct.

21. Myotonia is all of the following except:

    a. delayed relaxation after voluntary muscle contractions.
    b. prolonged depolarization of the muscle membrane.
    c. mostly inherited.
    d. unresponsiveness to neural stimulation.
    e. progressive atrophy of skeletal muscle.

Match the myopathy with its cause.

22. ____ McArdle disease
23. ____ acid maltase deficiency
24. ____ polymyositis

a. hypothyroidism
b. hyperparathyroidism
c. accumulation of glycogen in lysosomes
d. unable to catabolize glycogen
e. immune system abnormality

25. Rhabdomyosarcomas have:

    a. a poor prognosis.
    b. aggressive invasion.
    c. early, widespread dissemination.
    d. pleomorphic types.
    e. All of the above are correct.

Case Study

Mrs. B.B. is a 52-year-old homemaker who has complained of bilateral knee and hand pain for seven years. The pain has progressively worsened and persists during rest and limits her walking, climbing stairs, and weight bearing. Her physical examination showed slight ulnar deviation of the digits and swelling of the metacarpal, phalangeal, and proximal interphalangeal joints with limited range of motion and some instability of both knees.

Laboratory studies revealed:

CBC = normal, except for mild anemia
Rheumatoid factor = high titer
Synovial fluid analysis = turbid appearance
Radiographic examination of knees = joint narrowing on both knees, thinning of the articular cartilage, cystic areas, and bony spurs

Which arthritis is Mrs. B.B. experiencing? Explain your answer.

CHAPTER

37

Alterations of Musculoskeletal Function in Children

Foundational Objectives

Memory Check!

- See *Workbook*'s narrative for Foundational Objectives **a, b,** and **d** in Chapter 36.

Objectives

After studying this chapter, the learner will be able to:

1. Describe congenital musculoskeletal defects in children.
Study page 1072; refer to Figure 37-5.

Developmental dysplasia of the hip (DDH), formerly known as congenital hip dislocation, is an anomaly of the development of the proximal femur, acetabulum, or both. Risk factors include breech presentation, family history, first pregnancy, and oligohydramnios. Presence of other lower extremity deformities may increase the risk of DDH. Treatment generally consists of bracing the joint in flexion and abduction. Surgery is occasionally required.

Metatarsus adductus (MTA) is the most common congenital defect of the lower extremity and is believed to be due to intrauterine positioning of the feet. In this deformity, the bones of the forefoot are adducted. Most cases are self-correcting, but the more fixed forms require physical therapy or bracing. In **talipes equinovarus**, or **clubfoot**, the forefoot is abducted and the hindfoot is adducted and inverted. The entire foot points downward. The foot is in rigid fixation. Treatment consists of early serial casting and frequently requires surgery for full correction.

2. Describe the pathophysiology and clinical features of osteogenesis imperfecta.
Study page 1072.

Osteogenesis imperfecta is primarily a defect in collagen production resulting in easily fractured, "brittle" bones. It is usually inherited by the autosomal dominant route. Clinical features include bone fractures, osteoporosis, and bowed or deformed limbs. Short stature, curvature of the spine, or a bluish discoloration of the sclera also may be a feature. Four syndromes of varying severity have been identified: types II and III are the most severe; types I and IV are less severe but more common. Supplemental calcium, fluoride, vitamin C, and magnesium oxide, as well as orthopedic splinting, have all been treatments.

3. Describe major forms of scoliosis.
Study page 1072; refer to Figure 37-1.

Scoliosis, or lateral curvature of the spine, may be classified as (1) nonstructural occurring from causes extrinsic to the spine, such as posture, pain, or leg length discrepancy, or (2) structural that is associated with vertebral rotation. Adolescent idiopathic scoliosis is the most common; central nervous system abnormality may involve the balance mechanism in the midbrain in this type.

Pathophysiologic change includes shortening of ligaments on the concave side of the curve; this eventually results in vertebral deformity. The deformity is due to unequal stress on the epiphyseal centers of the vertebral bodies. Eventually, progressive deformity of the vertebral column and ribs develops.

Clinical manifestations include asymmetry of hip and shoulder height, rounded shoulder, and spiral curvature. Diagnosis is confirmed by x-ray. Treatment includes bracing, surgery, and transcutaneous muscle stimulation.

4. **Describe the pathophysiology of osteomyelitis in children.**
   Study pages 1072-1074; refer to Figure 37-2.

Osteomyelitis is an inflammation of the bone and bone marrow that occurs most frequently between 3 and 12 years of age with a predilection for boys. In this process, bacteria enter the bone through the bloodstream and lodge in the metaphysical side of the growth plate. This is frequently where the process is halted by phagocytes in this area. In other cases, however, bacteria invade the epiphyseal plate where phagocytes are absent, and resultant infection develops.

Osteomyelitis may be preceded by trauma which may then predispose to infection. The infection usually begins as a bloody abscess in the metaphysis of the bone that ruptures under the periosteum and spreads along the shaft or into the medullary cavity. The microorganism usually gains access to the subperiosteal space through the metaphysis, which is the path of least resistance because of the porous nature of the bone in that area.

If infection occurs near a joint, the accumulated pressure of inflammatory products may cause pus and bacteria to rupture through the bone and into the joint space, causing a **secondary suppurative arthritis**. The spread of infection into joint spaces is also aided because the epiphyseal plates in infants are penetrated by capillaries that communicate directly into joints. Severe infection in infants and young children rapidly leads to permanent damage of the joints and disruption of the blood supply to the bone with subsequent growth arrest. The most common etiologic agents in osteomyelitis vary and are related to the age of the child.

Clinical presentation of the illness tends to be somewhat variable. Osteomyelitis is frequently abrupt in onset in young children and infants as the child displays signs of toxicity, fever, and slow movement of the affected limb. This process may be more subacute in older children and adults; in young children and infants, osteomyelitis usually involves the long bones. Diagnosis is usually confirmed by an elevated white blood cell count and erythrocyte sedimentation rate. Treatment includes long-term, appropriate antibiotic therapy and surgical intervention where warranted.

5. **Describe the pathophysiology, evaluation, and treatment of Legg-Calve-Perthes disease.**
   Study page 1075; refer to Figure 37-3.

Legg-Calve-Perthes disease (LCP) is a process of interrupted blood supply to the femoral head. It commonly occurs between three and ten years of age with a peak incidence at six years of age. It is self-limiting in nature, running its course in two to five years. Interruption of blood flow to the femoral head results in necrosis of the femoral head. Inflammation and new bone formation follow over time with a resultant flattening of the femoral head. The first necrotic stage lasts only a few weeks; however, the healing phase lasts from two to four years. The etiology of LCP is unknown, although familial occurrence is known, as is a history of antecedent trauma. It is probable that an antecedent synovitis causes increased hydrostatic pressure within the joint and interferes with blood flow. Birth weight tends to be low in children with LCP disease, and skeletal maturation is delayed as well.

Presentation of LCP disease may be fairly incipient, with the child complaining of lower extremity pain for weeks to months. A limp known as the antalgic abductor lurch then follows. The child frequently demonstrates pain when the hip is externally rotated while in extension. Treatment is accomplished by bracing the legs in abduction or by surgical intervention if necessary.

6. **Describe the pathophysiology, evaluation, and treatment of Duchenne muscular dystrophy.**
   Study pages 1077-1078; refer to Figures 37-4 and 37-5 and Table 37-1.

Duchenne muscular dystrophy is an X-linked inherited disorder that is caused by a deletion of a segment of DNA. This deletion results in an absence of dystrophin, which is found in normal muscle cells. The lack of dystrophin apparently causes loss of muscle bulk and fibers. In the late stages, interstitial connective tissue and fat may replace muscle fibers.

The disease is frequently diagnosed at approximately three years of age when parents notice slow motor development, problems with coordination and walking, and generalized weakness. Weakness always begins in the pelvic girdle, and hypertrophy is present in the calf muscles of approximately 80 percent of affected children. Gower sign, a peculiar manner of standing from sitting by climbing up the legs, is often evident. Within three to five years, the shoulder girdle muscle becomes involved with constant progression of the illness. Pulmonary and cardiac failure may follow and, eventually, death usually results by age 20.

Diagnosis is confirmed by serum enzyme studies and electromyelography. Creatine phosphokinase (CPK) may be ten times normal, and histologic examination of biopsied muscle fibers will be abnormal as well. Treatment is chiefly supportive, with the goal being to preserve function of remaining muscle groups for as long as possible.

7. Characterize childhood osteosarcoma and Ewing sarcoma.
Study pages 1078-1080.

Osteosarcoma accounts for 60 percent of the bone tumors in children and originates in bone-producing mesenchymal cells. Three-fourths of these neoplasms occur between the ages of 10 and 25.

Osteosarcoma can be induced by ionizing radiation or by therapeutic radiation for other forms of cancer. It is more likely to occur if an individual has bilateral retinoblastoma. The link between retinoblastoma and subsequent osteosarcoma occurs whether or not radiation has been part of the treatment for retinoblastoma.

The most common complaint is pain. Symptoms may also include cough, dyspnea, and chest pain when lung metastasis occurs.

Surgery and chemotherapy are the primary treatments for osteosarcoma. Chemotherapy is an important component of treatment because as many as 80 percent of children treated with surgery alone eventually develop metastatic disease. The tumor is resistant to radiation.

Ewing sarcoma is the second most common but most lethal malignant bone tumor of childhood. It probably originates from cells within the bone marrow space and does not involve bone-forming cells. Its incidence is greatest between 5 and 15 years of age; it is rare after age 30. The most common site of this tumor is the marrow of the femur, followed by the marrow of the pelvis and then of the humerus.

The most common symptom is pain that increases in severity. A soft-tissue mass is often present. Ewing sarcoma metastasizes early to nearly every organ. The most common sites are the lung, other bones, lymph nodes, liver, spleen, and central nervous system.

Treatment is preoperative chemotherapy followed by radiation or surgical resection or both and continued chemotherapy for 12 to 18 months afterward. Involved sites with the best prognosis are the extremities; the worst prognosis involves tumors of the trunk and the pelvis.

8. Describe rhabdomyosarcoma of childhood.
Study pages 1080-1082; refer to Tables 37-2 and 37-3.

Rhabdomyosarcoma (RMS) is the most common sarcoma of childhood and accounts for more than 50 percent of soft-tissue tumors but less than 3 percent of all childhood cancers. Rhabdomyosarcoma arises from embryonal cells that normally differentiate into mature striated muscle; five different types have been identified.

Rhabdomyosarcomas are located, in descending order of frequency, in the (1) head and neck, (2) trunk, (3) extremities, and (4) genitourinary tract. More than two-thirds are diagnosed by ten years of age, with males affected more often than females. Rhabdomyosarcoma has been reported to be a complication of neurofibromatosis and has been associated with breast cancer and abnormalities in chromosomes 2, 11, and 13.

Rhabdomyosarcoma generally appears as firm, fleshy, grayish white masses. Depending on the phase of differentiation of the rhabdomyoblast, these tumors may have round or spindle-shaped, tadpole-shaped, or multinucleated giant cells. They spread by rapid local infiltration and via the bloodstream and lymphatic system. The sites of metastases include the lungs, lymph nodes, bone marrow, liver, brain, and bone. Twenty percent of children with RMS have metastatic disease at diagnosis.

The tumors are usually painless and are detected by the presence of a palpable or visible mass. Deep-seated tumors cause functional impairment.

Rhabdomyosarcoma is treated by a combination of surgery, radiation, and chemotherapy. Children with localized disease have long-term survival rates of 70 to 80 percent. In widespread disease, long-term survival rates drop to 20 percent.

Practice Examination

True/False

1. ____ In talipes equinovarus, the entire foot points upward.

2. ____ Developmental dysplasia of the hip is often noted shortly after birth due to a positive Gower sign.

3. ____ Osteogenesis imperfecta is a disease related to overcalcification of the bone that causes it to be brittle and break easily.

4. ____ Metatarsus abductus is a positional deformity of the foot that may be self-correcting.

5. ____ Legg-Calve-Perthes disease may be suspected when a positive Ortolani or Barlow maneuver is noted.

6. ____ Osteomyelitis is an infection of bone that can be spread to the site through the blood.

7. ____ Breech presentation is not a risk factor for developmental hip dysplasia because traction on the feet during the birth process negates undue pressure on the hip joint.

8. ____ Clubfoot is not self-limiting and requires casting with or without surgery for successful treatment.

9. ____ Muscular dystrophies are characterized by defective creatine metabolism.

10. ____ Treatment of clubfoot is usually delayed because the bones of the infant are generally not well ossified at birth and may be easily corrected later.

Fill-in-the-Blank

11. The process of Legg-Calve-Perthes disease is presumably produced by interruption of the blood supply to the __________ head.

12. A risk factor in developmental dysplasia of the hip may be __________ in utero.

13. Duchenne muscular dystrophy results from a lack of __________ in muscle cells.

14. DDH is treated by bracing the hips in __________ and __________.

15. Talipes equinovarus is also known as __________.

Match the outcome or circumstance with the alteration.

16. ____ fractures present at birth
17. ____ death by 20 years of age
18. ____ congenital abnormality in acetabulum
19. ____ Gower sign
20. ____ antalgic abductor lurch
21. ____ subluxed, dislocated, dislocatable
22. ____ pain in external rotation with affected limb
23. ____ long-term antibiotics required
24. ____ defect in collagen synthesis
25. ____ lateral curvature of the spine

a. scoliosis
b. osteogenesis imperfecta
c. osteomyelitis
d. Legg-Calve-Perthes disease
e. developmental hip dysplasia
f. Duchenne muscular dystrophy

Case Study

Bobby B. is a three-year-old white male visiting a pediatrician's office because of his mother's concern regarding his clumsiness, frequent falls, and difficulty in climbing stairs. On physical examination, Bobby B. tends to walk on his toes, exhibits a positive Gower sign, and appears to have hypertrophy of calf muscles.

What disease is suspected? How could the diagnosis be confirmed?

CHAPTER

38

Structure, Function, and Disorders of the Integument

Foundational Objectives

a. Describe the skin and its layers. Review page 1085; refer to Figure 38-1 and Table 38-1.

Memory Check!

- The skin has two major layers: a superficial epidermis and a deeper layer, the dermis. The subcutaneous tissue, or hypodermis, is an underlying layer of connective tissue that contains macrophages, fibroblasts, and fat cells.
- The dermal appendages include the nails, hair, sebaceous glands, and the eccrine and apocrine sweat glands. The nails are protective keratinized plates that appear at the ends of fingers and toes. Hair follicles arise from the matrix located deep in the dermis. Hair growth begins in the bulb, with cellular differentiation occurring as the hair progresses up the follicle. Hair is fully cornified by the time it emerges at the skin surface. The sebaceous glands open onto the surface of the skin through a canal and secrete sebum composed primarily of lipids, which oil the skin and hair and prevent drying.
- The eccrine sweat glands are distributed over the body and are important in cooling of the body through evaporation. The apocrine sweat glands are fewer in number and are located in the axillae, scalp, face, abdomen, and genital area.
- The blood supply to the skin is by the papillary capillaries or plexus of the dermis. Arteriovenous anastomoses in the dermis facilitate the regulation of body temperature. Heat loss can be regulated by varying blood flow through the skin by opening or closing the arteriovenous anastomoses to modify evaporative heat loss through sweat. The sympathetic nervous system regulates both vasoconstriction and vasodilation as there are only adrenergic receptors in the skin. The lymphatic vessels of the skin arise in the dermis and drain into larger subcutaneous trunks; these vessels remove cells, proteins, and immunologic mediators.

b. Identify the changes that occur in skin during aging. Review page 1087.

Memory Check!

- The skin becomes thinner, dryer, and wrinkled, and pigmentation changes during aging. Fewer melanocytes decrease the protection against ultraviolet radiation. Fewer Langerhans cells decrease the skin's immune response during aging. The thickness of the dermis decreases and the skin becomes translucent and assumes a paper-thin quality. Loss of the rete pegs gives the skin a smooth, shiny appearance. Atrophy of eccrine, apocrine, and sebaceous glands causes the skin to become drier with age. Loss of elastin fibers is associated with wrinkling. The collagen fibers become less flexible and decrease the ability of the skin to stretch and regain shape. Decreased cell generation and blood supply delay wound healing in aging skin. Graying of hair color is due to loss of melanocytes. Barrier function of the stratum corneum is reduced. There is increased permeability and decreased clearance of substances from the dermis. The accumulation of such substances can cause skin irritation. Temperature regulation is less effective in the elderly, and there is increased risk for both heatstroke and hypothermia. The pressure and touch receptors and free nerve endings all decrease in number and reduce sensory perception.

Objectives

After studying this chapter, the learner will be able to:

1. **Distinguish between skin lesions.**
   Refer to Tables 38-2 and 38-3.

Basic Lesions of the Skin

Type	Characteristics	Example/Disease
	Flat Lesions	
Macule	A flat, circumscribed, discolored lesion of any size	Hyperpigmentation, erythema, telangiectasia, purpura
Patch	A flat, irregular lesion larger than a macule	Vitiligo
Petechiae	A circumscribed area of blood less than 0.5 cm in diameter	Thrombocytopenia
Purpura	A circumscribed area of blood greater than 5.0 cm in diameter	Bruises
Telangiectasia	Dilated, superficial blood vessels	Rheumatoid arthritis, hepatitis

(Continued)

Basic Lesions of the Skin (cont'd)

Type	Characteristics	Example/Disease
	Elevated Lesions	
Papule	A lesion 1 cm or less in diameter because of infiltration or hyperplasia of the dermis	Verrucae (warts), lichen planus, nevus
Plaque	A lesion with a large surface area, larger laterally than in height	Psoriasis, eczema
Nodule	A palpable, circumscribed lesion 1-2 cm in diameter located in the epidermis, dermis, or hypodermis; smooth to ulcerated	Benign or malignant tumors, foreign body inflammation, calcium deposits
Wheal	A transient lesion with well-defined and often changing borders caused by edema of the dermis	Hives, angioedema
Vesicle and bulla	A fluid-filled, thin-walled lesion; a bulla is a vesicle greater than 0.5 cm in diameter	Herpes zoster, impetigo, pemphigus, second-degree burns
Pustule	A lesion containing an exudate of white blood cells	Acne, pustular psoriasis
Comedo	Plugged hair follicle	Blackhead, whitehead
Scale	Accumulation of loose stratum corneum from cellular retention or cellular overproduction	Psoriasis
Crust	Accumulation of dried blood or serum, size varies	Eczema, impetigo
Lichenification	Thickening, toughening of the skin with accentuation of skin lines caused by scratching	Chronic dermatitis
Cyst	An encapsulated mass of dermis or subcutaneous layers, solid or fluid-filled	Sebaceous cyst
Tumor	A well-demarcated solid lesion greater than 2 cm in diameter	Fibroma, lipoma, melanoma, hemangioma
Scar	Thin or thick fibrous tissue	Healed laceration, burn, surgical incision
	Depressed Lesions	
Atrophy	Thinning of the epidermis or dermis caused by decreased connective tissue	Thin facial skin of elderly, striae of pregnancy
Ulcer	Loss of epidermis and dermis	Pressure sores, basal cell carcinoma
Excoriation	Loss of epidermis with exposed dermis	Scratches
Fissure	Linear crack or break exposing dermis	Athlete's foot, cheilosis
Erosion	Moist, red break in epidermis, follows rupture of vesicle or bulla, larger than fissure	Chickenpox, diaper dermatitis

2. Describe keloids; identify stimuli for pruritus.
Study pages 1093-1094; refer to Figure 38-3.

Keloids are sharply elevated, irregularly shaped scars that progressively enlarge. They are caused by trauma to the skin and the excessive accumulation of collagen in the corneum during connective tissue repair. Burns incite this reaction more commonly than other types of injury. Even minor trauma may result in a keloidal reaction in blacks and Orientals. A familial tendency for keloid formation exists, with both autosomal recessive and autosomal dominant inheritance patterns present.

Keloids begin as pink or red, firm, well-defined, rubbery plaques that persist for several months after trauma. The fibrous tissue that accumulates in keloids is associated with increased cellularity and metabolic activity of fibroblasts. Injection of corticosteroids into the lesion is the treatment of choice.

Pruritus, or itching, is a symptom associated with many primary skin disorders and systemic diseases. The condition may be localized or generalized and may move from one location to another.

Multiple stimuli can produce itching, including substance P, histamine, heat, and electrical stimulation. Substance P, a neurotransmitter, causes histamine release and wheal formation with itching when injected into the skin. Lymphocytes present in itching skin may be involved in the pathogenesis of itching.

Management of pruritus depends on the cause; the primary condition must be treated. Symptomatic relief can be obtained from antihistamines and topical steroids in some cases. Some pruritus is resistant to any type of therapy.

3. Identify the causes and lesions of inflammatory and papulosquamous disorders of the skin.
Study pages 1094-1099; refer to Figures 38-4 through 38-12.

Inflammatory Skin Disorders

Disorder	Cause	Lesion
	Inflammatory Disorders	
Allergic contact dermatitis	Allergen binds to carrier protein to form a sensitizing antigen, T cell hypersensitivity	Pruritic (itching) vesicles
Irritant contact dermatitis	Nonimmunologic inflammation due to chemicals	As above
Atopic dermatitis	Mast cell and IgE, T lymphocytes, and monocytes interact	Red, weeping crusts, lichenification
Stasis dermatitis	Venous stasis and edema	Initial erythema and pruritus; then, scaling, petechiae, and hyperpigmentation
Seborrheic dermatitis	Unknown	Scaly plaques with mild pruritus
		(Continued)

Inflammatory Skin Disorders (cont'd)

Disorder	Cause	Lesion
	Papulosquamous Disorders	
Psoriasis	Unknown, genetic or immunologic	Thick, silvery, scaly, erythematous, plaque surrounded by normal skin; rapid shedding of epidermis
Pityriasis rosea	Unknown (virus?)	Pruritus, demarcated salmon-pink scale within a plaque
Lichen planus	Unknown (exposure to drugs?)	Nonscaling, violet-colored pruritic papules
Acne vulgaris	Increased activity of sebaceous glands or sebum inability to escape through the narrow opening	Comedones
Acne rosacea	Unknown, associated with chronic flushing and sensitivity to sun	Erythema, papules, pustules, and telangiectasis
Discoid lupus erythematosus	Immune response to unknown antigen	Cutaneous manifestations of elevated red plaque with brown scale, hair loss, urticaria (hives), telangiectasis

4. Contrast pemphigus and erythema multiforme.
Study pages 1099-1100.

Pemphigus is a rare, chronic, blister-forming disease of the skin and oral mucous membranes with several different types that include pemphigus vulgaris, pemphigus foliaceus, and pemphigus erythematosus. The blisters form in the epidermis and occur deeply in pemphigus vulgaris and superficially in pemphigus foliaceus and pemphigus erythematosus.

Pemphigus is an autoimmune disease caused by circulating IgG autoantibodies. Serum autoantibodies are formed which react with the intracellular cement of substance that holds the epidermal cells together. The antibody reaction likely causes the intraepidermal blister formation and acantholysis, or loss of cohesion between epidermal cells.

Pemphigus vulgaris is the most common form of the disease and begins with the formation of a blister in the mouth or on the scalp. Within six months to one year, flaccid bullous lesions appear that rupture easily and leave crusty, denuded skin. Pressure on the blister may cause it to spread to adjacent skin; this is the Nikolsky sign. In **pemphigus foliaceus** and **pemphigus erythematosus**, oral lesions are usually absent and erythema with localized crusting, scaling, and occasional bullae develop.

In the diagnosis of pemphigus, immunofluorescence demonstrates the presence of antibodies at the site of blister formation. The primary treatment for pemphigus is systemic corticosteroids usually in high doses to suppress the immune response during acute episodes or when there is widespread involvement.

Erythema multiforme is an acute, recurring, inflammatory disorder of the skin and mucous membranes. It is associated with allergic or toxic reactions to drugs or microorganisms such as *Mycoplasma pneumoniae* and herpes simplex. Immune complex formation and deposition of C3, IgM, and fibrinogen around the superficial dermal blood vessels, basement membrane, and keratinocytes can be observed in most individuals with erythema multiforme. The characteristic "bull's eye" lesion occurs on the skin surface with a central erythematous region surrounded by concentric rings or alternating edema and inflammation. A vesiculobullous form is characterized by mucous membrane lesions and erythematous plaques on the extensor surfaces of the extremities.

The most common form expressed in children and young adults is **Stevens-Johnson syndrome** wherein there are numerous erythematous, bullous lesions on both the skin and mucous membranes. The bullous lesions form erosions and crusts when they rupture. The mouth, air passages, esophagus, urethra, and conjunctiva may be involved. Mild forms of the disease require no treatment as they are self-limiting; underlying infections should be treated.

5. **Identify the causes and lesions of cutaneous infections.**
   Study pages 1100-1103; refer to Figures 38-13 through 38-16 and Tables 38-4 and 38-5.

Cutaneous Infections

Infection	Cause	Lesion
Folliculitis	Bacterial infection of hair follicles usually by *Staphylococcus aureus*	Pustules with surrounding erythema
Furuncle	Infection from folliculitis spreading into dermis	Deep, red, firm, painful nodule changes to fluctuant and tender cystic nodule
Carbuncle	Collection of infected hair follicles	Erythematous, painful mass that drains through many openings
Cellulitis	Infection of dermis and subcutaneous tissue; extension from skin wound, ulcer, furuncle, or carbuncle	Erythematous, swollen, and painful area
Erysipelas	Group A streptococci	Systemic manifestations, red spots progress to pruritic vesicles
Impetigo	Coagulase positive staphylococci; beta-hemolytic streptococci	Serous and purulent vesicles that rupture and crust
Herpes simplex virus type 1 (HSV-1)	Primary and secondary infections (sensory nerve ganglion latency) on nongenital sites such as cornea, mouth, and labia	Clusters of vesicles on an erythematous base that become purulent and crusty
HSV-2	Primary and secondary infection (sensory nerve ganglion latency) genital herpes	Vesicles that progress to painful ulceration, pruritus, and weeping
Varicella (chickenpox) primary Herpes zoster (shingles) secondary	Varicella-zoster virus	Varicella: pink papules with reddened halo that is dry and crusty Zoster: erythema followed by grouped vesicles along a unilateral dermatome that later crust

(Continued)

Cutaneous Infections (cont'd)

Infection	Cause	Lesion
Warts (verrucae)	Human papillomavirus	Round, elevated with a rough, grayish surface
Tinea capitis (scalp) Tinea pedis (athlete's foot) Tinea corporis (ringworm) Tinea cruris ("jock itch")	Dermatophytes (fungi) that invade and thrive on keratin	Scaling and erythema, vesicles and fissures
Candidiasis	*Candida albicans* (yeastlike fungus) changes from a skin and mucous membrane commensal to a pathogen	Thin-walled pustule with inflammatory pruritic base

6. Contrast vasculitis, urticaria, and scleroderma.
Study pages 1103-1105; refer to Figure 38-17.

Vasculitis, or angiitis, is an inflammation of the blood vessels. Cutaneous vasculitis develops from the deposit of immune complexes in small blood vessels as a response to drugs, allergens, or streptococcal or viral infection. The deposit of immune complex likely activates complement which is chemotactic for polymorphonuclear leukocytes. The lesions appear as palpable purpura and progress to hemorrhagic bullae with necrosis and ulceration because of occlusion of the vessel. Identifying and removing the antigen is the first step in treatment. Prednisone may be used if symptoms are severe.

Urticarial lesions are most commonly associated with type I hypersensitivity reactions to drugs, certain foods, intestinal parasites, or physical agents. The lesions are mediated by histamine release, which causes the endothelial cells of skin blood vessels to contract and increase their permeability. The fluid from the vessel appears as wheals, welts, or hives. Antihistamines usually reduce the hives and provide relief from itching. Corticosteroids may be required for treatment of severe attacks.

Scleroderma is sclerosis of the skin which may remain localized to the skin or affect the visceral organs. If systemic, scleroderma involves the connective tissue and affects the kidneys, gastrointestinal tract, and lungs. The cutaneous lesions can cover the entire skin but are most often on the face and hands, the neck, and the upper chest.

The lesions exhibit massive deposits of collagen with fibrosis, inflammatory reactions, vascular changes in the capillary network with decreased capillary loops, and dilation of the remaining capillaries. Autoimmunity and an immune reaction to toxic substances are possible initiating mechanisms of the disease. Autoantibodies often can be recovered from the skin and serum of individuals with scleroderma.

The skin is hard, hypopigmented, taut, and tightly connected to the underlying tissue. An immobile masklike appearance with incomplete opening of the mouth is due to the tightness of facial skin. The fingers become tapered and flexed and lose fingertips from atrophy. Calcium deposits develop in the subcutaneous tissue and erupt through the skin. When progression to body organs occurs, death is caused by subsequent respiratory failure, renal failure, cardiac dysrhythmias, or obstructions or perforations of the esophagus or intestine. There is no specific treatment, and 50 percent of individuals die within five years of the onset of scleroderma.

7. Identify diseases caused by insect bites.
Study pages 1105-1106.

Ticks are significant vectors of transmitted diseases, including Rocky Mountain spotted fever and other rickettsial diseases, tularemia, and Lyme disease. Ticks embed their heads in the skin to obtain blood. If mouth parts remain in the skin after tick removal, a persistent nodule may develop. As ticks feed, they enlarge to many times their normal size and may release toxins or transmit microorganisms. In most instances, tick bites cause only a papular urticaria.

Lyme disease is a multisystem inflammatory disease caused by *Borrelia burgdorferi* transmitted by tick bites. The disease occurs in stages. Soon after the bite, a rash with or without flulike illness occurs. Nine months later, secondary erythema migrans, arthralgias, meningitis, neuritis, and carditis develop. Persistent infection continues for years with arthritis, encephalopathy, and polyneuropathy. Serological tests may confirm the diagnosis subsequent to presence or history of tick bite. Antibiotics are used for treatment with good success in early stages, but the response may be slow.

Mosquitoes are responsible for malaria, yellow fever, dengue fever, filariasis, and St. Louis encephalitis. Mosquitoes can bite through thin, loose clothing and are attracted by warmth and perspiration. The edema, pruritus, and papular lesions are caused by insertion of a blood tube by a female mosquito. Irritating salivary secretions also contain anticoagulants. Reactions vary depending on the sensitivity of the victim.

Several species of flies are bloodsuckers. The bite of a small female fly produces immediate pain, erythema, and vesicles. Itching and vesicular reactions may persist for weeks. The fiercest bloodsuckers are the larger types like the horseflies and deerflies. These produce painful, bleeding bites because of their large mouth parts. The bites produce urticaria that may be accompanied by weakness, dizziness, and wheezing.

8. Compare the benign tumors of the skin.
Study page 1106; refer to Figure 38-18 and Table 38-6.

Seborrheic keratosis is a benign proliferation of basal cells that produces elevated smooth or warty lesions. Multiple lesions are seen on the chest, back, and face in older people. The color varies; it may be tan to waxy yellow, flesh-colored, or dark brown-black, and the lesions are often oval and greasy-appearing with a hyperkeratotic scale. Lesion size varies from a few millimeters to several centimeters. Cryotherapy with liquid nitrogen is an effective treatment, and the lesions usually slough in two to three weeks after treatment.

A **keratoacanthoma** is a benign, self-limiting tumor that arises from hair follicles. It usually occurs on sun-exposed surfaces and develops in individuals between 60 and 65 years of age. The lesion develops in stages. The proliferative stage produces a rapid-growing, dome-shaped nodule with a central crust. In the mature stage, the lesion is filled with whitish-colored keratin. The mature lesion requires differentiation from squamous cell carcinoma. The involution stage usually occurs over a three- to four-month period as the lesion regresses. Although the lesion will resolve spontaneously, it can be removed surgically.

Actinic keratosis is a premalignant lesion found on skin surfaces exposed to ultraviolet radiation of the sun. The lesions can progress to squamous cell carcinoma. The prevalence is highest in individuals with unprotected, light-colored skin. The lesions appear as pigmented patches of rough, adherent scale, and surrounding areas may have telangiectasia. Freezing with liquid nitrogen provides quick, effective treatment. Excisions provide tissue for biopsy.

Nevi, or moles, are pigmented or nonpigmented lesions that form from melanocytes beginning at ages three to five years. During early development, the melanocytes accumulate at the junction of the dermis and epidermis and become macular lesions. Over time, the cells move into the dermis and become nodular and palpable. Nevi may appear anywhere on the skin singly or in groups and vary in size. Nevi may undergo transition to malignant melanoma; if irritated, they can be excised.

9. Describe malignant skin lesions.
Study pages 1106-1110; refer to Figures 38-19 through 38-23.

(See box on page 329 of *Workbook.*)

10. Classify burns according to the extent of injury.
Study pages 1110-1113; refer to Figures 38-24 through 38-29 and 38-31 and Tables 38-7 and 38-8.

(See box on page 330 of *Workbook.*)

11. Characterize the edematous, cardiovascular, and cellular response to burn injury.
Study pages 1113-1115; refer to Figure 38-30.

Hypovolemic shock develops quickly following major burn injury. Within minutes of a major burn injury, the capillary bed opens not only in the burn area but also in the entire capillary system.

Cancerous Skin Lesions

Lesion	Cause	Growth Rate/ Metastasis	Appearance
Basal cell carcinoma	Sunlight-exposed skin	Slow growth; almost never metastasize, invasive destruction	Smooth surface with rolled border, depressed center, telangiectasis
Squamous cell carcinoma	Sunlight-exposed skin, arise from premalignant lesions	Moderate growth; some metastasize	Rough, firm nodule with an indurated base, ulcer, bleeding
Malignant melanoma	Genetic predisposition, solar radiation and steroid hormones, precursor nevi	Fast growth, highly invasive; rapid metastasis	Nevi that change color, size, or margins; pruritus, bleeding, nodule formation or ulceration
Kaposi sarcoma	Immunodeficient states, genetics—black, Jewish, or Italian males	Slow spread through skin, some aggressive change	Multifocal purplish, brown vascular macules that develop into plaques and nodules which may be painful

Note: Treatment consists of surgery, electrodesiccation, radiation, or cryosurgery. For malignant melanomas, wide and deep excisions and removal of lymph nodes is required. For basal cell and squamous cell skin cancers, cure is virtually assured with early detection and treatment. The survival is poor for malignant melanoma because it metastasizes quickly. The general response to treatment of Kaposi sarcoma is poor.

This increased capillary permeability is the mechanism for fluid, electrolyte, and protein loss into the interstitium; this leads to the ensuing hypovolemic shock and massive edema. If the profound hypovolemic shock is not treated, irreversible shock and death may occur within a few hours.

Burn shock resuscitation involves infusion of intravenous fluid at a rate faster than the loss of circulating volume fluid for 24 hours after burn injury. The most reliable criterion to determine adequate resuscitation of burn shock is the urine output. If the individual does not have adequate urine output, sufficient fluid is not being administered. As burn shock ends, fluid administered remains in the circulating volume and is reflected as increased urine output.

The cellular response to burn injury has a metabolic response and an immunologic response. In individuals surviving burn shock, **immunosuppression** and increased susceptibility to potentially fatal systemic burn wound sepsis develop. Phagocytosis is impaired and cellular and humoral immunity is abnormal. The burned individual has decreased opsonization of bacteria and less polymorphonuclear neutrophil chemotaxis. Individuals with altered immunocompetence who are burned are at additional risk for complications.

12. Characterize frostbite.

Study page 1116.

Frostbite is an injury to the skin caused by exposure to extreme cold. The mechanism of injury appears to be direct cold injury to cells, indirect injury from ice crystal formation, or impaired circulation from anoxia to the exposed area.

Frozen skin becomes white or yellowish, is waxy, and has no sensation of pain. With mild frostbite during rewarming, there is redness and discomfort followed by a return to normal in a few hours. Cyanosis and mottling develop, followed by redness, swelling, and burning pain on rewarming in more severe cases. The most severe cases result in gangrene and loss of the affected part. Frostbite

Burn Injury

Feature	First-Degree	Second-Degree		Third-Degree
		Superficial Partial-Thickness	Deep Partial-Thickness	Full-Thickness
Morphology	Destruction of epidermis only	Destruction of epidermis and some dermis	Destruction of epidermis and dermis	Destruction of epidermis, dermis, and subcutaneous tissue
Skin function	Yes	No	No	No
Tactile and pain sensors	Yes	Yes	Diminished	No
Blisters	Present after 24 hours	Present within minutes	May or may not appear, a flat dehydrated layer lifts off in sheets	Are rare, a flat dehydrated layer lifts off easily
Appearance of wound after initial debridement	Skin peels after 24 to 48 hours, normal or slightly red	Red to pale ivory, moist surface	Mottled with areas of waxy white, dry surface	White, cherry red, or black; may contain visible thrombosed veins; dry, hard leathery surface
Healing time	3 to 5 days	21 to 28 days	30 days to many months, excision and grafting	Will not heal, may close from edges as secondary healing if wound is small, excision and grafting
Scarring	None	May be present, influenced by genetic predisposition	Highest incidence, influenced by genetic predisposition	Scarring minimized by early excision and grafting, influenced by genetic predisposition

may be classified by depth of injury. Superficial frostbite includes partial skin freezing and is known as first-degree; full-thickness skin freezing is second-degree; full-thickness skin and subcutaneous freezing is third-degree.

Immersion in a warm water bath until frozen tissue is thawed is the best treatment. Pain during the thawing period is severe and should be treated with potent analgesics. Gentle cleansing and avoidance of pressure on the skin should be maintained during healing. Amputation of necrotic tissue is delayed until a clear line of demarcation appears.

13. Define terms used in disorders of the hair and nails.
Study pages 1116-1117.

Male-pattern alopecia is an inherited form of irreversible baldness in which hair is lost in the central scalp and recession of the temporofrontal hairline occurs. **Female-pattern alopecia** is a thinning of the central hair of the scalp that begins in women at 20 to 30 years of age. **Alopecia areata** is patchy loss of hair usually associated with stress or metabolic diseases; it is usually reversible. **Hirsutism** is a male pattern of hair growth in women; it may be normal or the result of excessive secretion of androgenic hormones. **Paronychia** is an inflammation of the cuticle that can be acute or chronic and is usually caused by staphylococci or streptococci or occasionally by *Candida.* **Onychomycosis** is a fungal infection of the nail plate; the plate turns yellow or white and accumulates hyperkeratotic debris.

Practice Examination

1. Which stratum of the epidermis contains dead keratinocytes?

   a. corneum
   b. lucidum
   c. granulosum
   d. spinosum
   e. germinativum

2. The dermis is composed of all of the following except:

   a. melanocytes.
   b. collagen.
   c. elastin.
   d. apocrine sweat glands.
   e. sebaceous glands.

3. Which does not occur as the skin ages?

   a. more melanocytes
   b. decreased Langerhans cells
   c. loss of rete pegs
   d. loss of elastin fibers
   e. depressed immune response

4. Arteriovenous anastomoses in the dermis:

   a. prevent skin drying.
   b. regulate vasoconstriction.
   c. oppose evaporative heat loss.
   d. facilitate the regulation of body temperature.
   e. None of the above is correct.

Match the lesion with its descriptor.

5. ____ macule
6. ____ nodule
7. ____ scale
8. ____ wheal

a. hardened, adherent serum
b. changed color, not raised or depressed
c. accentuated skin lines caused by scratching
d. palpable, elevated solid lesion
e. flaky, accumulated stratum corneum
f. ridgelike, reddened elevation caused by edema and congestion

9. The cause of atopic dermatitis is:

   a. unknown.
   b. venous stasis.
   c. increased activity of sebaceous glands.
   d. mast cell, T cells, and monocyte interaction.
   e. nonimmunologic inflammation to chemicals.

10. The skin lesion of psoriasis is a:

   a. nonscaling, violet-colored pruritic papule.
   b. comedo.
   c. pruritic vesicle.
   d. erythematous, butterfly-shaped rash.
   e. thick, scaly, erythematous plaque.

11. A circular, demarcated, salmon-pink scale within a plaque is characteristic of:

   a. psoriasis.
   b. seborrheic dermatitis.
   c. acne rosacea.
   d. pityriasis rosea.
   e. lichen planus.

12. The Nikolsky sign is seen in:

   a. herpes simplex.
   b. pemphigus.
   c. erythema multiforme.
   d. Stevens-Johnson syndrome.
   e. Both c and d are correct.

13. The cause of impetigo is:

   a. *Staphylococcus aureus.*
   b. group A streptococci.
   c. coagulase-positive staphylococci.
   d. beta-hemolytic streptococci.
   e. Both c and d are correct.

14. The usual transmission mode of herpes simplex type 2 is by:

   a. fomites.
   b. kissing and touching.
   c. sexual encounters.
   d. contaminated food or water.
   e. b, c, and d are correct.

15. Of the benign tumors of the skin, keratoacanthomas are characterized by:

   a. proliferation of basal cells.
   b. hyperkeratotic scales.
   c. origination from hair follicles.
   d. a proliferative stage that produces a nodule with a central crust.
   e. Both c and d are correct.

16. Which are most likely to undergo malignant transition?

   a. seborrheic keratosis and keratoacanthoma
   b. seborrheic keratosis and actinic keratosis
   c. nevi and keratoacanthoma
   d. nevi and actinic keratosis
   e. None of the above is correct.

17. The cause of Kaposi sarcoma likely is:

   a. solar radiation.
   b. steroidal hormones.
   c. precursor nevi.
   d. immunodeficiency.
   e. keratinization.

18. Squamous cell carcinoma of the skin is manifested as:

   a. irregular pigmentation.
   b. elevated, firm lesions.
   c. a smooth, pearly lesion with multiple telangiectasia.
   d. multifocal purplish, brown macules.

19. An untreated basal cell carcinoma:

   a. metastasizes frequently.
   b. often involves regional lymphatics.
   c. ulcerates and involves local tissue.
   d. grows rapidly.
   e. will eventually require removal of nearby lymph nodes.

20. Which malignant skin lesion metastasizes the earliest?

   a. basal cell carcinoma
   b. squamous cell carcinoma
   c. malignant melanoma
   d. Kaposi sarcoma

21. In which burn does skin function continue?

    a. first-degree
    b. superficial partial-thickness
    c. deep partial-thickness
    d. full-thickness

22. A burn that destroys the epidermis and dermis is a:

    a. first-degree burn.
    b. superficial partial-thickness burn.
    c. deep partial-thickness burn.
    d. full-thickness burn.

23. Hypovolemic shock in severely burned individuals is the result of:

    a. dilation of capillaries.
    b. increased capillary permeability.
    c. increased peripheral resistance.
    d. Both a and b are correct.
    e. a, b, and c are correct.

24. In individuals surviving burn shock, increased wound sepsis is due to:

    a. released inflammatory cytokines.
    b. fewer opsonins.
    c. inability of phagocytes to migrate to the site of infection.
    d. All of the above are correct.
    e. Both b and c are correct.

25. Onychomycosis is:

    a. a fungal infection of the nail plate.
    b. caused by staphylococci or streptococci.
    c. an inflammation of the cuticle.
    d. None of the above is correct.

Case Study

Mr. E. is a 26-year-old white male who sustained severe burns while welding an automobile gasoline tank that had been removed from a truck. Mr. E.'s friend, for whom the welding was being done, took him immediately to a regional burn center located 20 miles away.

Initial assessment revealed that Mr. E. had received full-thickness burns on his face, to both arms and hands bilaterally and circumferentially, and to the anterior trunk.

What are the immediate and major concerns of the burn unit?

CHAPTER 39

Alterations of the Integument in Children

Foundational Objective

a. Identify the structures of the integumentary system and describe their function. Review page 1085; refer to Figures 38-1 and 38-2 and Table 38-1.

> **Memory Check!**
>
> - See *Workbook*'s narrative for Foundational Objective **a** in Chapter 38.

Objectives

After studying this chapter, the learner will be able to:

1. Describe acne vulgaris.
Study page 1123; refer to Figure 39-1.

Acne vulgaris is the most common of the skin diseases and affects 85 percent of the population between the ages of 12 and 25. The incidence of acne is the same in both genders; severe disease affects males more often. Genetics may determine the susceptibility and severity of the disease.

Acne develops primarily on the face and upper parts of the chest and back from sebaceous follicles. The follicles have many large sebaceous glands, a small vellus hair, and a dilated follicular canal that is visible on the skin surface as a pore. In **noninflammatory acne**, the comedones are open (blackheads) and closed (whiteheads) and the accumulated material causes follicular distension and thinning of follicular canal walls. **Inflammatory acne** develops in closed comedones when follicular walls rupture and expel sebum into the surrounding dermis and initiate inflammation.

The causes are abnormal keratinization of follicular epithelium, excessive sebum production, and proliferation of *Propionibacterium acnes*. Androgenic hormones increase the size and productivity of the sebaceous glands. Sebum and bacterial accumulation produce inflammation of the dermis as the follicle ruptures.

Topical treatment, including benzoyl peroxide, salicylic acid, and tretinoin, is used because it is the least invasive. Use of systemic therapies, including antibiotics, sex hormones, and corticosteroids, may be limited because of side effects.

2. Differentiate between atopic and diaper dermatitis in infants and children.
Study pages 1123-1125; refer to Figures 39-2 and 39-3.

Atopic dermatitis, or eczema, is an inflammation of the skin of unknown etiology. There is, however, an increased incidence of 75 to 80 percent in individuals who have allergies and reactive airways. Onset usually is in infancy, with 85 percent of cases occurring by five years of age. Positive allergy tests, increased serum IgE levels, and eosinophilia are common findings. The face, scalp, trunk, and extensor surfaces of the extremities are commonly affected in younger children; the neck, hands, feet, and flexor surfaces are commonly affected in older children. In the infant, the characteristic rash is erythematous with weeping and crusting lesions. In older children, the rash is frequently erythematous with scaling and thick, leatherlike lesions. Pruritus or itching leads to rubbing and scratching and more damage to the skin. Scratching causes microscopic cracking in the skin that allows water loss and exposes the lower layers to irritants which, in turn, lead to increased pruritus and scratching.

Treatment includes avoiding known irritants, hydration of the skin, antihistamines to relieve pruritus, and topical steroids to decrease inflammation. Antibiotics or antifungal agents may be necessary for secondary skin infections.

Diaper dermatitis is an inflammation of the skin in the diaper area that is caused by many factors, including lengthy exposure to wet and soiled diapers. It mostly is localized in the perineal area but may extend from the abdomen to the thighs and usually affects infants and young children. Diaper dermatitis is characterized by an erythematous rash of varying degrees of severity and often is complicated by a secondary fungal infection caused by the microorganism *Candida albicans*. The characteristic rash of *C. albicans* is very erythematous and papular and is associated with **papulovesicular satellite lesions**.

The best treatment is preventive by keeping the perineal area clean and dry with frequent diaper changes and routine hygiene. Topical barriers may become necessary once the rash develops. If *C. albicans* is present, a topical antifungal agent should be included in the treatment.

3. Categorize and characterize the infectious processes of impetigo.
Study page 1125.

Impetigo is a common bacterial skin infection in children and is either bullous or vesicular. (See first box on page 337 of *Workbook*.)

4. Describe the etiology and pathophysiology of staphylococcal scalded-skin syndrome.
Study pages 1125-1126; refer to Figure 39-4.

Staphylococcal scalded-skin syndrome is a serious infection caused by group II staphylococci. The primary site of infection often is in the throat or chest, with the onset of lesions usually preceded by an upper respiratory infection that is characterized by fever, rhinorrhea, and malaise. This severe infection is an illness of children under ten years of age and is frequently seen in newborns because their immune systems are immature.

Manifestations are caused by an epidermolytic toxin produced by the staphylococcal microorganisms at the primary site of infection; the toxin circulates to the skin where it produces the classic effects. The toxin splits the epidermis away from the underlying layers. The first sign of skin involvement is the acute onset of generalized erythema and tenderness over the entire body except the palms, soles of the feet, and mucous membranes. Blisters and bullae form over the next several days which rupture and denude the skin, leaving the child at risk for dehydration and secondary infection. In severe cases, generalized skin sloughing may occur.

Diagnosis is confirmed by culture and histologic studies. Lesions are treated like severe burns and the primary infection is treated with oral or parenteral antibiotics. Healing in uncomplicated cases usually requires 10 to 14 days.

5. Compare tinea capitis and tinea corporis; describe thrush.
Study pages 1126-1127; refer to Figure 39-5.

Candida albicans is part of the normal skin flora in certain individuals that invades susceptible tissue sites if the predisposing factors are not eliminated. This organism penetrates the epidermal barrier because of its keratolytic proteases and other enzymes. *C. albicans* attracts neutrophils to skin sites of invasion and generates inflammation by activation of the complement system. **Thrush** is the presence of *Candida* in the mucous membranes of the mouth of infants and, less frequently, adults.

Thrush is characterized by white plaques or spots in the mouth that lead to shallow ulcers. The underlying mucous membrane is red and tender and may bleed when the plaques are removed.

Treatment is with oral antifungal washes. Simultaneous treatment of nipple infection or vaginitis in the mother is helpful in reducing *C. albicans* surface colonization of the infant.

(See second box on page 337 of *Workbook*.)

Impetigo

Feature	Bullous	Vesicular
Etiologic agent	*Staphylococcus aureus*	Streptococcus pyogenes or combined with staphylococci
Source	Other infected individuals or contaminated objects	Other infected individuals, contaminated objects, insect bites
Regional lymphadenitis	Uncommon	Common
Treatment	Systemic antibiotics	Systemic antibiotics
Potential complications	Uncommon	Acute glomerulonephritis

Fungal Infections

Feature	Tinea Capitis	Tinea Corporis
Etiologic agent	*Microsporum canis*, *Trichophyton tonsurans*	Microsporum canis, Trichophyton *mentagrophytes*
Source	*M. canis* from cats, dogs, or rodents *T. tonsurans* from humans	*M. canis* and *T. mentagrophytes* from kittens or puppies
Lesion	Circular, slight erythema, scaling raised border	Oval or round with scale, central clearing, mild erythema or ringworm
Diagnostic test	KOH examination	KOH examination
Treatment	Oral antifungals (topicals do not penetrate hair bulb)	Topical antifungals

6. **Describe the infections in children caused by poxviruses, papovaviruses, and herpesviruses.**
Study pages 1127-1130; refer to Figures 39-6 through 39-8 and Table 39-1.

Molluscum contagiosum is a contagious, viral disease characterized by a 1- to 5-mm-diameter pearlescent, dome-shaped lesion that may appear anywhere on the body but most frequently affects the face, trunk, and extremities. The lesions are not inflamed. No specific treatment is recommended because it is self-limiting, although recurrence is common.

Rubella, or three-day measles, is a common communicable disease of children and young adults caused by an RNA virus that enters the bloodstream through the respiratory tract. The incubation period is between 14 and 21 days. A faint-pink to red coalescing maculopapular rash develops on the face and spreads to the trunk and extremities one to four days after the prodromal symptoms. Women of childbearing age are immunized if their antibody titers are low, and pregnancy should be avoided for three months after vaccination because the attenuated virus may remain for this time period. Pregnant women who have rubella early in the first trimester may have a fetus develop congenital defects. There is no specific, only supportive, treatment. Recovery is spontaneous.

Rubeola, or red measles, is a contagious disease of children transmitted by direct contact with droplets from infected persons. Rubeola is caused by an RNA paramyxovirus having an incubation period of 7 to 12 days. Prodromal symptoms are followed within three to four days by an erythematous maculopapular rash over the head that spreads distally over the trunk, extremities, hands, and feet. Early lesions blanch with pressure, but do not do so as the rash fades. Pinpoint white spots surrounded by an erythematous ring develop over the buccal mucosa and are known as Koplik spots. Most children recover completely, but measles encephalitis occurs in about 1 in 800 cases. There is no specific treatment for measles.

Roseola likely is a viral infection; it is seen most often in infants between the ages of six months and two years. There is a sudden onset of fever that lasts for three to five days. After the fever, an erythematous macular rash lasts for about 24 hours; it is primarily over the trunk and neck. Usually there is no treatment.

Chickenpox is a highly contagious disease of early childhood and is primarily spread by droplet transmission from an infected person to others. Household infection rates approach 90 percent in susceptible individuals. The incubation period is approximately 14 days, with infected persons contagious for approximately 24 hours prior to the onset of the rash and for five to six days after the rash appears. Chickenpox is usually an illness of late winter or early spring. The first signs of illness are pruritus or itching or the appearance of vesicles. There may be no prodromal symptoms.

Characteristically, the rash undergoes a process of maturation with lesions starting as macules that progress to superficial papules and vesicles, which then rupture and heal. The rash lasts for four to five days and may consist of up to 300 lesions distributed over the body. Complications from chickenpox are fairly rare but may include pneumonia due to the varicella virus. Treatment is symptomatic and consists of cool baths, wet dressings, and oral antihistamines.

Herpes zoster (shingles) occurs mainly in adults, but approximately 5 percent of cases are in children younger than 15 years of age. The chickenpox virus persists for life in sensory nerve ganglia and reactivates to cause herpes zoster. The zoster consists of groups of vesicles situated on an inflammatory base that follows the course of a sensory nerve. The base of the lesion appears hemorrhagic, and some may become necrotic and ulcerative. In children, the thorax is the site of distribution of the lesions. Therapy is similar to that for chickenpox unless it is disseminated zoster or there is ophthalmic involvement; then, acyclovir is indicated.

7. Compare and contrast the infestations of scabies and lice.

Study pages 1130-1131; refer to Figure 39-9.

Insect Infestations

Feature	Scabies (mite)	Pediculosis (lice)
Etiologic agent	*Sarcoptes scabiei*	*Pediculus capitis* (head), *Pediculus corporis* (body), *Phthirius pubis* (pubic)
Transmission	Contact with infested person	Contact with infested person or object (hat, clothing)
Symptoms	Burrows, papules, and vesicles	Pruritus, ova (nits) may be seen on hair shafts, mature lice may be seen
Cause of symptoms	Sensitization to larva buried in the skin	Irritation from toxic saliva from louse bites
Treatment	Permethrin/lindane, treatment of exposed persons and infested objects	Permethrin/lindane, treatment of exposed persons and infested objects

8. Compare and contrast the congenital vascular disorders.
Study pages 1132-1133; refer to Figures 39-11 and 39-12.

Vascular Disorders

Feature	Strawberry Hemangioma	Cavernous Hemangioma	Salmon Patches	Portwine Stain
Description	Raised vesicular	Raised vesicular with larger mature vessels	Macular, most common	Flat, becomes papular and cavernous
Manifestation	At birth or in three to five weeks	At birth	At birth	At birth or in a few days
Color	Bright red (capillary projections)	Bluish, less distinct borders	Pink, distended dermal capillaries	Pink to dark reddish purple
Location	One lesion on head, neck, or trunk	Head, neck	Nape of neck, forehead, upper eyelid	Face and other body surfaces
Growth	Initially rapid, then at child's rate of growth	Rapid first six months, matures at one year	Fades in one year	Does not fade
Involution	Begins by 12 to 16 months, complete by five to six years	Begins by 6 to 12 months, complete by nine years	N/A	N/A
Treatment	None	May require surgery, laser surgery, or liquid nitrogen depending on location of lesion	None	Cryosurgery, laser surgery

Practice Examination

True/False

1. ____ Diaper dermatitis is caused by *Candida albicans*.
2. ____ Impetigo is contracted only by human-to-human contact.
3. ____ Molluscum contagiosum is a very painful viral infection.
4. ____ Atopic dermatitis is also called eczema.
5. ____ Staphylococcal scalded-skin syndrome is a contagious disease of the skin.

6. ____ Tinea capitis must be treated with systemic antifungal agents.

7. ____ Salmon patches are commonly called stork bites and fade over time.

8. ____ Portwine stains will involute by adulthood.

9. ____ Acute glomerulonephritis is a complication of bullous impetigo.

10. ____ The microorganism that causes bullous impetigo is *Streptococcus pyogenes*.

Match the description with the alteration.

11. ____ viral skin infection contracted during the first decade of life
12. ____ positive allergy tests, increased IgE, and eosinophilia
13. ____ erythematous lesions in the perineal area with secondary papulovesicular satellites
14. ____ raised, erythemic, scaling lesions on the scalp
15. ____ dome-shaped lesions ranging from 1 mm to 5 mm on the extremities without pruritus
16. ____ macules, fever, itching, papules, and rupturing and healing vesicules
17. ____ crusted lesion
18. ____ mite burrowing in the stratum corneum
19. ____ present at birth or shortly after birth
20. ____ entire skin sloughing
21. ____ nits on hair shaft
22. ____ chronic condition with acute exacerbations, pruritus
23. ____ oval or circular lesions, peripheral spreading, central clearing (ringworm)
24. ____ action of a epidermolytic toxin
25. ____ parasitic in nature, acquired by personal contact and sharing combs or hair brushes

a. staphylococcal scalded-skin syndrome
b. tinea capitis
c. atopic dermatitis
d. pediculosis
e. diaper dermatitis with *Candida albicans*
f. chickenpox
g. vascular disorders
h. impetigo
i. molluscum contagiosum
j. scabies
k. tinea corporis

Case Study

Lance D. is a five-year-old white male who visits the nurse practitioner's office with a "runny" nose that started about one week ago but has not resolved. He has been blowing his nose quite frequently and "sores" have developed on his face. His mother states that the sores started as "big blisters" that rupture; sometimes, a scab forms with a crust that looks like "dried maple syrup" but continues to weep and drain. She is worried because the lesions are now also on his forearm. Lance's past medical and family histories are normal. He has been febrile but is otherwise asymptomatic. The physical examination is unremarkable except for moderate, purulent rhinorrhea and 0.5- to 1-cm-diameter weeping lesions around the nose and mouth and on the radial surface of the right forearm. There is no regional lymphadenopathy.

What is the likely name and cause of these lesions? Why have these lesions spread to Lance's arm?

Answers

Chapter 1

1. c	6. a	11. g	16. b	21. a, b, c, d, e
2. a, c, e	7. b	12. e	17. b, d	22. a, b, c, d
3. a	8. d	13. f	18. b	23. b
4. e	9. h	14. j	19. e	24. c
5. d	10. d	15. i	20. c	25. d

Chapter 2

1. a	6. b	11. d	16. f	21. h
2. b	7. b	12. d	17. h	22. d
3. d	8. c	13. b	18. g	23. f
4. c	9. c	14. c	19. i	24. g
5. d	10. a	15. a	20. b	25. c

Chapter 3

1. d	6. b	11. d	16. c	21. c
2. c, d	7. d	12. b	17. b	22. a
3. d	8. a	13. a	18. d	23. d
4. e	9. c	14. d	19. a	24. b
5. d	10. e	15. d	20. e	25. e

Chapter 4

1. e	6. e	11. d	16. c	21. e
2. b	7. b	12. d	17. e	22. b
3. b	8. b	13. a, b, e	18. b	23. a
4. c	9. a	14. b	19. d	24. c
5. d	10. c	15. e	20. a	25. b

Chapter 5

1. c	6. e	11. d	16. d	21. c
2. a	7. b	12. e	17. a	22. a
3. d	8. d	13. d	18. b	23. a
4. e	9. d	14. e	19. c	24. b
5. f	10. a	15. d	20. f	25. a

Chapter 6

1. e	6. a	11. d	16. d	21. b
2. b	7. a	12. a	17. d	22. d
3. d	8. b	13. e	18. e	23. e
4. b	9. e	14. b	19. e	24. g
5. d	10. d	15. c	20. e	25. f

Chapter 7

1. b
2. c
3. a
4. c
5. d
6. b
7. d
8. c
9. d
10. d
11. d
12. e
13. c
14. d
15. a
16. a
17. d
18. e
19. c
20. b
21. e
22. e
23. d
24. a
25. d

Chapter 8

1. c
2. f
3. d
4. e
5. g
6. a
7. b
8. c
9. b
10. d
11. c
12. a
13. d
14. a
15. a
16. a
17. c
18. a
19. c
20. a
21. c
22. e
23. g
24. h
25. i

Chapter 9

1. c
2. e
3. f
4. e
5. c
6. a
7. d
8. e
9. b
10. f
11. c
12. d
13. e
14. c
15. e
16. b
17. e
18. e
19. a
20. d
21. e
22. c
23. d
24. a
25. f

Chapter 10

1. e
2. c
3. d
4. e
5. e
6. e
7. b
8. e
9. d
10. c
11. c
12. d
13. a
14. e
15. c
16. d
17. d
18. a
19. d
20. b
21. g
22. c
23. e
24. f
25. a

Chapter 11

1. c
2. d
3. c
4. b
5. e
6. a
7. c
8. a
9. b
10. b, d
11. a
12. c
13. a
14. c
15. a
16. c
17. a
18. d
19. c
20. a
21. a
22. b
23. a
24. d
25. c

Chapter 12

1. b
2. a
3. e
4. b
5. c
6. b
7. e
8. e
9. c
10. c
11. e
12. b
13. d
14. b
15. b
16. c
17. a
18. e
19. d
20. e
21. c
22. j
23. i
24. h
25. g

Case Study Discussion

Her history and response to medication were typical of *depression*. Depression causes sleep disturbances characterized by insomnia, early morning awakenings, or multiple awakenings during the night. The improvement in the quality of sleep following antidepressants often occurs before other appropriate behavioral changes are seen. It seems likely that her insomnia may return, and an appropriate course of action might involve seeking assistance from a sleep disorder center.

Chapter 13

1. c	6. c	11. c	16. c	21. l
2. e	7. e	12. b	17. a	22. b
3. b	8. d	13. a	18. e	23. e
4. a	9. e	14. b	19. j	24. f
5. b	10. d	15. c	20. k	25. g

Case Study Discussion

Normal laboratory values and the normal CSF likely exclude the possibility of an infection such as meningitis and other causes known to precipitate seizures. The skull x-ray ruled out the possibility of a skull fracture. A normal EEG likely excludes intracranial pressure from brain masses. Since an EEG may be normal between seizures, the episodal pattern suggests a *generalized grand mal seizure.* A judicious administration of anticonvulsant medications likely is indicated.

Chapter 14

1. d	6. d	11. a	16. d	21. b
2. b	7. e	12. b	17. b	22. d
3. e	8. a	13. c	18. c	23. g
4. c	9. b	14. e	19. b	24. c
5. b	10. e	15. c	20. a, c	25. f

Case Study Discussion

Mrs. B. exhibits risk factors for a CVA. She smokes cigarettes, is overweight, and is hypertensive. Her mother and siblings have histories of diabetes, CVA, and hypertension; all of these indicate a family history that increases the risk for CVA.

Her symptoms and signs suggest a *thrombotic stroke* with ischemia rather than a hemorrhagic or embolic stroke. The absence of blood in CSF rules out a hemorrhagic stroke. Since there was no fibrillation on the electrocardiogram, the heart was an unlikely source for emboli, thus ruling out an embolic stroke. Mrs. B.'s elevated blood pressure likely is caused by atherosclerosis, which can lead to a thrombus formation.

Chapter 15

1. False	6. True	11. False	16. Craniosynostosis	21. e
2. False	7. True	12. Reye, hepatic	17. i	22. d
3. False	8. True	13. posterior	18. h	23. c
4. True	9. False	14. anterior	19. g	24. b
5. False	10. False	15. meningitis	20. f	25. a

Case Study Discussion

X-rays reveal an absence of spinal processes on the vertebrae from L3 to L5. A *meningomyelocele* at the same level with tethering of the cord is revealed. A neurosurgical consultation is ordered and surgery is likely.

Chapter 16

1. a	6. b	11. b	16. d	21. a
2. e	7. a	12. d	17. e	22. c
3. c	8. c	13. e	18. b	23. e
4. b	9. d	14. c	19. d	24. d
5. d	10. c	15. d	20. e	25. f

Chapter 17

1. c	6. a	11. a	16. c	21. a, b, c
2. a	7. d	12. b	17. a	22. c
3. a	8. a	13. b	18. e	23. e
4. d	9. a	14. b	19. c	24. d
5. b	10. d	15. c	20. e	25. b

Case Study Discussion

Scott's symptoms, signs, and laboratory values are classic for *diabetes ketoacidosis.*The serum values indicated metabolic acidosis with some accompanying respiratory compensation. His elevated glycosylated hemoglobin showed that he likely had been hyperglycemic for several months. This diabetes is type I (IDDM) and will require insulin administration and personal instructions regarding recognition of future signs and symptoms of hyperglycemia and hypoglycemia, self–blood glucose monitoring, insulin therapy, diet, and exercise.

Chapter 18

1. e	6. c	11. d	16. b	21. e
2. b	7. c	12. e	17. c	22. e
3. e	8. c	13. e	18. a	23. b
4. d	9. d	14. d	19. a	24. d
5. a	10. e	15. d	20. b	25. d

Chapter 19

1. e	6. a	11. e	16. c	21. a
2. d	7. b	12. c	17. e	22. b
3. c	8. a	13. b	18. c	23. a
4. a	9. b	14. c	19. b	24. d
5. b	10. b	15. d	20. a	25. e

Case Study 1 Discussion

Three anemias have erythrocytes that are microcytic and hypochromic: iron deficiency, sideroblastic anemia, and thalassemia. Ann's history has some factors that could contribute to anemia from blood loss. The menorrhagia causes more iron loss than is normal with each menstrual period, and excessive aspirin intake irritates the gastrointestinal mucosa and can precipitate chronic mucosal microhemorrhage.

Iron deficiency anemia is most likely and can be verified by providing oral iron replacement and checking her hemoglobin values in one month. If the hemoglobin deficit is corrected, it is likely that the correct diagnosis was made. The source of bleeding should be corrected, if possible; a substitute for aspirin should be used; and iron supplementation should be used for at least one year.

Ann's homeostatic mechanisms are trying to compensate in several ways, including shunting blood to more critical organs, increasing erythropoiesis, increasing the heart rate to handle increased venous return, and increasing the respiratory rate to make oxygen available to the remaining erythrocytes. The last two signs are relevant compensation efforts in Ann's circumstance.

Case Study 2 Discussion

The physician likely would conclude that L.L. has *acute lymphocytic leukemia.* The pale skin with petechiae and ecchymoses is abnormal, as is the gingival bleeding from minor trauma. Although the abnormal values for RBCs, hemoglobin, total leukocyte count, and platelet count have many possible causes, the presence of leukocytic blasts in peripheral blood indicates a bone marrow dysfunction. At this time, the physician likely will refer L.L. to a pediatric oncologist for extensive diagnostic tests and treatment.

Chapter 20

1. False	6. False	11. d	16. b	21. e
2. True	7. False	12. c	17. e	22. c
3. True	8. a	13. e	18. e	23. d
4. False	9. b	14. d	19. a	24. c
5. True	10. e	15. e	20. b	25. d

Case Study Discussion

Steven has the typical manifestations of *idiopathic thrombocytopenic purpura* (ITP), although it has come to medical attention in a very circuitous manner.

Chapter 21

1. b	6. b	11. a	16. b, d, e	21. a
2. b	7. e	12. a	17. c	22. d
3. b	8. a	13. c	18. b	23. b
4. c	9. c	14. d	19. d	24. b
5. b, c	10. e	15. a	20. a	25. b

Chapter 22

1. d	6. b	11. e	16. f	21. a, b, c
2. e	7. d	12. a	17. b, d	22. d
3. c	8. e	13. b	18. c	23. b
4. b	9. c	14. c	19. a, c	24. c
5. a	10. b, d, e	15. e	20. b, d	25. b

Case Study Discussion

Alterable myocardial infarction risk factors for W.S. are essential hypertension and cigarette smoking. Unalterable risk factors for W.S. include advancing age, male sex, and family history of early cardiac death. Atherosclerosis in the anterior descending branch of the left coronary artery was the beginning process leading to this infarction. The location of infarction was verified by the electrocardiogram.

The precipitating event in this myocardial infarction was complete occlusion of the coronary artery. The history of hypertension also supports occlusion of the coronary artery as the cause for this myocardial infarction.

Pulmonary thromboembolism is a common cause of death from myocardial infarction as emboli disseminate from debris or clots from the infarcted endocardium. Prophylactic heparin therapy decreases the risk of pulmonary embolism by interfering with the conversion of prothrombin to thrombin so that thrombi are less likely to form.

Chapter 23

1. False	6. shunt	11. left, right	16. e	21. c
2. True	7. left, right	12. first weeks	17. a	22. e
3. False	8. right, left	13. pulmonary stenosis	18. a	23. d
4. True	9. oxygenated, unoxygenated	14. afterload, congestive heart failure	19. b	24. d
5. False	10. equal	15. coarctation of the aorta	20. c	25. a

Case Study Discussion

Following the consultation, the echocardiogram demonstrates a moderate *coarctation of the aorta* in the aortic arch. This discrepancy in the quality of upper and lower extremity pulses is due to well-developed collateral circulation to the descending aorta; the femoral pulses will be decreased as blood fills the collateral vessels.

Chapter 24

1. d	6. e	11. c	16. d	21. a
2. d	7. d	12. a	17. a	22. a
3. c	8. c	13. c	18. b	23. a
4. d	9. a	14. d	19. e	24. b
5. d	10. b	15. b	20. e	25. a

Chapter 25

1. g	6. d	11. c	16. d	21. a, b, d
2. c	7. e	12. e	17. e	22. d
3. h	8. f	13. d	18. b, c	23. e
4. l	9. j	14. e	19. b	24. b
5. i	10. m	15. a	20. a, b, d	25. a

Case Study Discussion

Mr. S. presents the classic symptoms and signs of *emphysema.* His long-term, extensive smoking is consistent with most cases of emphysema, as is his dyspnea on exertion progressing to dyspnea even at rest. Hyperinflation of lungs causes the anteroposterior chest diameter to increase. The chest radiograph is consistent with findings in emphysema. Prolonged forced expiratory volume, decreased tidal volume, and increased total lung capacity are also present in emphysema. These tests indicate that the walls of alveoli have been destroyed and the lungs have become more distended or less compliant and have less elastic recoil. Therefore, air is trapped and expiration flow is diminished.

Chapter 26

1. False	6. True	11. c	16. d	21. e
2. False	7. e	12. d	17. a	22. c
3. False	8. e	13. c	18. b	23. d
4. True	9. d	14. e	19. f	24. c
5. False	10. e	15. d	20. f	25. a

Case Study Discussion

Tyler has classic manifestations of *bronchiolitis*. The most likely etiologic agent in Tyler's illness is respiratory syncytial virus to which his parents likely exposed him during their "colds." He is displaying the classic signs of respiratory distress in an infant and is unable to feed due to this respiratory distress. His lethargy is probably due to mild hypoxia and hypercapnia, and his general fatigue is from prolonged ventilatory effort. He may suffer respiratory failure if left untreated. Hospitalization for rehydration and respiratory therapy should support him through the worst of his illness, and he should improve within a few days.

Chapter 27

1. c	6. b	11. e	16. d	21. b
2. a	7. b	12. b	17. a	22. c
3. d	8. c	13. b	18. c, d, e	23. c
4. a	9. d	14. d	19. d	24. c
5. d	10. d	15. b	20. a	25. d

Chapter 28

1. d	6. d	11. d	16. b	21. c
2. b	7. a, b, c	12. e	17. d	22. b
3. a	8. b	13. d	18. c	23. d
4. a	9. b	14. d	19. a	24. a
5. e	10. b, c, d	15. a, e	20. d	25. e

Case Study Discussion

Eddie's history of sore throat and back pain and his laboratory values suggest *poststreptococcal glomerulonephritis*. Proteinuria is a sensitive indicator of glomerular dysfunction. In glomerulonephritis, the glomerulus is injured and its permeability increased enough to permit protein to enter into the filtrate and urine. Blood and RBC casts also are seen in glomerulonephritis. BUN and creatinine are excreted entirely by the kidneys and therefore are directly related to renal excretion. Eddie's pediatrician most likely will place him on penicillin and may prescribe an antihypertensive medication and monitor his blood pressure, electrolyte balance, and BUN and creatinine levels.

Chapter 29

1. False	6. False	11. e	16. d	21. b
2. True	7. d	12. d	17. e	22. c
3. False	8. a	13. d	18. e	23. c
4. False	9. d	14. d	19. d	24. a
5. True	10. c	15. d	20. f	25. g

Case Study Discussion

The laboratory values reveal an anemia and thrombocytopenia; the child is losing red blood cells and platelets. Since she has not voided any urine, acute renal failure is very likely. These results suggest the diagnosis of *hemolytic uremic syndrome*. She will require hospitalization for blood transfusions and dialysis.

Chapter 30

1. b, d	6. d	11. a	16. c	21. a
2. a	7. a	12. e	17. e	22. c
3. e	8. b	13. b	18. c	23. c
4. d	9. e	14. c	19. e	24. e
5. c	10. b	15. a	20. a	25. a

Chapter 31

1. d	6. b	11. d	16. d	21. c
2. c	7. d	12. d	17. b	22. e
3. e	8. a	13. d	18. a	23. f
4. d	9. e	14. a	19. b	24. h
5. e	10. b	15. d	20. b	25. i

Case Study Discussion

Mrs. B.'s history and examination are indicative of *breast cancer* in her left breast. A positive familial history of breast cancer has a strong, confirmed causal link to breast cancer. A chromosome 17 defect has been implicated as a genetic causal factor in breast cancer as well. Other associated risk factors for breast cancer that Mrs. B. exhibits include late age at first delivery, early menarche, birth control pills, and benign breast tumors.

The cardinal manifestation of breast cancer was a hard, fixed mass palpable in Mrs. B.'s left breast. The freely moveable, soft masses of the right breast are likely benign, as they display fluctuating patterns of tissue proliferation different from those of the left breast. The palpation of the axillary lymph node indicated that cancer cells have metastasized through the lymphatic channels surrounding the breast.

Chapter 32

1. d	6. d	11. d	16. d	21. b
2. d	7. d	12. b	17. a	22. c
3. b	8. a	13. a	18. b	23. e
4. e	9. d	14. c	19. a	24. c
5. e	10. b	15. c	20. c	25. a

Chapter 33

1. b	6. d	11. b	16. d	21. b
2. d	7. c	12. e	17. e	22. e
3. a	8. e	13. b	18. e	23. d
4. e	9. a	14. a	19. a, b, c, d	24. a
5. e	10. b	15. c	20. a	25. d

Case Study Discussion

A *gastric ulcer* is likely. Factors associated with these ulcers include smoking, stress, and use of aspirin or other ulcerogenic drugs. Although the clinical manifestations of gastric ulcers are similar to those of duodenal ulcers, the pain of gastric ulcers is more likely to occur immediately after eating. Also, gastric ulcers tend to be chronic rather than alternate between periods of remission and exacerbation. An upper gastrointestinal study using barium sulfate as a contrast medium and endoscopy can detect the location of the ulcer and confirm that Dr. R. has a gastric ulcer.

Chapter 34

1. False	6. True	11. True	16. Rectal prolapse	21. e
2. True	7. True	12. Gastroesophageal reflux	17. a	22. d
3. False	8. False	13. biopsy	18. c	23. d
4. False	9. True	14. decrease	19. b	24. c
5. False	10. False	15. nasal, oral	20. a	25. c

Case Study Discussion

A *pyloric stenosis* is diagnosed on the basis of clinical manifestations. The standard treatment is a pyloromyotomy to separate the muscles of the pylorus.

Chapter 35

1. a, c, d	6. b	11. d	16. d	21. c
2. d	7. b	12. d	17. a	22. e
3. d	8. d	13. a	18. b	23. e
4. e	9. b	14. c	19. d	24. e
5. b	10. b	15. a	20. b	25. c

Chapter 36

1. a	6. e	11. a	16. a	21. d
2. b	7. c	12. e	17. a, b	22. d
3. d	8. c	13. b	18. a, b, d, e	23. c
4. b	9. e	14. d	19. e	24. e
5. d	10. a	15. e	20. b	25. e

Case Study Discussion

The presenting symptoms of Mrs. B.B. are compatible with either osteoarthritis or rheumatoid arthritis. The laboratory studies support a diagnosis of *rheumatoid arthritis.* The presence of rheumatoid factor is helpful in the diagnosis of rheumatoid arthritis. It is positive in about 80 percent of individuals who have rheumatoid arthritis. Although other diseases may show a positive test, osteoarthritis will not. Synovial fluid analysis showing inflammatory exudates satisfies the diagnostic criteria for rheumatoid arthritis. The radiograph is more representative of rheumatoid arthritis than osteoarthritis. In osteoarthritis, deformity of articular cartilage, bone sclerosis, cystic areas, and bony spurs would be likely observations.

Chapter 37

1. False	6. True	11. femoral	16. b	21. e
2. False	7. False	12. breech position	17. f	22. d
3. False	8. True	13. dystrophin	18. e	23. c
4. True	9. True	14. abduction, flexion	19. f	24. b
5. False	10. False	15. clubfoot	20. d	25. a

Case Study Discussion

Bobby B. displays the clinical manifestations of *Duchenne muscular dystrophy.* The diagnosis can be confirmed by measurement of serum creatine phosphokinase (CPK) levels, electromyography, and muscle biopsy. The CPK level in Duchenne muscular dystrophy will be increased more than ten times normal. Histologic examination of the biopsy will show muscle degeneration, with fat and connective tissue replacing muscle fibers.

Chapter 38

1. a	6. d	11. d	16. d	21. a
2. a	7. e	12. b	17. d	22. c
3. a	8. f	13. e	18. b	23. d
4. d	9. d	14. c	19. c	24. d
5. b	10. e	15. e	20. c	25. a

Case Study Discussion

Adults with burns involving large surface areas require cardiovascular support through intravenous fluid since *hypovolemic shock* develops quickly following major burn injury. Within minutes of a major burn injury, the capillary bed not only at the site of the burn but throughout the entire body becomes more permeable to water, sodium, and proteins. This leads to fluid loss from the intravascular spaces into the interstitial spaces and massive edema; the blood volume and cardiac output diminish. The infusion of intravenous fluid or burn shock resuscitation for the first 24 hours must be faster than the rate of loss of circulatory volume. To determine adequate levels of infusion, urine output must be measured, so Mr. E. will require placement of a catheter into his bladder.

Although hypovolemic shock is the immediate concern for major burn patients, other alterations are very important; monitoring and maintenance of electrolytes are required. The hypermetabolic rate of burned individuals requires adequate nutrition. Finally, early excision and grafting procedures are required.

Chapter 39

1. False
2. False
3. False
4. True
5. False
6. True
7. True
8. False
9. False
10. False
11. f
12. c
13. e
14. b
15. i
16. f
17. h
18. j
19. g
20. a
21. d
22. c
23. k
24. a
25. d

Case Study Discussion

This is a fairly classic case of *bullous impetigo* caused by a *Staphylococcus aureus* infection in Lance's nasopharynx. Abrasion from blowing and wiping his nose frequently has opened the skin and allowed the bacteria to enter the skin and cause the lesions. The infection spread to his arm because he has been wiping his nose on his arm.